Prevention and treatment of suicidal behaviour

Prevention and treatment of suicidal behaviour:

from science to practice

Edited by
Keith Hawton
Centre for Suicide Research,
Oxford University, Oxford, UK

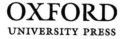

OXFORD
UNIVERSITY PRESS

Great Clarendon Street, Oxford OX2 6DP

Oxford University Press is a department of the University of Oxford.
It furthers the University's objective of excellence in research, scholarship,
and education by publishing worldwide in

Oxford New York

Auckland Cape Town Dar es Salaam Hong Kong Karachi
Kuala Lumpur Madrid Melbourne Mexico City Nairobi
New Delhi Shanghai Taipei Toronto

With offices in

Argentina Austria Brazil Chile Czech Republic France Greece
Guatemala Hungary Italy Japan South Korea Poland Portugal
Singapore Switzerland Thailand Turkey Ukraine Vietnam

Oxford is a registered trade mark of Oxford University Press
in the UK and in certain other countries

Published in the United States
by Oxford University Press Inc., New York

© Oxford University Press 2005

The moral rights of the author have been asserted

Database right Oxford University Press (maker)

First published 2005

A catalogue record for this title is available from the British Library

Library of Congress Cataloging in Publication Data
Prevention and treatment of suicidal behaviour: from science to pratice / edited by Keith Hawton.
Includes bibliographical references and index.
1. Suicidal behaviour–Prevention.   2. Suicidal behavior–Treatment.
3. Suicide–Psychological aspects.   1. Hawton, Keith, 1942- .
[DNLM: 1. Suicide–prevention & control.   2. Health Policy.   3. Suicide
–psychology. HV 6545 P9438 2005]
RC569.P73 2005   362.28–dc22   2005016390
ISBN 0–19–852975–9 (Hardback: alk. paper)   978–0–19–852975–0 (Hardback: alk. paper)
ISBN 0–19–852976–7 (Pbk.: alk. paper)   978–0–19–852976–7 (Pbk.: alk. paper)

Typeset by SPI Publisher Services, Pondicherry, India
Printed in Great Britain
on acid-free paper by
Biddles Ltd, King's Lynn

About the editor

Professor Keith Hawton DSc

Professor Hawton is Director of the Centre for Suicide Research at Oxford University Department of Psychiatry, Professor of Psychiatry at Oxford University, and Consultant Psychiatrist at Oxfordshire Mental Healthcare Trust. After studying at Cambridge and Oxford Universities he trained in psychiatry in Oxford. In addition to working as a consultant psychiatrist he has been very active in research throughout his career. For 30 years he and his research group have been conducting investigations concerning the causes, treatment, and prevention of suicidal behaviour. They have taken a particular interest in suicidal behaviour in young people, the epidemiology of deliberate self-harm, psychological autopsy studies of groups at high risk of suicide, media influences on suicidal behaviour, treatment of suicide attempters, systematic reviews in relation to prevention of suicidal behaviour, and the evaluation of suicide prevention strategies. He has received the Stengel Research Award from the International Association for Suicide Prevention (1995), the Dublin Career Research Award from the American Association of Suicidology (2001), and the Research Award of the American Foundation for Suicide Prevention (2002). He is co-editor of *The international handbook of suicide and attempted suicide* (Wiley, 2000) and also co-author of *Attempted suicide: A practical guide* (Oxford University Press, 1982, 1987) and author of *Suicide and attempted suicide in children and adolescents* (Sage, 1986). Other books include *Cognitive behaviour therapy for psychiatric problem: A practical guide* (co-editor, Oxford University Press, 1989).

Acknowledgements

As others who have been in a similar position will be well aware, editing a major book can be a painful process. However, this has mostly not been my experience with this book. I have been delighted by the enthusiastic collaboration of all the contributors. I wish to thank them most sincerely and trust that they will feel that their efforts have been rewarded in terms of having played their part in the production of a work that I hope will be a significant contribution to the field of both treatment and prevention of suicidal behaviour.

I also wish to thank my colleagues, especially Sue Simkin who, in addition to her general support over many years of our work at the Centre for Suicide Research, has helped me a great deal with getting some of the chapters of this book into their final form. In addition, I thank my personal assistant, Tania Castro-Martinez, for helping in the production of some of the chapters, and dealing with other matters necessary for the completion of the book.

Finally, I thank my wife, Joan, for her longstanding support of my work, and especially for tolerating many late evenings where I have been working on this volume.

The following publications are acknowledged:

American Journal of Psychiatry to publish Table 2.1, which is a modified version of a table in Qin, P., Agerbo, E., and Mortensen, P.B. (2003) Suicide risk in relation to socioeconomic, demographic, social, and familial factors: a national register-based study of all suicides in Denmark, 1981–1997. *American Journal of Psychiatry*, **160**, 765–772.

Lancet to publish Figure 3.5, which is a modified version of a figure in Gunnell, D. and Middleton, N. (2003) National suicide rates as an indicator of the effect of suicide on premature mortality. *Lancet*, **362**, 961–962.

Epidemiology and Community Medicine to publish Figures 16.1 and 16.2, which are modified versions of figures in Kreitman, N. (1976) The coal gas story. United Kingdom rates, 1960–1971. *Journal of Preventive Medicine*, **30**, 86–93.

Suicide and Life-Threatening Behavior to publish Table 19.2, which is a modified version of a table in Lester, D. (1997) The effectiveness of suicide prevention centers: a review. *Suicide and Life-Threatening Behavior*, 27, 304–310.

Keith Hawton
September 2005

Contents

Contributors

Esben Agerbo
National Center for Register-based Research,
University of Aarhus, Denmark

Louis Appleby
National Confidential Inquiry into
Suicide and Homicide by People with
Mental Illness,
Centre for Suicide Prevention,
University of Manchester,
Manchester, England

Simon Armson
Samaritans,
London, England

Thorsten Barnhofer
Centre for Suicide Research,
Department of Psychiatry,
University of Oxford,
Oxford, England

Yeates Conwell
Center for the Study and Prevention
of Suicide,
University of Rochester School
of Medicine and Dentistry,
Rochester, New York, USA

Catherine Crane
Centre for Suicide Research,
Department of Psychiatry,
University of Oxford,
Oxford, England

Paul Duberstein
Center for the Study and Prevention
of Suicide,
University of Rochester School of
Medicine and Dentistry,
Rochester, New York, USA

Danielle Duggan
Centre for Suicide Research,
Department of Psychiatry,
University of Oxford,
Oxford, England

Robert D. Goldney
Department of Psychiatry,
University of Adelaide,
Adelaide, Australia

Onja Grad
University Psychiatric Hospital,
Ljubljana, Slovenia

David Gunnell
Department of Social Medicine,
University of Bristol,
Bristol, England

Keith Hawton
Centre for Suicide Research,
Department of Psychiatry,
University of Oxford,
Oxford, England

Kees van Heeringen
Unit for Suicide Research,
University of Ghent,
Ghent, Belgium

Kay Redfield Jamison
Johns Hopkins University
School of Medicine,
Baltimore, Maryland, USA

Rachel Jenkins
WHO Collaborating Centre,
Institute of Psychiatry,
Kings College,
London, England

Navneet Kapur
National Confidential Inquiry into
Suicide and Homicide by People
with Mental Illness,
Centre for Suicide Prevention,
University of Manchester,
Manchester, England

Preben Bo Mortensen
National Center for Register-based
Research,
University of Aarhus,
Denmark

Andrej Marušič
Institute of Public Health of the
Republic of Slovenia,
Ljubljana, Slovenia

Peter McGuffin
MRC Social, Genetic and
Developmental Psychiatry Centre,
Institute of Psychiatry,
King's College, London,
England

Lars Mehlum
Suicide Research and
Prevention Unit,
University of Oslo,
Oslo, Norway

Fiona O'May
Faculty of Health and
Social Sciences,
Queen Margaret University College,
Edinburgh, Scottland

Jo Paton
Safer Custody Group,
National Offender Management
Service,
London, England

Stephen Pavis
Information and Statistics Division,
Common Services Agency,
NHS Scotland,
Edinburgh, Scotland

Stephen Platt
Research Unit in Health,
Behaviour and Change,
School of Clinical Sciences and
Community Health,
University of Edinburgh,
Scotland

Ping Qin
National Center for Register-based
Research,
University of Aarhus, Denmark

Ingeborg Rossow
Norwegian Institute for Alcohol
and Drug Research,
Oslo, Norway

Michael Sharpe
School of Molecular and Clinical Medicine,
University of Edinburgh,
Edinburgh, Scotland

Nicola Swinson
National Confidential Inquiry into Suicide and Homicide by People with Mental Illness,
Centre for Suicide Prevention,
University of Manchester,
Manchester, England

Herman M. van Praag
Department of Psychiatry and Neuropsychology,
Academic Hospital,
Maastricht University,
Maastricht, The Netherlands

Lakshmi Vijayakumar
SNEHA,
Chennai, India

J. Mark G. Williams
Centre for Suicide Research,
Department of Psychiatry,
University of Oxford,
Oxford, England

Kathryn Williams
Centre for Health Service Development,
University of Wollongong,
New South Wales, Australia

Abbreviations

ADP	average daily population		LEIDS	Leiden Index of Depression Sensitivity
AIDS	acquired immunodeficiency syndrome		MBCT	mindfulness-based cognitive therapy
AVP	arginine vasopressin		MEPS	means ends problem-solving task
CI	confidence interval		OCD	obsessive–compulsive disorder
CRH	corticotrophin-releasing hormone		PAR	population attributable risk
CSA	childhood sexual abuse		PET	positron emission tomography
CSF	cerebrospinal fluid		PTSD	post-traumatic stress disorder
DAS	Dysfunctional Attitudes Scale		PYLL	potential years of life lost
DSH	deliberate self-harm		SIRI	Suicide Intervention Response Inventory
GABA	gamma-aminobutyric acid		SMR	standardized mortality ratio
GDP	gross domestic product		SNRI	selective serotonin reuptake inhibitor
5-HIAA	5-hydroxyindoleacetic acid			
HIV	human immunodeficiency virus		SPAN	Suicide Prevention Advocacy Network
HPA	hypothalamic–pituitary–adrenal (axis)		SPECT	single photon emission computed tomography
5-HT	serotonin		SSRIs	selective serotonin reuptake inhibitors
5-HTT	serotonin transporter			
IRR	incidence risk ratio		TCA	tricyclic antidepressant
MAO	monoaminoxidase		TPH	tryptophan hydroxylase
MRI	magnetic resonance imaging			

Introduction and overview

Keith Hawton

In recent years there has been increasing recognition of the extent and global burden of suicide. This is partly because more countries are now providing national suicide statistics. The World Health Organization (2004) estimated that about 1 million people die by suicide each year, although the true figure may be considerably higher. This number exceeds the number of deaths due to homicide and war combined (World Health Organization 2004). In most European countries the number of suicides is greater than the number of deaths due to road traffic accident fatalities.

Suicide rates differ greatly between countries, with high rates in Eastern Europe and in some Asian countries, notably China and Sri Lanka. Relatively low rates are found in Latin America and certain Muslim countries. In Europe, rates tend to be higher in countries in the north, and lower in countries around the Mediterranean. Relatively little information is available on suicide in many African countries. The general gender pattern for suicide is that rates in males considerably exceed those of females. Rural China is an exception—here suicide is more common in females than in males.

In many countries suicide rates increase with age, although the actual numerical burden and years of life lost to suicide may be greater in young people. In the past two or three decades there has been a very marked increase in suicide rates in young people, especially in males. This pattern was reported from, for example, the USA, Australia, and New Zealand, and several countries in Europe. It was this development, as well the greater recognition of the extent of suicide and the potential for prevention, that has stimulated a major focus on suicide prevention in many countries of the world (United Nations 1996). A large number of countries now have national suicide prevention strategies. The first major national programme was established in Finland and, importantly, was based on the findings of a major research programme. Several other European countries have followed this lead. In 2001 the Surgeon General oversaw the publication of the suicide prevention strategy for the USA (US Department of Health and Human Services 2001). Australia and New

Zealand have also formulated strategies, with a particular emphasis on suicide prevention in young people. Now a strategy is being developed for China, where the numerical burden of suicide is huge.

Non-fatal suicidal acts and other acts of deliberate self-harm occur far more frequently than suicides. International estimates are of a ratio of some 10–20 such acts for every suicide (World Health Organization 2004). For the UK, because of its relatively high rate of deliberate self-harm, this ratio would be more like 30–40 times. These are crude estimates based on hospital statistics. It is increasingly recognized that much more deliberate self-harm occurs in the community and does not result in presentation to hospital or receive other medical attention. The overall burden of distress and misery represented by the extent of this phenomenon is clearly enormous. Of crucial importance in relation to suicide prevention is that this behaviour is the strongest predictor of eventual suicide. Therefore, national suicide prevention strategies rightly include a focus on non-fatal suicidal behaviour and other acts of deliberate self-harm, including their prevention and treatment.

For initiatives aimed at suicide prevention and treatment of suicidal behaviour to be effective, it is essential that they are based, whenever feasible, on sound research. This includes research into the epidemiology and causes of the problem, as well as the results of treatment and preventive initiatives. This is the reason for this book. Leading scientists and practitioners in the field were asked to present strategies for prevention and treatment of suicidal behaviour, based, wherever this is available, on firm scientific evidence. Thus each chapter includes a strong evidence base as well as clear practical guidance. Most essential components of a comprehensive suicide prevention strategy are covered, as well as guidance on effective clinical practice.

Part of the inspiration for this book was the Ninth European Symposium on Suicide and Suicidal Behaviour, held in the UK at Warwick University in September 2002. This was jointly organized by the Centre for Suicide Research at Oxford University and Samaritans. It provided the setting for the launch of the *National suicide prevention strategy for England* (Department of Health 2002). The conference was attended by researchers and clinicians in the field of suicidal behaviour from 39 nations. Many of the authors of chapters in this book gave keynote lectures at the conference. Other authors were enlisted to contribute in order to provide more comprehensive coverage of important topics, and because of their recognized expertise.

One approach to gaining evidence relevant to understanding which factors contribute to suicide is through the use of large-scale epidemiological registers. Very few countries have national registers, which is unfortunate as these provide an extremely powerful means of examining factors associated with a relatively rare event such as suicide. The Danish case registers are a prime example of such a database. In Chapter 2 Pin Qin and colleagues describe the use of various longitudinal registers for the whole Danish population, to investigate a range of factors in terms of their relative contribution to suicide. For example, they have been able to link information on family structure, to examine how marriage and parenthood influence suicide, including the potential protective aspects of these factors, and the different impacts these have on men and women. They have also investigated the impact of loss of a child on parental suicide risk. Other examples of uses of these registers include studying the influence of unemployment, disability, and income on suicide risk. Because the registers include information of psychiatric history, it has been feasible to determine how this moderates other influences. Further evidence from the registers that Qin and colleagues discuss includes the risk of suicide associated with living in rural compared with urban areas, the degree of contribution of psychiatric and physical disorders, and the role of family history of suicidal behaviour and psychiatric disorder. The results of this work have made a very considerable contribution, not only to an understanding of important risk and protective factors for suicide, but also pointing the way for preventive initiatives.

In Chapter 3 David Gunnell has used the national mortality register on suicide in England and Wales to review socio-economic influences on rates of suicide, and how rates have changed in relation to availability of certain methods used for suicide. He has highlighted the important fact that years of life lost to suicide need to be borne in mind, especially when assessing the impact of temporal changes in suicide rates, where rates in specific age groups change over time. He also addresses the evidence from national statistics of the influences of alcohol, socio-economic deprivation, and social fragmentation on suicide risk. In addition, Gunnell examines the important topic of variation in suicide rates between countries, and factors that may underly these. As he explains, the evidence he considers in this chapter has significant implications for national prevention policies.

A very different, but complementary approach to examining influences on suicide is taken by Stephen Platt and colleagues in Chapter 4. They move from the macro-level approach taken by the authors of the two previous chapters to using qualitative research methodology to investigate how personal disadvantage, negative early life experiences, and processes that lead to social exclusion interact with poor socio-economic and other adverse environmental conditions to lead to suicidal behaviour. Qualitative research methods have not been used a great deal so far in this field and one of the contributions of Platt and colleagues is to highlight how they may be applied to enhance our understanding of, and indeed to question, some of the findings based on quantitative research. Their results also help to put the role or function of non-fatal suicidal behaviour (and, by implication, suicide) in context in a way that may come as a surprise to some readers. The findings that they present have very important implications for the design of services and the content of treatments offered to patients who present to clinical agencies because of deliberate self-harm, especially those living in deprived and disrupted social environments.

The psychological basis of suicidal behaviour has been clarified further in recent years with the development of a model in which the role of a sense of entrapment has become central. Entrapment results from a person perceiving that they are defeated and/or humiliated, feeling that they must escape, and sensing that their present situation will continue indefinitely. Suicidal acts are viewed as a means of an individual escaping from this position. Mark Williams has principally been responsible for elucidating this model. In Chapter 5 he and his colleagues explain the basis of this theory in detail, including how deficiencies in problem solving, related to abnormalities of autobiographical memory, may contribute to a person feeling entrapped, and how a tendency to experience hopelessness may add to this. They also consider how differential activation—that is the tendency for patterns of moods, thoughts and bodily sensations all to be activated by changes in a single modality—may explain why some people rapidly and repeatedly experience thoughts of suicidal behaviour. They use this model as a basis for proposing how mindfulness-based cognitive therapy, already shown to be effective in preventing relapse of mood disorders, might have a significant role to play in the prevention of repetition of suicidal acts.

In Chapter 6 Kees van Heeringen also considers what makes some people vulnerable to suicidal behaviour, starting with the entrapment model and then considering how biological factors may provide a basis for understanding this. He draws on research findings concerning brain neurotransmitters, especially in the serotonergic and noradrenergic systems, and the hypothalamic–pituitary–adrenal axis, and of functional imaging of these systems, to postulate a bio-psychological model. While there remain gaps in our knowledge, the model van Heeringen proposes fits well with the psychological explanations by Williams and co-workers. It points to treatment innovations, particularly including combined psychological and pharmacological therapies aimed at having a maximal effect on suicidal predisposition.

It has long been recognized that suicide and deliberate self-harm may cluster in families, and that this may be due to inheritance of specific personality traits which may predispose people to suicidal behaviour. In Chapter 7, Andrej

Maruŝic and Peter McGuffin consider genetic vulnerability to suicidal behaviour. They outline the methods used for studying genetic influences and then focus on how these influences may affect the most well-studied biological substrate of suicidal phenomena, the serotonergic system. Maruŝic and McGuffin consider how genetic vulnerability may vary at the international level and hence influence differences in suicide rates between countries. Finally, they raise the important question of how the ethical aspects of our rapidly advancing knowledge of genetic factors in this field should be addressed.

In explaining suicide and deliberate self-harm there has long been emphasis on the impact of loss and conflict as key contributory factors. In Chapter 8 Lars Mehlum focuses instead on the role of traumatic stress. After explaining what traumatic stress is, including the differences in impact between acute and chronic stress, he examines the evidence for an association of suicidal behaviour with various stress experiences, including those related to childhood abuse, violence, and war. Mehlum then examines the mechanisms that may explain these associations. Finally, he considers the implications of the strong association between stress and suicidal behaviour for prevention and treatment, and especially for the clinician dealing with traumatized patients.

In Chapter 9 Louis Appleby and colleagues take a broad view on prevention, addressing the question of how the risk of suicide in patients in contact with psychiatric services could be reduced. They use data from the National Confidential Inquiry into Suicide (and Homicide) by People with Mental Illness, a clinical database of people who have died by suicide while in current or recent psychiatric care in the UK, together with findings from other related research studies, to identify key factors that should be addressed in a comprehensive programme for preventing suicide in psychiatric patients. These include developments in training, clinical services, use of medication, and management of patients with co-morbidity of psychiatric disorders, as well as specific means of making the environment of psychiatric in-patient units safer. These developments are central to one of the principal goals of the National Suicide Prevention Strategy for England (Department of Health 2002). They are also reflected in national suicide prevention strategies of some other nations.

One of the major obstacles to evaluation of initiatives to prevent suicide is the relatively low base rate of suicide. This limits our ability to evaluate many preventive initiatives using the gold standard of the randomized controlled trial. In Chapter 10 Robert Goldney explores interventions that have been evaluated largely pragmatically, not necessarily involving the rigour of randomized controlled trials but which he, none the less, rightly believes contribute to our knowledge base regarding prevention strategies. Some of these studies are based on longitudinal research methodology. Goldney also uses evidence from epidemiological and clinical studies to highlight important opportunities for effective suicide prevention.

A key factor in the recent focus of many nations on prevention of suicide has been the recognition of the extent of the burden of suicide in the context of overall causes of death. In Chapter 11 Kay Jamison and Keith Hawton illustrate this with a striking comparison of how numbers of suicides compare with those due to other causes of death, especially war and HIV/AIDS. They also underline the necessity of not just using rates to identify populations most at risk but also numerical burden, which may be concealed within rates due to differences in base populations across the age span. They then focus on the contribution of psychiatric disorders to risk of suicide, especially in young people for whom the early stages of these disorders often pose the greatest risk. Jamison and Hawton go on to make specific suggestions of how risk may be reduced during this period, especially in relation to the psychiatric disorders that carry the most serious suicide risk.

Deliberate self-harm (or attempted suicide) is the most important risk factor for eventual suicide. Risk is increased further when the behaviour is repeated. Also, the numbers of people who present to clinical services because of deliberate self-harm are very large, and in several countries the numbers are known to be increasing, especially in young people. Therefore much attention is being focused on how to treat patients more effectively, and especially how to reduce their risk of repetition. In Chapter 12 Keith Hawton considers the characteristics and needs of deliberate self-harm patients that should be addressed if treatments are to be effective. He then reviews the range of psychosocial interventions that have been evaluated in randomized controlled trials, and what conclusions can be reached to inform clinical practice. Finally, he outlines how treatments might be improved and what is required to develop a more informative evidence base in this field.

In most countries suicide rates are highest in older people. In Chapter 13 Yeates Conwell and Paul Duberstein review what is known about factors that contribute to suicide in older people, based on a series of psychological autopsy studies and community surveys from several countries. The evidence includes the role of psychiatric disorders, certain personality traits, specific symptoms that can prove particularly troubling in older people, physical disorders and impaired physical functioning, neurobiological changes, socio-cultural factors, and availability of means for suicide. Conwell and Duberstein then use this information to propose a comprehensive approach to suicide prevention in this segment of the population, and highlight evidence of the effectiveness of specific strategies.

Perhaps the most important contemporary controversy around suicide prevention is whether or not antidepressants prevent suicide or whether they can increase suicide risk (or indeed both). Given the high rates of depression found in all psychological autopsy studies of suicides, it may seem strange to suggest that the increasing use of antidepressants could do other than reduce suicide rates. Yet, as Herman van Praag correctly argues in Chapter 14, there is a surprising paucity of evidence that antidepressants are effective in this respect. He puts forward a series of possible explanations for why this might be, including a suggestion that predisposition to suicidality might be, to some extent, independent of depression. Van Praag's arguments present some important challenges for suicide prevention initiatives through the treatment of depression specifically by means of antidepressants. It is necessary to highlight the fact that other authors have argued in the opposite direction, for example putting forward evidence which they believe indicates that increased prescribing of antidepressants, especially selective serotonin reuptake inhibitors (SSRIs), has contributed to the reversal of the rising trend in suicides in both young people (e.g. Olfson *et al.* 2003) and in adults (Grunebaum *et al.* 2004). At the same time, the Committee on Safety of Medicines in the UK (Committee on Safety of Medicines 2004b) and the Federal Drugs and Foods Agency in the USA (Food and Drug Administration 2004) have issued specific warnings about use of SSRI antidepressants in young people, because of little evidence of efficacy, and indications that risk of adverse effects, including self-harm and suicidal thoughts, may be increased. A subsequent report on adults from a Committee on Safety of Medicines Expert Working Group, while not finding a specific association of suicide risk with SSRI antidepressants, has nevertheless urged greater care in prescribing of all antidepressants (Committee on Safety of Medicines 2004a). Clearly, we are at a very difficult point in time for clinicians and their patients with depression. Probably the best advice is that whenever antidepressants are prescribed there should be very careful monitoring, especially during the early stages of treatment when risk of suicide is greatest (Jick *et al.* 2004), and that other types of therapy should usually be considered, either as alternatives or to be combined with drug treatment.

Alcohol misuse has long been strongly linked to risk of suicide and deliberate self-harm. In Chapter 15 Ingeborg Rossow reviews the extensive evidence for this association. She also considers the association between drug abuse and suicidal behaviour. She then examines the specific factors that may make certain substance misusers more at risk than others and reviews the explanations for the specific impact of substance misuse on suicide risk. She also considers important gender, social, and cultural influences on alcohol and drug misuse, and how these are therefore relevant to population levels of suicidal behaviour. Finally, she reviews the key directions for prevention of risk related to substance misuse, with particular emphasis on national alcohol policy measures.

Reduction of access to commonly used methods of suicide is a key element in all national suicide prevention strategies. In Chapter 16 Keith Hawton reviews the reasons for this, including evidence that availability of means increases risk for suicide, the often transient nature of periods of high risk for suicidal actions, and examples of where changed availability of common methods of suicide has produced a reduction in rates of suicide. He then highlights specific methods of suicide for which tackling availability and access might further help reduce the burden of suicide.

Media influences on suicidal behaviour are also included as a target in many national suicide prevention strategies. In Chapter 17 Keith Hawton and Kathryn Williams summarize the results of a systematic review that they have conducted on the international research literature regarding studies of the influence of reporting of suicide in the news via newspapers and television, of portrayal of suicide and suicidal acts, both fictional and non-fictional, on film and television and in books. They also consider the influence of music on suicidal behaviour. They examine the role of increasingly available suicide instructions. In addition, they highlight the potential role of the Internet, which is causing alarm at the present time, especially with dramatic reports of strangers meeting through websites and arranging to die by suicide together. After considering the limited evidence on efforts to reduce such media influences, Hawton and Williams make proposals for future preventive activities in this area.

Suicide rates are thought to be high in prisons in many countries. In Chapter 18 Jo Paton and Rachel Jenkins consider the evidence for this, and then review what types of prisoners are most at risk and the environmental factors that may increase this problem. They also consider the extent and nature of suicide attempts in the prison population. Prevention of suicidal behaviour in the prison setting presents a considerable challenge. Paton and Jenkins describe the range of approaches that have been used, review the evidence of their effectiveness, and review other potential approaches.

In some countries voluntary agencies have led suicide prevention efforts. Samaritans, which started in London under the visionary lead of Chad Varah, represents probably the most well-known example of such an agency. In Chapter 19, Lakshmi Vijayakumar, leader of Sneha, an Indian volunteer agency, and Simon Armson, who was until recently Chief Executive of Samaritans in the UK, describe the nature of volunteer work, the characteristics of effective volunteers, and the evidence that voluntary services can make a difference. They are modest in their claims, yet the potential contribution of volunteers to national suicide efforts must be very considerable.

One of the most tragic aspects of death by suicide is that it usually has devastating and long-lasting effects on relatives, friends, and workmates. It has been suggested that each suicide has a major impact on approximately six living individuals. Also, it is well recognized that risk of suicide in people close to those who have died is greatly increased. The worldwide burden of those affected by such deaths is enormous. In the final chapter of this book Onja Grad considers in detail the impact of suicide, issues societies have in assisting the bereaved, and, most importantly, how this problem can be addressed in a humane and beneficial way.

This book is not intended to be a comprehensive textbook—other books fulfil this function (e.g. Hawton and van Heeringen, 2000; Maris *et al.*, 2000). Rather, it is intended to provide a major source for all who have an interest in prevention and treatment of suicidal behaviour, including psychiatrists, psychologists, social scientists, public health doctors and policy makers, general practitioners, psychiatric nurses, social workers, and workers in voluntary agencies.

As stated at the beginning of this chapter, the primary reason for preparing this book was to bring together the main sources of evidence that underpin efforts to effectively prevent suicide and treat those who survive suicidal acts. It is also intended to provide a rich source of ideas for all concerned with designing and implementing such prevention efforts. It is hoped that readers of this book will feel that these aims have been fulfilled—or at least that they will return to their important task with some new ideas which they can carry forward in their future work.

References

Committee on Safety of Medicines (2004a). Report of the CSM Expert Working Group on the safety of selective serotonin reuptake inhibitor antidepressants. Available at website http://www.mhra.gov.uk/news/2004/SSRIfinal.pdf (accessed 19 January 2005).

Committee on Safety of Medicines (2004b). Selective serotonin reuptake inhibitors (SSRIs): overview of regulatory status and CSM advice relating to major depressive disorder (MDD) in children and adolescents including a summary of available safety and efficacy data. Available at website http://medicines.mhra.gov.uk/ourwork/monitorsafequalmed/safetymessages/ssrioverview%5F101203.htm (accessed 14 January 2005).

Department of Health. (2002). *National suicide prevention strategy for England.* Department of Health, London.

Food and Drug Administration (2004). Antidepressant use in children, adolescents, and adults. Available at website http://www.fda.gov/cder/drug/antidepressants/default.htm (accessed 18 January 2005).

Grunebaum, M. F., Ellis, S. P., Li, S., Oquendo, M. A., and Mann, J. J. (2004). Antidepressants and suicide risk in the United States, 1985–1999. *Journal of Clinical Psychiatry,* 65, 1456–62.

Hawton, K. and Van Heeringen, K. (2000). *The international handbook of suicide and attempted suicide.* Wiley, Chichester.

Jick, H., Kaye, J. A., and Jick, S. S. (2004). Antidepressants and the risk of suicidal behaviors. *Journal of the American Medical Association,* 292, 338–43.

Maris, R. W., Berman, A. L., and Silverman, M. M. (2000). *Comprehensive textbook of suicidology.* Guilford, New York.

Olfson, M., Shaffer, D., Marcus, S. C., and Greenberg, T. (2003). Relationship between antidepressant medication treatment and suicide in adolescents. *Archives of General Psychiatry,* 60, 978–82.

United Nations (1996). *Prevention of suicide: Guidelines for the formulation and implementation of national strategies.* United Nations, New York.

US Department of Health and Human Services (2001). *National strategy for suicide prevention: Goals and objectives for action.* US Department of Health and Human Services, Public Health Service, Rockville, Maryland.

World Health Organization (2004). Suicide huge but preventable public health problem, says WHO (press release).

2

Factors contributing to suicide: the epidemiological evidence from large-scale registers

Ping Qin, Esben Agerbo, and Preben Bo Mortensen

The use of data from registers for suicide research

In the literature, most studies investigating risk factors for suicide have involved interviewing informants to collect data from a defined population. This may have advantages in yielding more detailed and complete information, for example in the context of psychological autopsy studies. However, one limitation of this method is that it may easily lead to recall bias or other information bias, because informants may have differential awareness of the problems in suicide victims and controls, respectively, or may not remember detailed information after a certain period after the suicide, or may have limited knowledge about the deceased, for example regarding family history of suicide and mental disorders. Another limitation of this method is often limited statistical power for analysis regarding less common risk factors, due to insufficient study cases. Fortunately, such shortcomings can be overcome in register-based studies.

Suicide research that uses data from large-scale registers has been developed in countries such as the USA (Herrell *et al.* 1999; Sernyak *et al.* 2001; Fu *et al.* 2002), Australia (Cantor *et al.* 1995), the UK (Hawton *et al.* 2003) and, in particular, in Nordic countries with a well-developed population registration system (Storm *et al.* 1992; Kyvik *et al.* 1994; Heikkinen *et al.* 1995; Stenager *et al.* 1996; Juel *et al.* 1999; Helweg-Larsen and Juel 2000; Koivumaa-Honkanen *et al.* 2001; Teasdale and Engberg 2001; Nilsson *et al.* 2002; Rasanen *et al.* 2002; Runeson and Åsberg 2003).

The main advantage of using large-scale registers for suicide research is the possibility of obtaining a large study population, thereby increasing the statistical power, which makes it possible to produce precise estimates, and to study rare events. For instance, in a Danish study (Qin *et al.* 2003), a large sample of more than 21 000 suicides during a 17-year period was obtained from the Danish Cause-of-Death Register, which made this study the largest case-control study in suicide research so far, and made it possible to include some very uncommon factors in the analysis, such as suicidal deaths in parents, children, and siblings. Another advantage is that data in registers are often collected systematically and uniformly, and without the purpose of any specific research project, which may reduce the risk of differential mis-classification bias. Moreover, through the well-established registers, it is pos-sible to obtain precise data concerning, for example, individual annual gross income, wealth, degree of unemployment, as well as the exact date of admis-sion to and discharge from a hospital, etc., which are generally difficult to obtain through interview.

On the other hand, there are also some limitations of using register data for suicide research. One is that the information in registers is sometimes limited. Since the variables included in studies largely depend on the availability of the data in source register databases, information on some desirable factors is likely to be missing. For instance, a previous suicide attempt has been noted as an important predictor for completed suicide, but such information is rarely available in a register that covers a nationwide or large community popula-tion. Also, non-differential information bias may be introduced because of the poor quality of data on some study variables in source registers. For example, alcohol and substance abuse are often variables of interest for suicide research, but it may be difficult to obtain precise information about them for individ-uals through a register.

Despite these limitations, the availability of registered individual data cov-ering a large, or even entire, national population has great potential for suicide research. This includes, for example, simple studies on prevalence, exploration of the longitudinal course of people who die by suicide, and record linkage studies on risk factors for suicide.

Denmark is one of the few countries in the world where various longitudinal registers containing data on individuals for a wide range of factors (e.g. family structure and history, income, hospital contacts) are available for the entire national population. The unique personal identification number, assigned to each individual born or residing in Denmark, is used in all national registers. This has made linkage of personal information across registers possible and accurate. In this chapter, we summarize the findings from register-based studies on risk factors for suicide, mainly from work done by our group, while drawing together findings from other large-scale studies.

Factors contributing to suicide

There have been few previous studies addressing suicide risk in large population-based samples while taking many risk factors into account simultaneously. The possibility of retrieving data from various Danish longitudinal registers has enabled us to conduct some of the largest studies on suicide, in terms of both the number of suicide cases and the range of study variables included. It has also enabled us to estimate the relative importance of a large range of factors associated with suicide (Table 1). In order to provide a clear picture, we group these variables into five major categories, including family structure, socio-economic and demographic factors, health status, and family history.

Family structure

Family structure could affect a person's decision to commit suicide through several factors, including marriage itself, parenthood, and, probably, factors relevant to the spouse.

Marital status has a strong influence on completed suicide (Kreitman 1988; Smith *et al.* 1988; Cantor and Slater 1995; Heikkinen *et al.* 1995; Kposowa 2000). Compared with married people, our study (Qin *et al.* 2003) demonstrated a significantly increased risk of suicide in single people [incidence risk ratio (IRR): 1.9, 95% confidence interval (CI): 1.8–1.9]. The risk was also increased in those who were cohabiting (IRR: 1.3, 95%CI: 1.2–1.4) even though cohabitation is almost equivalent to an officially certified marital relationship in the eyes of most people in Denmark. We also found that registered partners (i.e. homosexual couples living under the same legal status as a married couple) were more than 3.6 times (95%CI: 1.7–7.7) as likely to commit suicide in the full analysis after adjusting for differences in socio-economic status and psychiatric history.

The lower risk of suicide associated with married status may result from the protective effect of marriage itself, such as through promotion of motivation to remain alive, or through spousal supports when suffering setbacks or difficulties, while it may also result from the selection effect of marriage (Waldron *et al.* 1996)—that persons in better health or leading a happier life are more likely to marry, while persons with ill health are less likely to marry. Moreover, the finding that suicide risk incrementally increased between the categories of married, cohabiting, single, and registered homosexual relationship, suggests that family structure and coherence is associated with suicide, possibly because people with a traditional family orientation are less likely to

Table 2.1 Conditional logistic regression analysis of variables predicting risk of suicide among all persons who committed suicide in Denmark, 1981–1997, derived from comparison with live subjects matched for age, gender, and calendar year of suicide[a] (source: Qin et al. (2003). *American Journal of Psychiatry*, **160**, 765–72)

Variable	Crude Analysis[b] All subjects		Joint analysis[c] All subjects		Male subjects		Female subjects		Test of sex interaction[d]	
	IRR	95% CI	IRR	95% CI	IRR	95% CI	IRR	95% CI	χ²	P-value
Family structure										
Marital status									32.25	<0.0001
Married[e]	1.00		1.00		1.00		1.00			
Cohabiting	1.54*	1.45–1.63	1.32*	1.24–1.41	1.31*	1.22–1.41	1.19*	1.05–1.35		
Single	3.17*	3.08–3.27	1.87*	1.80–1.94	1.93*	1.84–2.03	1.55*	1.45–1.67		
Parenthood status									30.90	<0.0001
No young child[e]	1.00		1.00		1.00		1.00			
Child <2 years old	0.50*	0.45–0.55	0.64*	0.57–0.72	0.72*	0.64–0.82	0.41*	0.31–0.53		
Child 2–3 years old	0.65*	0.60–0.71	0.91	0.83–1.01	1.04	0.93–1.15	0.53*	0.41–0.68		
Child 4–6 years old	0.70*	0.65–0.75	0.95	0.88–1.03	1.00	0.91–1.09	0.77*	0.65–0.92		
Link to first-degree relatives[f]									2.75	0.0975
No[e]	1.00		1.00		1.00		1.00			
Yes	0.64*	0.61–0.66	0.99	0.95–1.04	1.02	0.96–1.07	0.93	0.85–1.01		
Economic factors										
Employment									69.29	<0.0001
Fully employed[e]	1.00		1.00		1.00		1.00			
<20% unemployed[g]	1.55*	1.45–1.64	1.14*	1.06–1.22	1.11*	1.03–1.20	1.23*	1.06–1.43		
20–80% unemployed	2.15*	2.05–2.27	1.19*	1.12–1.27	1.18*	1.10–1.27	1.15#	1.01–1.31		

(Continued)

Table 2.1 (continued) Conditional logistic regression analysis of variables predicting risk of suicide among all persons who committed suicide in Denmark, 1981–1997, derived from comparison with live subjects matched for age, gender, and calendar year of suicide[a] (source: Qin et al. (2003). *American Journal of Psychiatry*, **160**, 765–72).

Variable	Crude Analysis[b] All subjects		Joint analysis[c] All subjects		Male subjects		Female subjects		Test of sex interaction[d]	
	IRR	95% CI	IRR	95% CI	IRR	95% CI	IRR	95% CI	χ^2	P-value
81–100% unemployed	2.13*	1.95–2.32	1.24*	1.12–1.37	1.21*	1.07–1.36	1.19	0.97–1.46		
Full-time student	1.57*	1.36–1.81	0.78*	0.67–0.92	0.74*	0.61–0.89	0.91	0.67–1.24		
Age pensioner	2.15*	2.00–2.31	1.59*	1.47–1.73	1.42*	1.30–1.56	2.22*	1.89–2.61		
Disability pensioner	5.90*	5.59–6.22	1.42*	1.32–1.53	1.24*	1.12–1.36	1.85*	1.63–2.09		
Receipt of other benefits	5.97*	5.45–6.55	0.92	0.81–1.05	0.81*	0.70–0.95	1.25#	1.00–1.58		
Out of labour market	2.13*	1.99–2.28	0.69*	0.63–0.76	0.86#	0.76–0.98	0.72*	0.62–0.83		
Income									70.61	<0.0001
Highest quartile[e]	1.00		1.00		1.00		1.00			
Second quartile	1.66*	1.59–1.73	0.96	0.91–1.00	1.05	0.99–1.11	0.79*	0.72–0.87		
Third quartile	2.43*	2.32–2.54	0.94#	0.89–0.99	1.03	0.96–1.10	0.76*	0.68–0.84		
Lowest quartile	5.52*	5.24–5.81	2.66*	2.46–2.88	3.26*	2.97–3.57	1.88*	1.63–2.18		
Wealth									17.81	0.0005
Highest quartile[e]	1.00		1.00		1.00		1.00			
Second quartile	1.17*	1.12–1.21	0.81*	0.78–0.85	0.82*	0.78–0.87	0.80*	0.74–0.87		
Third quartile	2.09*	2.00–2.18	1.14*	1.08–1.20	1.24*	1.16–1.33	1.04	0.95–1.14		
Lowest quartile	1.05#	1.01–1.10	0.88*	0.84–0.93	0.93*	0.88–0.98	0.78*	0.70–0.86		
Other demographic factors										
Ethnicity										
Danish citizens born in Denmark[e]	1.00		1.00		1.00				9.95	0.0190

(Continued)

Table 2.1 (continued) Conditional logistic regression analysis of variables predicting risk of suicide among all persons who committed suicide in Denmark, 1981–1997, derived from comparison with live subjects matched for age, gender, and calendar year of suicide[a] (source: Qin et al. (2003). American Journal of Psychiatry, **160**, 765–72).

Variable	Crude Analysis[b] All subjects		Joint analysis[c] All subjects		Male subjects		Female subjects		Test of sex interaction[d]	
	IRR	95% CI	IRR	95% CI	IRR	95% CI	IRR	95% CI	χ²	P-value
Danish citizens born in Greenland	3.69*	2.95–4.62	2.65*	2.01–3.49	2.67*	1.89–3.78	2.68*	1.69–4.25		
Danish citizens born abroad	1.23*	1.12–1.34	1.15*	1.03–1.27	1.05	0.91–1.20	1.29*	1.10–1.51		
Non-Danish citizens	0.86*	0.77–0.95	0.86*	0.76–0.97	0.74*	0.64–0.85	1.07	0.86–1.34		
Place of residence										
Other areas[e,h]	1.00		1.00		1.00		1.00		59.83	<0.0001
Large city	1.06*	1.01–1.11	0.96	0.91–1.01	0.86*	0.81–0.91	1.21*	1.11–1.33		
Capital area	1.31*	1.27–1.35	1.01	0.98–1.05	0.92*	0.88–0.97	1.22*	1.14–1.29		
Health-related factors										
Sickness absence from work >3 weeks										
No[e]	1.00		1.00		1.00		1.00			
Yes	2.52*	2.42–2.64	1.96*	1.86–2.08	1.87*	1.76–2.00	2.19*	1.96–2.45	3.13	0.770
Psychiatric admission										
None[e]	1.00		1.00		1.00		1.00			
Currently admitted	57.07*	52.17–62.42	43.08*	39.22–47.33	28.23*	24.96–31.94	77.77*	66.93–90.38	279.69	<0.0001
Discharged <8 days	278.30*	217.56–365.01	226.02*	175.72–290.73	137.48*	101.13–186.90	493.45*	313.62–776.38		
Discharged 8–30 days	132.84*	112.51–156.83	107.22*	90.28–127.33	78.30*	62.88–97.51	172.42*	130.14–228.45		
Discharged 1–6 months	61.48*	56.40–67.02	44.05*	40.26–48.20	33.20*	29.56–37.30	66.32*	57.37–76.67		
Discharged 7–12 months	33.55*	30.44–36.99	22.89*	20.67–25.36	16.84*	14.71–19.27	34.75*	29.61–40.78		

(Continued)

Table 2.1 (continued) Conditional logistic regression analysis of variables predicting risk of suicide among all persons who committed suicide in Denmark, 1981–1997, derived from comparison with live subjects matched for age, gender, and calendar year of suicide[a] (source: Qin et al. (2003). American Journal of Psychiatry, **160**, 765–72).

Variable	Crude Analysis[b] All subjects		Joint analysis[c] All subjects		Male subjects		Female subjects		Test of sex interaction[d]	
	IRR	95% CI	IRR	95% CI	IRR	95% CI	IRR	95% CI	χ^2	P-value
Discharged >1 year	8.50*	8.16–8.85	6.02*	5.75–6.29	4.86*	4.58–5.15	8.28*	7.72–8.89	5.98	0.0145
Clinical history of first-degree relatives										
Suicide										
None[e]	1.00		1.00		1.00		1.00			
At least one	3.50*	3.03–4.04	2.14*	1.79–2.57	1.90*	1.53–2.36	2.95*	2.10–4.13		
No link to first-degree relatives[i]	1.58*	1.52–1.65								
Psychiatric admission									0.12	0.7312
None[e]	1.00		1.00		1.00		1.00			
At least one	2.19*	2.07–2.31	1.27*	1.19–1.36	1.29*	1.19–1.39	1.24*	1.10–1.41		
No link to first-degree relatives[i]	1.67*	1.61–1.74								

[a] Data were drawn from four Danish Longitudinal registers. Subjects included 21 169 suicides (13 681 men, 7488 women) and 423 128 live controls matched for age, sex and calendar time of suicide using a nested case-control design.

[b] Incidence risk ratios (IRR) were adjusted for age, sex, and calendar year of suicide through matching.

[c] Incidence risk ratios were adjusted for age, sex, calendar year of suicide, and all other variables shown in the table.

[d] Test of sex interaction was carried out by means of likelihood ratio test.

[e] Reference category.

[f] Link to first-degree relatives (mother, father, siblings, children) was identified by means of the Danish Civil Registration System.

[g] Degree of unemployment was measured as the proportion of weeks in the year for which unemployment benefits were paid.

[h] Large cities were those with more than 100 000 inhabitants; the capital area encompassed the Copenhagen and Frederiksberg municipality and its suburbs.

[i] Reference category for link to relatives was excluded from the joint analysis.

* $P < 0.01$; * $P < 0.05$.

practice some negative health behaviours (Joung *et al.* 1995) associated with suicide risk, such as substance abuse.

Some studies have suggested that parenthood is associated with a reduced risk of suicidal behaviour (Linehan *et al.* 1983; Hoyer and Lund 1993; Jobes and Mann 1999). Our study on the impact of parental status on the risk of completed suicide in the context of other risk factors (Qin and Mortensen 2003) showed that the protective effect of parenthood existed independently of individual marital, socio-economic, and psychiatric status in both fathers and mothers, and that having a child of young age appeared to protect parents from suicide to a higher degree than having several children of older age. These results indicate that child-related concerns strongly affect a parent's decision about ending life. The presence of a young child may be particularly likely to raise the parents' perception of being needed, thus preventing them from committing suicide.

Moreover, marriage and parenthood seem to have different impacts on suicide risks of men and women. Our studies indicated that being married was more protective against suicide in men than in women, whereas parenthood was more protective against suicide in women than in men (Qin *et al.* 2000, 2003; Qin and Mortensen 2003). At the same time, our work also showed that the effect of parenthood (i.e. having children and/or having a young child) on risk of suicide did not differ according to marital status in women, whereas it differed significantly by marital status in men. Being a parent reduced suicide risk for men who were married or cohabiting, whereas it increased the risk for men who were living singly (Qin and Mortensen 2003). These combined results support the hypothesis first suggested by Durkheim (1966) that the protective effect of marriage for suicide risk of women is largely an effect of having children. They are also concordant with the so-called 'attachment effect' suggested by Adam (1990). The results, in other words, may imply that being a parent of a young child appears to explain the apparent protective effect of marriage for women rather than married status *per se*, whereas in men marriage appears to be a protective factor in its own right (Hawton 2000). However, this does not conflict with the protective impact of parenthood on suicide in men. The negative effect of having children on fathers living singly may largely be because fewer fathers than mothers have the custody of their children when separated or divorced.

On the other hand, our research also showed that loss of a child markedly increased suicide risk for both men and women, and that the relative risk was even increased when adjusted for other risk factors (Qin and Mortensen 2003). The effect was particularly marked in parents who had had a child die during early childhood [the odds ratio was 5.2 (95%CI: 3.2–8.4) for men and 4.7 (95%CI: 2.1–10.4] for women, respectively, if a child had died between the ages of 1 and 6 years). The relative risk decreased somewhat when a child had died at an older age, but the suicidal death of an adult child also showed a strong impact on parental, especially maternal, suicide risk. These findings suggest that the loss of a child may contribute more than other factors to provoking parents to want to die, and that this is especially the case when they lose a young child who is likely to be strongly attached to, and dependent upon, the parents. Moreover, our work further demonstrated that parents were at an extremely high risk for suicide during the first month after losing a child (IRR: 34.7, 95%CI: 19.3–62.3 for men; IRR: 76.1, 95%CI: 26.6–217.1 for women) (Qin and Mortensen 2003). This result strongly suggests that familial and social support is necessary and important for parents who lose a child, especially during the first month after the death.

However, it is unclear how children's health status affects parent's perception of dying. From our work, we found that having a child admitted for a psychiatric disorder significantly raised suicide risk in parents, but that its effect was reduced when adjusted for parents' own psychiatric history. Also, the increased risk was confined to parents who themselves had never had a psychiatric illness (Qin and Mortensen 2003). If psychiatric illness in children increases suicide risk in parents through the great likelihood of there being psychiatric illness in the parents, one may hypothesis that parents with a physically sick child may be less likely to commit suicide because of being needed. However, no study has so far addressed the risk of suicide among parents of children with physical illness.

For married people, suicide risk is also associated with their spousal conditions, such as psychiatric status and death. In a recent study, we included information on spouses for people aged 25–60 years, with the goal of investigating the non-genetic association between mental illness, suicide, or death, and suicide of the other spouse (Agerbo 2003). This study showed that individuals whose spouses had been first admitted to hospital with a psychiatric illness within the previous 2 years, had a fivefold increased risk of suicide. It also showed that conjugal bereavement has an impact on mortality among surviving spouses, and that suicide bereavement increases the risk of suicide more than bereavement following other causes of death.

Economic factors

The risk of suicide is generally high among people suffering from economic stressors, such as being unemployed, having a low income, or facing financial problems. In a recent systematic review of the literature from 1984 onward, Platt and Hawton (2000) concluded that unemployment significantly increased the risk of suicide at an individual level.

Our studies demonstrated significantly high risks for suicide associated with unemployment, receipt of disability pension, low income, and low wealth status, while adjusting only for age and sex (Mortensen *et al.* 2000; Qin *et al.* 2003). These results are as expected and are compatible with many other reports (Cantor *et al.* 1995; Johansson and Sundquist 1997; Lewis and Sloggett 1998). However, the increased risks associated with these variables were decreased markedly, or even reversed, after further adjusted for psychiatric and other factors. This suggests that the effects of socio-economic factors on suicide tend to be overestimated when the contribution of psychiatric disorders is not taken into account. This may explain why our estimates of relative risks and attributable risk associated with unemployment are lower than in other studies (e.g. Lewis and Sloggett 1998).

Indeed, in another of our studies we found a contrary pattern of the influence of income on suicide according to psychiatric status (Agerbo *et al.* 2001). For people without a psychiatric history, suicide risk increased with decreasing income, whereas for people with a psychiatric history, the risk of suicide fell significantly with decreasing income. However, this study could not resolve whether this was a 'healthy worker effect' (Li *et al.* 1999), or a true effect caused by stigma or other factors associated with the combined effect of being richer and suffering from a mental illness.

In addition, our studies indicated that the impacts of labour market status, income, and wealth on suicide risk differed significantly by sex (Mortensen *et al.* 2000; Qin *et al.* 2003). For instance, the risk of suicide rose with increasing degree of unemployment in men, while there was no such trend in women; compared with people whose annual incomes were in the highest quartile, men with lower-quartile income were at an increased risk whereas women with the middle level of income were at a reduced risk of suicide. Our results, which show that economic stressors or disadvantage, such as unemployment and low income, increased suicide risk more in men than in women, support the hypothesis that men respond more strongly to poor economic conditions than do women (Crombie 1990). The different roles and expectations of men and women in society may affect their propensity to commit suicide. Although economic stressors are common to both genders, one could hypothesize that the roles and expectations of men in family and society may more easily lead to loss of self-esteem if they are unable to live up to expectations, and then they may be more vulnerable to suicide.

Other demographic factors

Suicide rates are generally higher in urban than in rural areas in most countries, although there are important exceptions, such as in China (Qin and Mortensen 2001). Our finding of suicide risk increasing with the degree of urbanicity in univariate analysis (Qin *et al.* 2003) is concordant with some studies from Western countries reporting that people living in large urban areas were at an increased risk of suicide (Heikkinen *et al.* 1994; Johansson *et al.* 1997). However, when further adjusted for other risk factors, the result showed that living in a more urbanized area increased suicide risk in women but reduced suicide risk in men. One explanation could be that living in a big city may entail, for example, better job opportunities that may benefit men more, whereas women may be more vulnerable in a competitive environment than their male counterparts.

Furthermore, our finding of a higher risk of suicide for Danish citizens born abroad is consistent with a Swedish study by Johansson *et al.* (1997), but this effect is prominent only for women after adjusting for other factors in our study (Qin *et al.* 2003). At the same time, our study (Qin *et al.* 2003) shows that male non-Danish citizens have a lower risk of suicide than male Danish citizens born in Denmark. Reasons for this may include cultural differences in attitudes toward suicidal behaviour between countries, the different spectrum of countries that male and female immigrants come from, as well as different purposes of immigration between men and women.

Health status

Psychiatric illness has been demonstrated to be the most prominent risk factor for suicide. Our studies showed that a history of hospitalization for psychiatric disorder was the risk factor associated with the highest relative risk and the highest attributable risk for suicide in both men and women, and that the risk was extremely high for people recently discharged from hospital (Mortensen *et al.* 2000; Agerbo *et al.* 2002; Qin *et al.* 2003). This finding is consistent with many previous studies reporting a higher suicide risk for individuals diagnosed with mental disorders (Moscicki 1994; Dennehy *et al.* 1996; Harris and Barraclough 1997; Heikkinen *et al.* 1997). Also, the finding of an extremely high suicide risk for people recently discharged from hospital (e.g. discharged within 7 days, IRR: 226.0, 95%CI: 175.7–290.7) is in line with other studies using data from the Danish Psychiatric Central Register (Mortensen and Juel 1993; Rossau and Mortensen 1997; Emborg 1999; Hoyer *et al.* 2000), as well as studies from other countries (Goldacre *et al.* 1993; Appleby *et al.* 1999; Lawrence *et al.* 1999).

Moreover, we noted a significant gender difference in the influence of a previous psychiatric hospitalization on suicide (Qin *et al.* 2000, 2003), which, in connection with the results of adjusted analyses for men and women, means that a history of psychiatric hospitalization increased suicide risk significantly more in women than in men. However, it should be noted that this finding does not mean that women with a psychiatric disorder leading to hospitalization had higher suicide mortality than their male counterparts, because the suicide mortality in the general population is lower in women than in men.

In our studies, about 43% male and 60% female suicides had ever been admitted to hospital because of psychiatric illness (Qin *et al.* 2003), which are much lower figures than the often-reported 90% of all completed suicides fulfilling the criteria for a psychiatric diagnosis (Rich *et al.* 1986; Cheng 1995; Conwell *et al.* 1996; Foster *et al.* 1997). This is probably because we were only able to take in-patients into account and were unable to get information for those with disorders not leading to admission. It is likely that the effect of hospitalized psychiatric illness in our studies was underestimated because the excluded patients, for example outpatients, who are generally also at a higher risk of suicide than people without psychiatric illness, were placed in the reference group. However, in the context of the overall effect of psychiatric illness, it is difficult to say whether its effect was overestimated or underestimated, because on the one hand in-patients are probably more suicidal than other people suffering from mental illness, but on the other hand, a large proportion of people with mental disorders not leading to hospitalization were not counted as exposed to the risk factor of psychiatric illness (as defined by admission to hospital). Nevertheless, this means that our estimates of the population attributable risk associated with psychiatric illness, that is that psychiatric illness accounted for 33.0% of male suicides and 53.6% of female suicides (Qin *et al.* 2003), are likely to be underestimated.

Other indicators concerning health status that we have studied are receipt of disability pension and sickness absence from job due to illness. Although a history of either of these two variables might result from mental illness, the analyses showed that their effects remained highly significant even after adjusting for psychiatric status and other factors (Qin *et al.* 2003). This may indicate that poor health status due to other illnesses, rather than psychiatric disorders, is also a significant risk factor for suicide. This would be consistent with the finding summarized in two reviews (Harris and Barraclough 1994; Stenager and Stenager 2000) that physical illness could increase the risk of suicide.

Family history of suicide and psychiatric illness

It has been demonstrated in many studies that suicide risk is associated with familial psychopathology (Egeland and Sussex 1985; Shafii *et al.* 1985; Gould *et al.* 1996; Wagner 1997) and suicidal behaviours (Murphy and Wetzel 1982; Gould *et al.* 1996; Runeson 1998). Our study, based on the general population data, indicated that both a family history of completed suicide (IRR: 2.1. 95%CI: 1.8–2.6) and a family history of hospitalized psychiatric disorders (IRR: 1.3, 95%CI: 1.2–1.4) raised the risk of suicide even after further adjusted for the person's own psychiatric admission status and other risk factors (Qin et al. 2003). Moreover, the impact of family history seems to be stronger for adolescents and young adults. For instance, in our study on young people under 21 years old we found that the risk of suicide was 4.8 (95%CI: 2.1–10.8) times more likely in the offspring of mothers who had completed suicide and 2.3 (95%CI:1.1–4.8) times as common in the offspring of fathers who had committed suicide, while the equivalent risks associated with a history of psychiatric admission in mothers and fathers, respectively, were 1.7 (95%CI: 1.3–2.3) and 1.6 (95%CI: 1.1–2.2) (Agerbo et al. 2002).

A further study in which we focused on suicide in relation to family history provides more insights into this matter (Qin et al. 2002). This study demonstrated that completed suicide and a history of hospitalized psychiatric illness in mothers, fathers, and/or siblings acted independently as risk factors for suicide in the general population, and that their effects could not be explained by differences in socio-economic, demographic, and psychiatric status. Moreover, this study also showed that a family history of psychiatric illness significantly interacted with psychiatric status of probands, increasing suicide risk only in persons without a history of psychiatric hospitalization, whereas a family history of completed suicide significantly increased suicide risk independently of a family history of psychiatric disorder or mental illness in probands. These results strongly suggest that suicide clusters in families independently of familial clustering of psychiatric disorder, and that a family history of psychiatric illness only increases suicide risk through increasing the risk for developing a mental disorder, while a family history of completed suicide significantly increases suicide risk in its own right.

Implications

The findings and interpretation of risk factors identified in our studies, as well as other register-based studies, may have implications for the choice of strategies for suicide prevention in the general population, and, in turn, may also assist in predicting the potential effects of different suicide prevention strategies.

There are basically two approaches to suicide prevention: one aims to influence the risk in the general population while the other aims to influence the risk in individuals at high risk of suicide. The detailed strategies developed and implemented in different countries share many common themes (Taylor *et al.* 1997), but the effectiveness of these intervention strategies is poorly documented in the literature (Lewis *et al.* 1997).

Based upon the findings from our studies, we believe, as also suggested by the others (Rihmer 1996; Appleby 2000; Jenkins and Singh 2000), that mental illness should be a focus for preventive interventions and assessment of these interventions. This approach has been included in health programmes in some countries, such as Finland, UK, Canada, USA, and Australia (Jenkins and Singh 2000). Although, so far, there is no strong evidence to demonstrate the efficiency of such an approach, the study on Gotland in Sweden indicated that systematic postgraduate education of general practitioners could explain the reduction of suicide rate after the implementation of the programme (Rutz *et al.* 1989). However, it is difficult to know to what extent this can be generalized to other regions in Sweden or other countries, because Gotland is an island with a small population. As most patients with psychiatric illness do not commit suicide, we think that better training of mental health professionals and general practitioners about the diagnosis and management of mental disorders, and improved psychopathological assessment and post-discharge treatment in psychiatric departments, should be seen as measures generally to improve psychiatric services, with the added potential of decreasing suicide rates, rather than having the sole aim of suicide prevention. Also, improvement of health-service care for the general population, and maintaining care beyond the point of clinical recovery, may be important in protecting high-risk individuals.

Although suggestions of improving social cohesion to make suicide less likely may not be realistic and efficient, we should not discount the possiblity that approaches such as social and economic policies, for example, reducing unemployment (as suggested by Lewis *et al.* 1997), might well have some impact on suicide rates, even though only to a limited extent.

Our results concerning the significant gender differences in risk factors for suicide suggest that both population-based and high-risk group prevention strategies should take gender differences in risk factors into account, and that the effects of interventions may differ by gender. The different roles of men and women in family and society may affect their reactions when exposed to risk factors. Men may generally be more unwilling to seek help and to recognize their own depression and helplessness, whereas women generally have better coping strategies, such as the use of supportive social networks (Haste *et al.* 1998). The educational programme for general practitioners in Gotland actually indicated that the benefits were mostly confined to women (Rutz 2001). However, replications are needed, especially on the basis of large population samples.

References

Adam, K.S. (1990). Environmental, psychosocial, and psychoanalytic aspects of suicidal behavior. In *Suicide over the life cycle: risk fators, assessment, and treatment of suicidal patients*, (ed. S.J. Blumental and D.J. Kupfer), pp. 39–97. American Psychiatric Press, Washington, DC.

Agerbo, E. (2003). Spousal psychiatric illness, suicide and other causes of death in relation to risk of suicide: nested case-control study. *British Medical Journal*, 327, 1025–6.

Agerbo, E., Mortensen, P.B., Eriksson, T., Qin, P., and Westergaard-Nielsen, N. (2001). Risk of suicide in relation to income level in people admitted to hospital with mental illness: nested case-control study. *British Medical Journal*, 322, 334–5.

Agerbo, E., Nordentoft, M., and Mortensen, P.B. (2002). Familial, psychiatric, and socioeconomic risk factors for suicide in young people: nested case-control study. *British Medical Journal*, 325, 74.

Appleby, L. (2000). Prevention of suicide in psychiatric patients. In *The international handbook of suicide and completed suicide*, (ed. K. Hawton and K. van Heeringen), pp. 617–30. Wiley, Chichester.

Appleby, L., Shaw, J., Amos, T., McConnell, R., Harris, C., McCann, K., *et al.* (1999). Suicide within 12 months of contact with mental health services: national clinical survey. *British Medical Journal*, 318, 1235–9.

Cantor, C.H. and Slater, P.J. (1995). Marital breakdown, parenthood and suicide. *Journal of Family Studies*, 1, 91–102.

Cantor, C.H., Slater, P.J., and Najman, J.M. (1995). Socioeconomic indices and suicide rate in Queensland. *Australian Journal of Public Health*, 19, 417–20.

Cheng, A.T. (1995). Mental illness and suicide. A case-control study in east Taiwan. *Archives of General Psychiatry*, 52, 594–603.

Conwell, Y., Duberstein, P.R., Cox, C., Herrmann, J.H., Forbes, N.T., and Caine, E.D. (1996). Relationships of age and axis I diagnoses in victims of completed suicide: a psychological autopsy study. *American Journal of Psychiatry*, 153, 1001–8.

Crombie, I.K. (1990). Can changes in the unemployment rates explain the recent changes in suicide rates in developed countries? *International Journal of Epidemiology*, 19, 412–16.

Dennehy, J.A., Appleby, L., Thomas, C.S., and Faragher, E.B. (1996). Case-control study of suicide by discharged psychiatric patients. *British Medical Journal*, 312, 1580.

Durkheim, E. (1966). *Suicidei* (trans. J.A. Spaulding and G. Simpson). The Free Press, New York.

Egeland, J.A. and Sussex, J.N. (1985). Suicide and family loading for affective disorders. *Journal of the American Medical Association*, 254, 915–18.

Emborg, C. (1999). Mortality and causes of death in eating disorders in Denmark 1970–1993: a case register study. *International Journal of Eating Disorders*, 25, 243–51.

Foster, T., Gillespie, K., and McClelland, R. (1997). Mental disorders and suicide in Northern Ireland. *British Journal of Psychiatry*, 170, 447–52.

Fu, Q., Heath, A.C., Bucholz, K.K., Nelson, E.C., Glowinski, A., Goldberg, J., *et al.* (2002). A twin study of genetic and environmental influences on suicidality in men. *Psychological Medicine*, 32, 11–24.

Goldacre, M., Seagroatt, V., and Hawton, K. (1993). Suicide after discharge from psychiatric inpatient care. *Lancet*, 342, 283–6.

Gould, M.S., Fisher, P., Parides, M., Flory, M., and Shaffer, D. (1996). Psychosocial risk factors of child and adolescent completed suicide. *Archives of General Psychiatry*, 53, 1155–62.

Harris, E.C. and Barraclough, B.M. (1994). Suicide as an outcome for medical disorders. *Medicine*, 73, 281–96.

Harris, E.C. and Barraclough, B. (1997). Suicide as an outcome for mental disorders. A meta-analysis. *British Journal of Psychiatry*, 170, 205–28.

Haste, F., Charlton, J., and Jenkins, R. (1998). Potential for suicide prevention in primary care? An analysis of factors associated with suicide. *British Journal of General Practice*, 48, 1759–63.

Hawton, K. (2000). Sex and suicide. Gender differences in suicidal behaviour. *British Journal of Psychiatry*, 177, 484–5.

Hawton, K., Zahl, D., and Weatherall, R. (2003). Suicide following deliberate self-harm: long-term follow-up of patients who presented to a general hospital. *British Journal of Psychiatry*, 182, 537–42.

Heikkinen, M., Aro, H., and Lonnqvist, J. (1994). Recent life events, social support and suicide. *Acta Psychiatrica Scandinavica (Suppl)*, 377, 65–72.

Heikkinen, M.E., Isometsa, E.T., Marttunen, M.J., Aro, H.M., and Lonnqvist, J.K. (1995). Social factors in suicide. *British Journal of Psychiatry*, 167, 747–53.

Heikkinen, M.E., Henriksson, M.M., Isometsa, E.T., Marttunen, M.J., Aro, H.M., and Lonnqvist, J.K. (1997). Recent life events and suicide in personality disorders. *Journal of Nervous and Mental Disease*, 185, 373–81.

Helweg-Larsen, K. and Juel, K. (2000). Sex differences in mortality in Denmark during half a century, 1943–92. *Scandinavian Journal of Public Health*, 28, 214–21.

Herrell, R., Goldberg, J., True, W.R., Ramakrishran, V., Lyons, M., Eisen, S., and Tsuang, M.T. (1999). Sexual orientation and suicidality: a co-twin control study in adult men. *Archives of General Psychiatry*, 56, 867–74.

Hoyer, E.H., Mortensen, P.B., and Olesen, A.V. (2000). Mortality and causes of death in a total national sample of patients with affective disorders admitted for the first time between 1973 and 1993. *British Journal of Psychiatry*, 176, 76–82.

Hoyer, G. and Lund, E. (1993). Suicide among women related to number of children in marriage. *Archives of General Psychiatry*, 50, 134–7.

Jenkins, R. and Singh, B. (2000). General population strategies of suicide prevention. In *The international handbook of suicide and attempted suicide* (ed. K. Hawton and K. van Heeringen), pp. 597–625. Wiley, Chichester.

Jobes, D.A. and Mann, R.E. (1999). Reasons for living versus reasons for dying: examining the internal debate of suicide. *Suicide and Life-Threatening Behavior*, 29, 97–104.

Johansson, L.M., Sundquist, J., Johansson, S.E., and Bergman, B. (1997). Ethnicity, social factors, illness and suicide: a follow-up study of a random sample of the Swedish population. *Acta Psychiatrica Scandinavica*, 95, 125–31.

Johansson, S.E. and Sundquist, J. (1997). Unemployment is an important risk factor for suicide in contemporary Sweden: an 11-year follow-up study of a cross-sectional sample of 37,789 people. *Public Health*, 111, 41–5.

Joung, I.M., Stronks, K., Van de Mheen, H., and Mackenbach, J.P. (1995). Health behaviours explain part of the differences in self reported health associated with partner/marital status in The Netherlands. *Journal of Epidemiology and Community Health*, 49, 482–8.

Juel, K., Mosbech, J., and Hansen, E.S. (1999). Mortality and causes of death among Danish medical doctors 1973–1992. *International Journal of Epidemiology*, 28, 456–60.

Koivumaa-Honkanen, H., Honkanen, R., Viinamaki, H., Heikkila, K., Kaprio, J., and Koskenvuo, M. (2001). Life satisfaction and suicide: a 20-year follow-up study. *American Journal of Psychiatry*, 158, 433–9.

Kposowa, A.J. (2000). Marital status and suicide in the National Longitudinal Mortality Study. *Journal of Epidemiology and Community Health*, 54, 254–61.

Kreitman, N. (1988). Suicide, age and marital status. *Psychological Medicine*, 18, 121–8.

Kyvik, K.O., Stenager, E.N., Green, A., and Svendsen, A. (1994). Suicides in men with IDDM. *Diabetes Care*, 17, 210–12.

Lawrence, D.M., Holman, C.D., Jablensky, A.V., and Fuller, S.A. (1999). Suicide rates in psychiatric in-patients: an application of record linkage to mental health research. *Australian and New Zealand Journal of Public Health*, 23, 468–70.

Lewis, G. and Sloggett, A. (1998). Suicide, deprivation, and unemployment: record linkage study. *British Medical Journal*, 317, 1283–6.

Lewis, G., Hawton, K., and Jones, P. (1997). Strategies for preventing suicide. *British Journal of Psychiatry*, 171, 351–4.

Li, C.Y., Du, C.L., Chen, C.J., and Sung, F.C. (1999). A registry-based case-control study of risk factors for the development of multiple non-fatal injuries on the job. *Occupational Medicine*, 49, 331–4.

Linehan, M.M., Goodstein, J.L., Nielsen, S.L., and Chiles, J.A. (1983). Reasons for staying alive when you are thinking of killing yourself: the reasons for living inventory. *Journal of Consulting and Clinical Psychology*, 51, 276–86.

Mortensen, P.B. and Juel, K. (1993). Mortality and causes of death in first admitted schizophrenic patients. *British Journal of Psychiatry*, 163, 183–9.

Mortensen, P.B., Agerbo, E., Erikson, T., Qin, P., and Westergaard-Nielsen, N. (2000). Psychiatric illness and risk factors for suicide in Denmark. *Lancet*, 355, 9–12.

Moscicki, E.K. (1994). Gender differences in completed and attempted suicides. *Annals of Epidemiology*, 4, 152–8.

Murphy, G.E. and Wetzel, R.D. (1982). Family history of suicidal behavior among suicide attempters. *Journal of Nervous and Mental Disease*, 170, 86–90.

Nilsson, L., Ahlbom, A., Farahmand, B.Y., Åsberg, M., and Tomson, T. (2002). Risk factors for suicide in epilepsy: a case control study. *Epilepsia*, 43, 644–51.

Platt, S. and Hawton, K. (2000). Suicide behaviour and the labour market. In *The international handbook of suicide and attempted suicide*, (ed. K. Hawton and K. van Heeringen), pp. 309–84. Wiley, Chichester.

Qin, P. and Mortensen, P.B. (2001). Specific characteristics of suicide in China. *Acta Psychiatrica Scandinavica*, 103, 117–21.

Qin, P. and Mortensen, P.B. (2003). The impact of parental status on the risk of completed suicide. *Archives of General Psychiatry*, 60, 797–802.

Qin, P., Mortensen, P.B., Agerbo, E., Westergard-Nielsen, N., and Eriksson, T. (2000). Gender differences in risk factors for suicide in Denmark. *British Journal of Psychiatry*, 177, 546–50.

Qin, P., Agerbo, E., and Mortensen, P.B. (2002). Suicide risk in relation to family history of completed suicide and psychiatric disorders: a nested case-control study based on longitudinal registers. *Lancet*, 360, 1126–30.

Qin, P., Agerbo, E., and Mortensen, P.B. (2003). Suicide risk in relation to socioeconomic, demographic, psychiatric, and familial factors: a national register-based study of all suicides in Denmark, 1981–1997. *American Journal of Psychiatry*, 160, 765–72.

Rasanen, P., Hakko, H., Jokelainen, J., and Tiihonen, J. (2002). Seasonal variation in specific methods of suicide: a national register study of 20,234 Finnish people. *Journal of Affective Disorder*, 71, 51–9.

Rich, C.L., Young, D., and Fowler, R.C. (1986). San Diego suicide study. I. Young vs old subjects. *Archives of General Psychiatry*, 43, 577–82.

Rihmer, Z. (1996). Strategies of suicide prevention: focus on health care. *Journal of Affective Disorders*, 39, 83–91.

Rossau, C.D. and Mortensen, P.B. (1997). Risk factors for suicide in patients with schizophrenia: nested case-control study. *British Journal of Psychiatry*, 171, 355–9.

Runeson, B.S. (1998). History of suicidal behaviour in the families of young suicides. *Acta Psychiatrica Scandinavica*, 98, 497–501.

Runeson, B. and Åsberg, M. (2003). Family history of suicide among suicide victims. *American Journal of Psychiatry*, 160, 1525–6.

Rutz, W. (2001). Preventing suicide and premature death by education and treatment. *Journal of Affective Disorders*, 62, 123–9.

Rutz, W., von Knorring, L., and Walinder, J. (1989). Frequency of suicide on Gotland after systematic postgraduate education of general practitioners. *Acta Psychiatrica Scandinavica*, 80, 151–4.

Sernyak, M.J., Desai, R., Stolar, M., and Rosenheck, R. (2001). Impact of clozapine on completed suicide. *American Journal of Psychiatry*, 158, 931–7.

Shafii, M., Carrigan, S., Whittinghill, J.R., and Derrick, A. (1985). Psychological autopsy of completed suicide in children and adolescents. *American Journal of Psychiatry*, 142, 1061–4.

Smith, J.C., Mercy, J.A., and Conn, J.M. (1988). Marital status and the risk of suicide. *American Journal of Public Health*, 78, 78–80.

Stenager, E.N. and Stenager, E. (2000). Physical illness and suicidal behaviour. In *The international handbook of suicide and attempted suicide*, (ed. K. Hawton and K. van Heeringen), pp. 405–20. Wiley, Chichester.

Stenager, E.N., Koch-Henriksen, N., and Stenager, E. (1996). Risk factors for suicide in multiple sclerosis. *Psychotherapy and Psychosomatics*, 65, 86–90.

Storm, H.H., Christensen, N., and Jensen, O.M. (1992). Suicides among Danish patients with cancer: 1971 to 1986. *Cancer*, 69, 1507–12.

Taylor, S.J., Kingdom, D., and Jenkins, R. (1997). How are nations trying to prevent suicide? An analysis of national suicide prevention strategies. *Acta Psychiatrica Scandinavica*, 95, 457–63.

Teasdale, T.W. and Engberg, A.W. (2001). Suicide after a stroke: a population study. *Journal of Epidemiology and Community Health*, 55, 863–6.

Wagner, B.M. (1997). Family risk factors for child and adolescent suicidal behavior. *Psychological Bulletin*, 121, 246–98.

Waldron, I., Hughes, M.E., and Brooks, T.L. (1996). Marriage protection and marriage selection–prospective evidence for reciprocal effects of marital status and health. *Social Science and Medicine*, 43, 113–23.

3

Time trends and geographic differences in suicide: implications for prevention

David Gunnell

Introduction

Two of the most striking features of the epidemiology of suicide are the large variations in its incidence over time and the tenfold international differences in rates. Explanations for these patterns may provide insights not only into the causes of suicide but also into possible approaches to its prevention. An understanding of the influences on time trends in suicide is also important when judging the success or failure of national prevention strategies (US Department of Health and Human Services 2001; Department of Health 2002). Any beneficial effect of preventive activities on suicide may be masked by changes in other factors, such as economic recession, which health strategists cannot influence.

This chapter is divided into two sections. The first reviews influences on time trends in suicide. The second section describes regional and international differences in suicide.

Secular trends in national suicide rates

Secular trends in Britain in the twentieth century

Figure 3.1, based on data for England and Wales, clearly shows the marked temporal variability in the incidence of suicide in the 20th century. In males its incidence was highest in the first 30 years of the century, in females rates peaked in the 1960s. Rates of suicide are considerably lower in females than males, but both sexes exhibited similar twofold variations in incidence over the past century.

The incidence of suicide in England and Wales has declined over the past 100 years and is currently at its lowest recorded level (Fig. 3.1). Close inspection of Fig. 3.1 reveals three other features. The first is the downturn in suicide rates during the First World War (1914–1918) and Second World

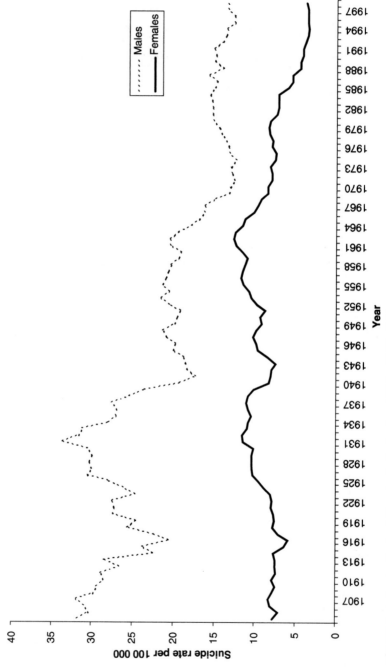

Fig. 3.1 Age-standardized suicide rates in England and Wales 1905–1999.

War (1939–1945). Similar reductions occurred at these times in many other countries (Sainsbury *et al.* 1979) and during periods of conflict in the nineteenth century (Durkheim, 1897). Durkheim argued that such downturns may be due to the greater sense of societal integration and common purpose in times of war.

The second prominent feature of twentieth-century trends in suicide in England and Wales is the rise in suicide in the late 1920s and 1930s (Fig. 3.1). This rise coincided with a period of profound economic recession. The third feature is the reduction in male and female suicides beginning in the mid-1960s and continuing through to the 1970s. The cause of this decline has been much debated. The most coherent explanation is that this was due to changes in the lethality—due to reduced carbon monoxide content—of domestic gas poisoning. In the 1960s this was the most commonly used method of suicide in the UK. The effects on patterns of suicide of (1) economic recession and (2) the ease of availability of lethal methods of suicide and their implications for prevention are discussed in the following sections.

Economic recession, unemployment, and suicide

The marked increase in suicide at the time of the inter-war recession in England (Fig. 3.1) parallels the rise in unemployment that occurred at this time (Swinscow 1951). Similar rises in suicide occurred in other countries affected by the Great Depression (Morrell *et al.* 1993; Webb *et al.* 2002). Periods of economic recession lead to increases in unemployment. Unemployment, in turn, is associated with an increased risk of suicide (Johansson and Sundquist 1997; Lewis and Sloggett 1998; Qin *et al.* 2000), although the pathways linking unemployment to suicide are uncertain (Platt 1984; Platt and Hawton 2000). Possible contributory factors include the loss of social ties in the workplace, the effects of financial difficulties on domestic relationships, and mental illness increasing the risk of both unemployment and suicide. The relative importance of the different contributory factors is likely to differ depending upon prevailing levels of unemployment.

Profound changes in levels of an important risk factor for suicide understandably influence its incidence. The influence of prevailing economic conditions on suicide has three important consequences for suicide prevention. First, national governments should consider the consequence of periods of economic recession on suicide and population health when they are determining their economic policies. Secondly, during periods of economic recession, interventions aimed at mitigating the ill-effects of unemployment and poverty on mental health should be supported (see Proudfoot *et al.* 1997). Thirdly, any beneficial effects of suicide prevention initiatives on the incidence of suicide may be imperceptible if such initiatives coincide with periods of economic recession, and a false impression of benefit or disbenefit could occur if the initiatives occur at a time of economic change.

The influence of changes in the availability of lethal methods of suicide

Declines in the carbon monoxide content of domestic gas in Britain in the 1960s and early 1970s were paralleled by a marked reduction in domestic gas suicides (Kreitman 1976). Overall suicide rates also decreased as there was no immediate compensatory rise in the use of other methods (Fig. 3.1). While some suicidal individuals turned to overdose as an alternative means of suicide (Gunnell *et al.* 2000), the overall impact on population suicide rates was striking. This phenomenon has been used as evidence to support restricting access to means of suicide as a strategy to reduce suicide rates (Clarke and Lester 1989; Gunnell and Frankel 1994; Department of Health 2002). Such an approach is supported by evidence from Australia where restrictions on the prescribing of barbiturates had a beneficial impact on national suicide rates (Oliver and Hetzel 1972). Similarly, temporal and geographical variations in the availability of other commonly used methods have been shown to influence patterns of firearm suicide in the USA (Cantor and Slater 1995; Miller *et al.* 2002), car-exhaust gas suicides in Britain and the USA (Clarke and Lester 1987; Amos *et al.* 2001) and suicide using paracetamol (acetaminophen) in the UK and Denmark (Lomholdt and Mosbech 1995; Gunnell *et al.* 1997).

Why does restricting access to means of suicide influence its incidence? In many people suicidal impulses occur in the context of acute emotional distress and are short lasting. If time can be 'bought', by restricting ease of access to readily available and lethal methods then, in some cases, suicidal impulses will pass without fatal consequences. People deterred from using one method of suicide do not necessarily turn to other methods. This is a crude approach to prevention. It does not alleviate the mental suffering of the suicidal. Furthermore, restricting access to some methods, e.g. guns and medicines, may inconvenience the many safe users of particular products (the population paradox; Rose 1992). Nevertheless in a field with a limited evidence base (Gunnell and Frankel 1994), it is one of the few approaches where some consensus exists.

Based on the above evidence, restrictions on the sales of paracetamol were introduced in Britain in 1998 and early evidence suggests that these have led to a reduction in serious overdoses and deaths (Hawton *et al.* 2001). What are the implications for other more commonly used methods of suicide? A current problem in a number of industrialized countries is the rise in suicide by hanging (Fig. 3.2) (Kosky and Dundas 2000; Langley *et al.* 2000; Middleton

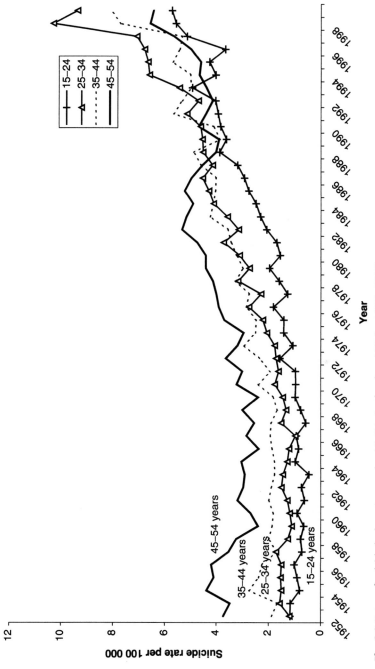

Fig. 3.2 Rates of suicide by hanging: males 15–54, England and Wales 1952–1998.

and Gunnell 2000). Approaches aimed at limiting access to ligatures and suspension points, which are a common feature of everyday life, seem unlikely to succeed except in controlled environments such as hospitals and prisons. Alternative approaches to preventing hanging suicides are urgently needed, as is a greater understanding of the reason for the epidemic rise in its use, especially among young people.

From a global perspective, one of the most commonly used methods of suicide is pesticide ingestion (Eddleston 2000). This accounts for an estimated 300 000 suicides worldwide each year (Gunnell and Eddleston 2003). The size of the problem is such that deaths from pesticide poisoning may distort conventional patterns of suicide in countries where it is commonplace (Gunnell and Eddleston 2003). In China and Sri Lanka there is a peak in suicide rates amongst 20–25-year-olds, who have higher rates than most other age groups except the elderly (Berger 1988; Phillips *et al.* 2002*a*). This peak coincides with the age when, in industrialized countries, rates of non-fatal (often impulsive) self-harm are highest (Schmidtke *et al.* 1996). Efforts to minimize access to toxic pesticides and improve the management of pesticide self-poisoning are likely to have great impacts on rates of suicide worldwide (Eddleston *et al.* 2002; Phillips *et al.* 2002*b*). This suggestion is highlighted (1) by the impact of the changing availability of pesticides in Western Samoa on overall rates of suicide (Fig. 3.3) (Bowles 1995); and (2) the effects of the availability of specific antidotes on mortality from yellow oleander seed poisoning in Sri Lanka (Eddleston *et al.* 2003). Rises in paraquat imports in Samoa were paralleled by increases in paraquat poisoning deaths, leading to a threefold increase in overall suicides. Subsequent reduction in imports, hence restricted availability, had the opposite effect (Bowles 1995). Reasons for global inaction despite over 30 years of evidence concerning the use of pesticides for suicide are complex and immediate action is required on this critical issue.

Age and cohort effects

A comparison of Figs 3.1 and 3.4 shows that trends in overall suicide rates may mask complex, and sometimes diverging, temporal trends in the young and the old, or in males compared to females (Gunnell *et al.* 2003*b*). The reduction in overall male suicide rates since 1950 (Fig. 3.1) masks a doubling of rates in males aged <45 years (Fig. 3.4). Furthermore, trends in suicide within particular age-groups may differ depending on an individual's place of residence. For example in Scotland between 1981–1983 and 1991–1993 the greatest rises in young male suicides occurred amongst those living in deprived areas (McLoone 1996). In Britain (Middleton *et al.* 2003), Australia (Dudley *et al.*

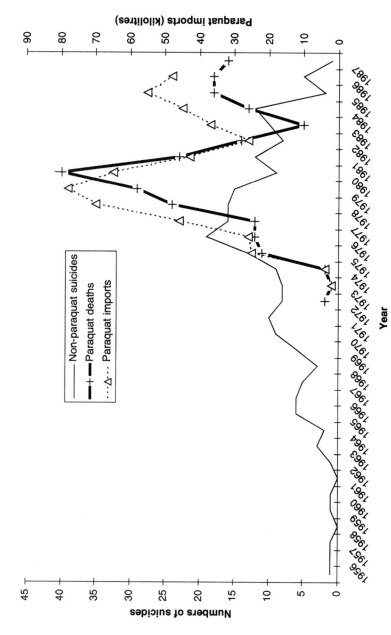

Fig. 3.3 Paraquat sales and suicide in Western Samoa 1956–1988. (Modified from Bowles, 1995.)

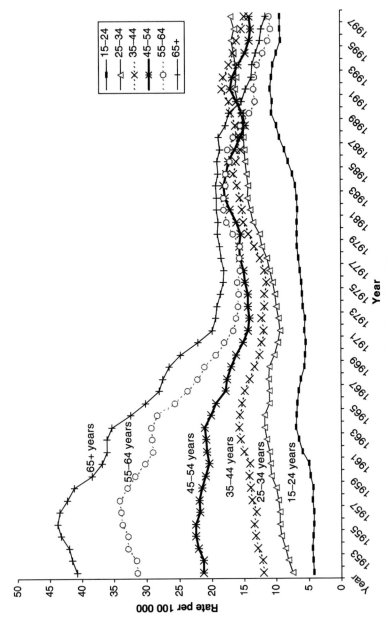

Fig. 3.4 Age-specific suicide rates in males: England and Wales 1950–1998.

1998), and Norway (Mehlum *et al.* 1999) some of the greatest rises in suicide in young adults have occurred amongst those living in rural areas.

Birth cohort effects arise when a group of people born around the same time carry with them an increased (or diminished) susceptibility to disease throughout their lives. For example, recent generations of males appear to have higher levels of suicide at all ages than preceding birth cohorts (Skegg and Cox 1991; Allebeck *et al.* 1996; Snowdon and Hunt 2002; Gunnell *et al.* 2003*a*). Possible explanations for such effects include the long-term impact of changing levels of childhood exposure to environmental influences—such as parental divorce or substance misuse—which may have a long-term impact on a generation's mental health. The increased influence of the media may also be important. Media portrayals of idealized lifestyles in films, television dramas and advertising may give young people unrealistic expectations from life. Such mismatches between expectation and reality may lead to disappointment and, in a few, suicide. Furthermore, changes in the media portrayal of suicide (as relatively commonplace and acceptable) may permanently influence the attitudes of young viewers regarding its cultural normality, and hence their likelihood of committing suicide, in times of crisis. Working with the media should form an important strand of suicide prevention strategies (Hawton and Williams 2002).

There are several implications of differing trends in suicide in the young and the old. First, overall reductions in national suicide rates may mask an increase in potential years of life lost (PYLL) from suicide because of the increase in rates amongst younger people (Fig. 3.5) (Gunnell and Middleton 2003). Measures of PYLL provide an alternative means of quantifying the impact of premature mortality for health outcomes with relatively high incidence in young people. This is because they take account of the age at which death occurred and thereby give more weight to deaths amongst young people. National targets for suicide prevention might usefully include either age-specific targets for those demographic groups experiencing adverse trends or targets based on PYLL as well as overall suicide rates. Secondly, the effects of risk factors such as unemployment and living alone appear to differ in different age groups (Dorling and Gunnell 2003). For this reason interventions may need to be tailored to different sections of the population, and epidemiological research should study risk factor associations separately in the young and old, males and females. Finally, as described above, recent evidence of a cohort effect of increased suicide rates in recent generations may herald an increased predisposition to suicide which today's young adults may carry with them as they age. This would lead to a rise in overall population suicide rates as current generations of young men enter middle and old age (Gunnell *et al.* 2003*a*).

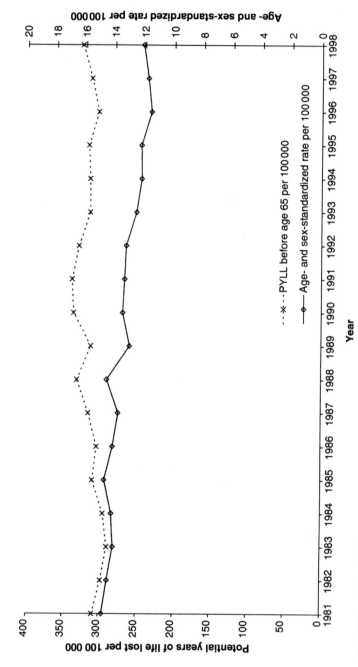

Fig. 3.5 Trends in suicide and undetermined mortality rate (aged 15+) and potential years of life lost (PYLL) (before the age of 65), England and Wales, 1981–1998. (Source: Gunnell and Middleton (2003): reprinted from the *Lancet* **362**, 961–2; with permission from Elsevier.)

Other influences on secular trends in suicide—alcohol, health care, socio-economic deprivation, and social fragmentation

The previous sections highlighted the factors that had the most striking impact on patterns of suicide in England and Wales over the past century. Other factors may also influence temporal trends. For example, stringent legislative restrictions on alcohol sales are thought to have influenced patterns of suicide in the former USSR (Wasserman and Varnik 1998) and Denmark (Skog 1993).

In view of the complex influences on suicide it is crucial that analyses investigating causes for changes in population suicide rates take account of all possible contributory factors, including temporal trends in the availability of lethal suicide methods (Low *et al.* 1981; Kreitman and Platt 1984; Gunnell *et al.* 1999a). Many studies have assessed the effects on suicide rates of changes in single factors such as unemployment (Crombie, 1990; Gunnell *et al.* 1999a) or alcohol intake (Yip *et al.*, 2000). Furthermore, most previous assessments of the causes of recent changes in national suicide rates have investigated factors associated with time-trends in overall population suicide rates (i.e. all age-groups combined) (Low *et al.*, 1981; Lester and Yang 1991; Weyerer and Wiedenmann 1995). Such analyses cannot elucidate factors underlying the markedly different time trends in males and females or in different age groups (see below). Inconsistent findings have emerged from time series studies carried out to date and, because many proposed risk factors are highly inter-correlated, it may not be possible to identify the specific factors underlying trends.

In a recent time series analysis that attempted to overcome some of the deficiencies of previous studies, post-war trends in suicide in Britain were associated with a range of social and health-care factors (Gunnell *et al.* 2003b). Rises in young male suicides were most consistently associated with increases in divorce, declines in marriage and increases in income inequality. These changes appeared to have little effect on suicide in young females—possibly because their rates were favourably influenced by the declining toxicity of drugs commonly taken in overdose—their favoured method of suicide (Gunnell *et al.* 1999b). Declines in suicide in older people were associated with increases in gross domestic product (GDP), the size of the female workforce and the prescribing of antidepressants (Gunnell *et al.* 2003b).

It is possible that some of the patterns observed are due to declining levels of social integration. Durkheim hypothesized that national suicide rates are influenced by the extent to which individuals are integrated within society. He argued: 'There is, in short, in a cohesive and animated society a constant inter-change of ideas and feelings from all to each and each to all, something like a mutual moral support, which instead of throwing the individual on his own resources, leads him to share in the collective energy and supports his own when exhausted' (Durkheim 1897, p. 210). Researchers have used various readily available measures of factors thought to identify environments conducive to social integration to investigate these theories. Population mobility, the proportion of people living alone, voting abstention, divorce, illegitimate births and religious book sales have all been used as measures of area levels of social integration (Sainsbury et al. 1979; Congdon 1996; Makinen 1997; Fernquist and Cutright 1998; Whitley et al. 1999). Findings from studies in this area to date are inconclusive. Based on an analysis of changing suicide rates between 1961–1963 and 1972–1974 in 18 European countries Sainsbury and colleagues (1979) reported that changes in the social environment—most particularly changes in the status of women, anomie, and socioeconomic conditions—were associated with changes in suicide rates. This finding was not confirmed in a more recent analysis of suicide trends in the same countries between 1977–1979 and 1988–1990 (Makinen 1997). Both studies are limited by their use of overall (all ages) suicide rates. Such an approach may mask age-specific effects of changes in particular risk factors. In a recent analysis of British data, geographic areas experiencing the greatest increase in social fragmentation (between 1981 and 1991) experienced the largest rises in suicide (Whitley et al. 1999). Effects were most marked in younger age groups.

Recent interest has focused on rises in antidepressant prescribing as a possible explanation for declines in suicide in some countries (Isaacson 2000, Hall et al. 2003). Analyses looking at this issue have either investigated associations of prescribing with overall (all-age) population suicide rates, restricted the analysis to single age groups, used inappropriate analytic approaches, or have not controlled for possible confounding factors which also vary over time (Isaacson 2000; Hall et al. 2003; Olfson et al. 2003). Of note, age-specific UK prescribing (Middleton et al. 2001) and suicide data, suggest that although rises in antidepressant prescribing have paralleled falls in suicide rates in older males, this has not been the case amongst those aged under 45, in whom increases in prescribing have been accompanied by increases in suicide (Fig. 3.6). This finding accords with meta-analyses of antidepressant trials which report, if anything, that those randomized to antidepressants have higher rates of non-fatal self-harm than those in the placebo arm, although the numbers of suicides are too small to detect important influences on suicide deaths (Fergusson et al. 2005; Gunnell et al. 2005). The impact of the increased prescribing of antidepressants on overall population suicide rates remains unclear.

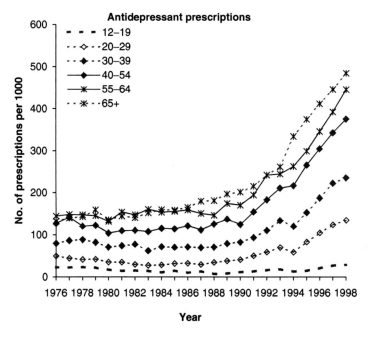

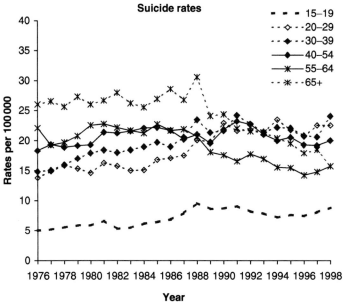

Fig. 3.6 Trends in antidepressant prescribing per 1000 (in the UK) males and age-specific male suicide rates per 100,000 (in England and Wales), 1976–1998.

International differences in trends in suicide

In the past two decades considerable policy and research attention has focused on the rise in suicide rates in young males. As Table 3.1 shows, while many industrialized nations experienced rises in young male suicides similar to those seen in England and Wales, patterns were far from uniform. The majority of countries listed in Table 3.1 experienced rises in young female as well as male suicide, whereas in Germany, Denmark, Austria, and Japan there have been declines in both young male and female suicide. Many of these countries have experienced similar changes in unemployment, divorce, and substance misuse, and so other factors are clearly important. A better

Table 3.1 Change in suicide rates in 25–34 year-old males and females in selected countries, 1960–1990

	Change in male rates 1960–1990	Change in female rates 1960–1990
Countries in which male and female suicide rates increased		
Ireland	+513%	+390%
Netherlands	+166%	+109%
Belgium	+155%	+68%
Canada	+119%	+64%
New Zealand	+104%	+81%
France	+101%	+80%
Norway	+96%	+154%
Spain	+91%	+21%
Portugal	+62%	+7%
Finland	+58%	+9%
Hungary	+42%	+13%
Poland	+33%	+20%
Sweden	+8%	+3%
Countries in which male rates increased and female rates decreased		
Iceland	+95%	−72%
Italy	+89%	−0.4%
USA	+63%	−12%
Australia	+51%	−11%
England and Wales	+46%	−41%
Switzerland	+35%	−15%
Greece	+9%	−52%
Countries where male and female rates decreased		
Japan	−39%	−57%
West Germany	−9%	−34%
Austria	−7%	−36%
Denmark	−3%	−32%

Source: WHO Website and Statistical Annuals 1992 ff. WHO, Geneva.
+: number or percentage increases;
−: number or percentage declines.

understanding of these factors will provide important insights into appropriate interventions to tackle rises in youth suicide.

Most research investigating factors associated with changing rates of suicide in different countries has focused on factors influencing overall (all-age) suicide rates (Sainsbury *et al.* 1979; Crombie 1990; Makinen 1997; Fernquist and Cutright 1998). As the effect of many of these risk factors may vary in different age- and sex-groups, more detailed studies are required to improve understanding of potentially modifiable influences on suicide.

Summary of temporal trends and suicide prevention

Fluctuations in the incidence of suicide point to the importance of potentially modifiable influences. A better understanding of these factors will contribute to national suicide prevention strategies. Evidence to date highlights the importance of: (1) restricting the lethality of, or access to, commonly used methods; (2) improving the medical management of those who self-poison in developing countries; (3) preventive activities to counter the effects on suicide risk of economic recession; (4) the social environment, in particular changing levels of social integration; and (5) setting age-specific suicide reduction targets and focusing on trends in potential years of life lost as well as overall suicide rates.

Inter- and intra-national variations in the incidence of suicide

International variations in suicide

One of the most remarkable features of the epidemiology of suicide is the magnitude of international differences in its incidence (Fig. 3.7). Some neighbouring countries, such as (1) the UK and France or (2) Austria and Italy, have twofold differences in their rates. Some of these differences may be explained by reporting and recording differences between countries. However, studies in the USA and Australia, comparing suicide rates of immigrants from different countries, assessed under the death registration system of a single country, confirm that these international differences reflect real variations in suicide risk depending on country of origin (Sainsbury 1983). Such differences are one of the great puzzles in suicide epidemiology. A greater understanding of their origins, and the extent to which their causes are modifiable, offers great potential for suicide prevention.

As well as variations in the absolute risk of suicide between countries, there are also international differences in the ratio of male:female suicide. In some Asian countries rates of suicide in females approach, and in case of China

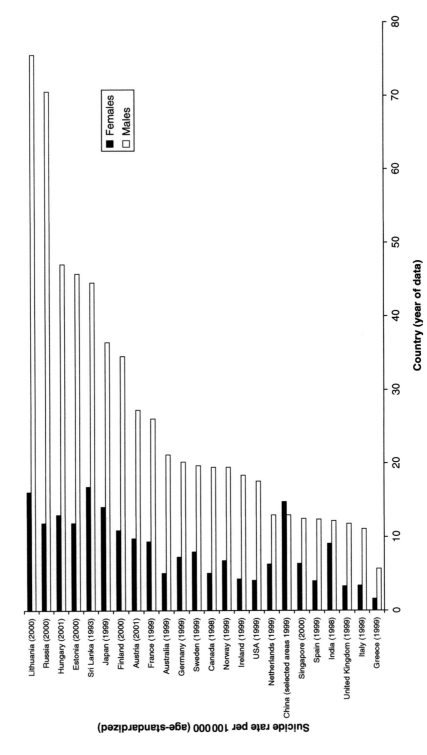

Fig. 3.7 International variations in suicide rates (source: WHO website, August 2003).

exceed, those of males (Canetto and Lester 1995). The lower ratio of male: female suicide in these Asian countries may reflect, amongst other factors, fewer legal or religious sanctions against suicide, the lower social status of women, and the high toxicity of women's favoured method of suicide in these countries—pesticide ingestion (Phillips *et al.* 2002*a*).

There are many possible explanations for the international differences in suicide (Table 3.2). It is likely that a combination of these factors contributes to observed patterns. The effect of some risk factors may vary depending on national context; for example, single parenthood or divorce may be associated with greater suicide risk in countries where these states are more socially stigmatized.

One area that has attracted particular interest over the course of the past century has been the importance of the dominant state religion and differences in levels of religious beliefs between countries (Durkheim 1897). Evidence indicates that countries with higher levels of religious belief have lower suicide rates (Stack 1983; Neeleman *et al.* 1997; Neeleman and Lewis 1999).

Possible genetic differences between people of different nationalities is an appealingly straightforward contributor to the observed international differences, particularly when geographically remote nations, such as Finland and Hungary, share both high suicide rates and a common ancestry (Marusic and Farmer 2001). Preliminary studies of the distribution of serotonergic gene

Table 3.2 Factors that may contribute to international differences in suicide rates

Under-reporting in countries where suicide is stigmatized

Differences in popular methods of suicide—countries where more lethal methods are favoured (e.g. firearms in the USA, pesticides in Sri Lanka) have higher self-harm fatality rates

Cultural/religious attitudes towards suicide: suicide rates may be higher in nations where suicide is less stigmatized, as it is a more acceptable option in times of acute emotional distress

Differences in levels of social integration—rates higher in less integrated societies

Economic differences—rates higher in countries experiencing economic recession

Differences in the availability and effective delivery of primary and secondary health-care services for mental illness

Levels of particular risk/protective factors—drug and alcohol misuse, divorce, parenthood, unemployment

Fictional portrayal and media reporting of suicide deaths—rates may be higher in nations where suicide is more frequently/differently reported both in fiction and in factual accounts of actual suicides. This affects the cultural acceptability of suicide and may provoke imitative behaviour

Genetic differences between populations

polymorphisms possibly associated with susceptibility to depression have failed to show similarities in Finnish and Hungarian populations (Hrdina 2002). Distinguishing the effects of shared genes from those of shared culture presents an important challenge over the next decade.

A clearer understanding of the relative importance of the various factors listed in Table 3.2, together with an understanding of the extent to which any of these factors are modifiable, will help underpin national and international suicide prevention strategies.

Geographic variations in suicide within countries

The incidence of suicide also varies between different regions of the same country. Such variations have been reported both at the relatively large geographic scale between populations of over 100 000 (Bunting and Kelly 1998) and within considerably smaller population groups of 10 000–30 000 people (Gunnell et al. 1995; Middleton et al. 2004). Surprisingly, the few studies examining the association of regional suicide rates with area levels of mental disorder or measures of mental health have found no strong evidence for an association (Zonda et al. 1992; Bartlett et al. 2002).

Regional variations in suicide were noted over 100 years ago by Morselli (1881) and Durkheim (1897), and over the past 80 years a number of sociological and epidemiological studies have investigated the causes of such spatial patterning (Cavan 1928; Sainsbury 1955; Lönnqvist 1977). A common finding is that districts characterized by markers of low social integration (social fragmentation)—such as the proportion of single-person households, divorced people, and population mobility in an area—have the highest rates of suicide. In keeping with this, recent analyses of small area variations in England and Wales show that the strongest predictors of the suicide risk in an area appear to be those encapsulated by Durkheim's notion of social integration (Congdon 1996; Whitley et al. 1999; Davey Smith et al. 2001; Middleton et al. 2004). Associations are independent of the (weaker) relationship of suicide with poverty (Whitley et al. 1999; Middleton et al. 2004). Recent research also suggests that associations with social fragmentation are independent of levels of severe psychiatric illness, as indexed by psychiatric admission rates (Evans et al. 2004). The specific contextual indicators of social fragmentation most strongly associated with risk are the proportion of single-person households and levels of population mobility (Ashford and Lawrence 1976; Middleton et al. 2004).

The above findings accord with Durkheim's notions concerning the influence of levels of social integration on suicide risk: 'The number of suicides occurring in a population is not simply the sum of a series of independent events, but may be seen as a 'social phenomenon'—indicative, in part, of the social fabric' (Durkheim 1897). However, to date no studies in this area have identified whether these associations are due to high concentrations of at-risk individuals living in particular areas (compositional effects) or—in accordance with Durkheim's hypothesis—discrete area (contextual) influences on suicide.

It is also possible that contextual (area) effects may affect particular residents differently, depending on their personal characteristics. The only study to have examined this issue formally in relation to suicide is Neeleman and Wessely's London-based study of suicide and ethnicity. They found that as the proportion of an area's population who came from ethnic minority groups increased, so the suicide risk of people from ethnic minorities living in that area decreased, whereas that for white residents increased (Neeleman and Wessely 1999). Similar associations have been reported with attempted suicide (Neeleman et al. 2001). These findings indicate that suicide risks are higher amongst people whose social and demographic characteristics differ from those of the majority of the population living in their neighbourhood.

The other specific measures associated with area differences in suicide rates are: levels of socio-economic deprivation (Gunnell et al. 1995; Congdon 1996; Whitley et al. 1999), rurality (Saunderson and Langford 1996; Middleton et al. 2003), levels of self-harm (Gunnell et al. 1995), and levels of gun ownership in the USA (Miller et al. 2002).

Conclusions

Suicide is an important contributor to global mortality patterns, with an estimated 849 000 deaths each year (World Health Organization 2002). Due to the very large sample sizes required (Gunnell and Frankel 1994), conducting randomized controlled trials of interventions aimed at preventing this important contributor to global mortality presents major challenges. Therefore observational studies, such as those summarized in this chapter, provide evidence to inform preventive activities.

In developing countries, prevention of pesticide poisoning and improved medical management of cases of self-poisoning may, potentially, have profound effects on rates of suicide worldwide (Eddleston et al. 2002, 2003).

Changes in the social and economic environment, as well as the availability of commonly used methods of suicide, have influenced national trends in suicide. Evidence of the beneficial effects of recent increases in the prescribing of antidepressants is not clear-cut. The importance of considering social and economic influences on suicide rates is borne out by the observation that only around half of all individuals who commit suicide are in contact with health services in the 4 weeks prior to their death, and fewer still (25%) are in contact with specialist mental health services (Foster *et al.* 1997).

The health sector's capacity to address possible social influences on suicide risk, such as substance misuse, divorce, social integration, and employment patterns, is limited. However, it is important that the effect of changing distributions of these factors is taken into account when assessing the success or failure of suicide prevention strategies. Importantly, health and social researchers should continue to remind policy makers of the consequences of social and health policy on suicide, and support policies most conducive to population mental health.

References

Allebeck, P., Brandt, L., Nordstrom, P., and Asgard, U. (1996). Are suicide trends among the young reversing? *Acta Paediatrica Scandinavica*, **93**, 43–8.

Amos, T., Appleby, L., and Kiernan, K. (2001). Changes in rates of suicide by car exhaust asphyxiation in England and Wales. *Psychological Medicine*, **31**, 935–9.

Ashford, J.R. and Lawrence, P.A. (1976). Aspects of the epidemiology of suicide in England and Wales. *International Journal of Epidemiology*, **5**, 133–44.

Bartlett, C., Gunnell, D., Harrison, G., and Moore, L. (2002) Neurotic symptoms, stress or deprivation: which is most closely associated with the incidence of suicide: An ecological study of English Health Authorities. *Psychological Medicine*, **32**, 1131–6.

Berger, L.R. (1988). Suicides and pesticides in Sri Lanka. *American Journal of Public Health*, **78**, 826–8.

Bowles, J.R. (1995). Suicide in Western Samoa: an example of a suicide prevention program in a developing country. In *Preventative strategies of suicide*, (ed. R.F.W. Diekstra *et al.*), pp. 173–206. E.J. Brill, Leiden.

Bunting, J. and Kelly, S. (1998). Geographic variations in suicide mortality, 1982–96. *Population Trends*, **93**, 7–18.

Canetto, S.S. and Lester, D. (1995). Gender and the primary prevention of suicide mortality. *Suicide and Life-Threatening Behavior*, **25**, 58–69.

Cantor, C.H. and Slater, P.J. (1995). The impact of firearm control legislation on suicide in Queensland: preliminary findings. *Medical Journal of Australia*, **162**, 583–5.

Cavan, R.S. (1928). *Suicide*. University of Chicago, Chicago.

Clarke, R.V. and Lester, D. (1987). Toxicity of car exhausts and opportunity for suicide: comparison between Britain and the United States. *Journal of Epidemiology and Community Health*, **41**, 114–20.

Clarke, R.V. and Lester, D. (1989). *Suicide: Closing the exits*. Springer-Verlag, New York.

Congdon, P. (1996). Suicide and parasuicide in London: A small-area study. *Urban Studies*, **33**, 137–58.

Crombie, I.K. (1990). Can changes in the unemployment rates explain the recent changes in suicide rates in developed countries? *International Journal of Epidemiology*, **19**, 412–16.

Davey Smith, G., Whitley, E., Dorling, D., and Gunnell, D. (2001). Area based measures of social and economic circumstances. *Journal of Epidemiology and Community Health*, **55**, 149–50.

Department of Health (2002). *National suicide prevention strategy for England.* Department of Health, London.

Dorling, D. and Gunnell, D. (2003). Suicide: the spatial and social components of despair in Britain 1980–2000. *Transactions of the Institute of British Geographers,* 28, 442–60.

Dudley, M.J., Kelk, N.J., Florio, T.M., Howard, J.P., and Waters, B.G. (1998). Suicide among young Australians, 1964–1993: an interstate comparison of metropolitan and rural trends. *Medical Journal of Australia,* 169, 77–80.

Durkheim (1897). *Suicide.* Republished 1952, Routledge and Kegan Paul, London.

Eddleston, M. (2000). Patterns and problems of deliberate self-poisoning in the developing world. *Quarterly Journal of Medicine,* 93, 715–31.

Eddleston, M., Karalliedde, L., Buckley, N., Fernando, R., Hutchinson, G., Isbister, G., *et al.* (2002). Pesticide poisoning in the developing world—a minimum pesticides list. *Lancet,* 360, 1163–7.

Eddleston, M., Senarathna, L., Mohamed, F., Buckley, N., Juszczak, E., Sheriff, M.H.R., *et al.* (2003). Deaths due to absence of an affordable antitoxin for plant poisoning. *Lancet,* 362, 1041–4.

Evans, J., Middleton, N., and Gunnell, D. (2004). Social fragmentation, severe mental illness and suicide. *Social Psychiatry and Psychiatric Epidemiology,* 39, 165–70.

Fergusson, D., Doucette, S., Cranley Glass, K., Shapiro, S., Healy, D., Herbert, P., *et al.* (2005). Association between suicide attempts and selective serotonin re-uptake inhibitors: systematic review of randomised controlled trials. *British Medical Journal,* 330, 396–9.

Fernquist, R. and Cutright, P. (1998). Societal integration and age-standardized suicide rates in 21 developed countries, 1955–1989. *Social Science Research,* 27, 109–27.

Foster, T., Gillespie, K., and McClelland, R. (1997). Mental disorders and suicide in Northern Ireland. *British Journal of Psychiatry,* 170, 447–52.

Gunnell, D. and Eddleston, M (2003). Suicide by intentional ingestion of pesticides: a continuing tragedy in developing countries. *International Journal of Epidemiology,* 32, 902–9.

Gunnell, D. and Frankel, S. (1994). Prevention of suicide: aspirations and evidence. *British Medical Journal,* 308, 1227–33.

Gunnell, D. and Middleton, N. (2003). National suicide rates as an indicator of the effect of suicide on premature mortality. *Lancet,* 362, 961–2.

Gunnell, D., Peters, T., Kammerling, M., and Brooks, J. (1995). The relation between parasuicide, suicide, psychiatric admissions and socio-economic deprivation. *British Medical Journal,* 311, 226–30.

Gunnell, D., Hawton, K., Murray, V., Garnier, R., Bismuth, C., Fagg, J., *et al.* (1997). Use of paracetamol for suicide and non-fatal self poisoning in the UK and France: are restrictions on availability justified? *Journal of Epidemiology and Community Health,* 51, 175–9.

Gunnell, D., Lopatatzidis, A., Dorling, D., Wehner, H., Southall, H., and Frankel, S. (1999*a*). Suicide and unemployment in young people. Analysis of trends in England and Wales, 1921–1995. *British Journal of Psychiatry,* 175, 263–70.

Gunnell, D., Wehner, H., and Frankel, S. (1999*b*). Sex differences in suicide trends in England and Wales. *Lancet,* 353, 556–7.

Gunnell, D., Middleton, N., and Frankel, S. (2000). Method substitution and the prevention of suicide – a reanalysis of secular trends in Britain 1950–1975. *Social Psychiatry and Psychiatric Epidemiology,* 35, 437–44.

Gunnell, D., Middleton, N., Whitley, E., Dorling, D., and Frankel, S. (2003a). Influence of cohort effects on patterns of suicide in England and Wales, 1950–1999. *British Journal of Psychiatry*, 182, 164–70.

Gunnell, D., Middleton, N., Whitley, E., Dorling, D., and Frankel, S. (2003b). Why are suicide rates rising in young men but falling in the elderly? A time-series analysis of trends in England and Wales 1950–1998. *Social Science and Medicine*, 57, 595–611.

Gunnell, D., Saperia, J., and Ashby, D. (2005). Selective serotonin re-uptake inhibitors and suicide in adults: a meta-analysis of drug company data from placebo-controlled randomised controlled trials submitted to the MHRA's safety review. *British Medical Journal*, 330, 385–8.

Hall, W.D., Mant, A., Mitchell, P.B., Rendle, V.A., Hickie, I.B., and McManus, P. (2003). Association between antidepressant prescribing and suicide in Australia, 1991–2000: trend analysis. *British Medical Journal*, 326, 1008–11.

Hawton, K. and Williams, K. (2002). Influences of the media on suicide. *British Medical Journal*, 325, 1374–5.

Hawton, K., Townsend, E., Deeks, J., Appleby, L., Gunnell, D., Bennewith, O., and Cooper, J. (2001). Effects of legislation restricting pack sizes of paracetamol and salicylate on self poisoning in the United Kingdom: before and after study. *British Medical Journal*, 322, 1203–7.

Hrdina, P. (2002). Genetic variation in European suicide rates. *British Journal of Psychiatry*, 181, 350.

Isaacson, G. (2000). Suicide prevention – a medical breakthrough? *Acta Psychiatrica Scandinavica*, 102, 113–17.

Johansson, S.E. and Sundquist, J. (1997) Unemployment is an important risk factor for suicide in contemporary Sweden: an 11-year follow-up study of a cross-sectional sample of 37789 people. *Public Health*, 111, 41–5.

Kosky, R.J. and Dundas, P. (2000). Death by hanging: implications for prevention of an important method of youth suicide. *Australian and New Zealand Journal of Psychiatry*, 34, 836–41.

Kreitman, N. (1976). The coal gas story. United Kingdom suicide rates, 1960–71. *British Journal of Preventive and Social Medicine*, 30, 86–93.

Kreitman, N. and Platt, S. (1984). Suicide, unemployment, and domestic gas detoxification in Britain. *Journal of Epidemiology and Community Health*, 38, 1–6.

Langley, J., Nada-Raja, S., and Alsop, J. (2000). Changes in methods of male youth suicide: 1980–95. *New Zealand Medical Journal*, 113, 264–5.

Lester, D. and Yang, B. (1991) The relationship between divorce, unemployment and female participation in the labour force and suicide rates in Australia and America. *Australian and New Zealand Journal of Psychiatry*, 25, 519–23.

Lewis, G. and Sloggett, A. (1998). Suicide, deprivation, and unemployment: record linkage study. *British Medical Journal*, 317, 1283–6.

Lomholdt, J.D. and Mosbech, J. (1995). Death due to paracetamol poisoning in Denmark 1979–1992. *Ugeskrift for Laeger*, 157, 874–6.

Lönnqvist, J. (1977). *Suicide in Helsinki*, Vol. 8. Monographs of Psychiatrica Fennica, Helsinki.

Low, A.A., Farmer, R.D., Jones, D.R., and Rohde, J.R. (1981). Suicide in England and Wales: an analysis of 100 years, 1876–1975. *Psychological Medicine*, 11, 359–68.

Makinen, I. (1997). Are there social correlates to suicide? *Social Science and Medicine*, 44, 1919–29.

Marusic, A. and Farmer, A. (2001). Genetic risk factors as possible causes of the variation in European suicide rates. *British Journal of Psychiatry*, 179, 194–6.

McLoone, P. (1996). Suicide and deprivation in Scotland. *British Medical Journal*, 312, 543–4.

Mehlum, L., Hutten, K., and Gjersten, F. (1999). Epidemiological trends of youth suicide in Norway. *Archives of Suicide Research*, 5, 193–205.

Middleton, N. and Gunnell, D. (2000). Trends in suicide in England and Wales. *British Journal of Psychiatry*, 176, 595.

Middleton, N., Gunnell, D., Whitley, E., Dorling, D., and Frankel, S. (2001). Secular trends in antidepressant prescribing in the UK, 1975–1997. *Journal of Public Health Medicine*, 23, 262–7.

Middleton, N., Gunnell, D., Whitley, E., Frankel, S., and Dorling, D. (2003). Urban–rural differences in suicide trends in young adults: England and Wales, 1981–1998. *Social Science and Medicine*, 57, 1183–94.

Middleton, N., Whitley, E., Frankel, S., Dorling, D., Sterne, J.A.C., and Gunnell, D. (2004). Suicide risk in small areas of England and Wales 1991–1993. *Social Psychiatry and Psychiatric Epidemiology*, 39, 45–52.

Miller, M., Azrael, D., and Hemenway, D. (2002). Household firearm ownership and suicide rates in the United States. *Epidemiology*, 13, 517–24.

Morrell, S., Taylor, R., Quine, S., and Kerr, C. (1993). Suicide and unemployment in Australia 1907–1990. *Social Science and Medicine*, 36, 749–56.

Morselli, H. (1881). *Suicide: An essay on comparative moral statistics*. Kegan Paul, London.

Murphy, G.E. and Wetzel, R.D. (1980). Suicide risk by birth cohort in the United States, 1949–1974. *Archives of General Psychiatry*, 37, 519–23.

Neeleman, J. and Lewis, G. (1999). Suicide, religion, and socioeconomic conditions. An ecological study in 26 countries, 1990. *Journal of Epidemiology and Community Health*, 53, 204–10.

Neeleman, J. and Wessely, S. (1999). Ethnic minority suicide: a small area geographical study in south London. *Psychological Medicine*, 29, 429–36.

Neeleman, J., Halpern, D., Leon, D., and Lewis, G. (1997). Tolerance of suicide, religion and suicide rates: an ecological and individual study in 19 Western countries. *Psychological Medicine*, 27, 1165–71.

Neeleman, J., Wilson-Jones, C., and Wessely, S. (2001). Ethnic density and deliberate self harm; a small area study in South East London. *Journal of Epidemiology and Community Health*, 55, 85–90.

Olfson, M., Shaffer, D., Marcus, S.C., and Greenberg, T. (2003). Relationship between antidepressant medication treatment and suicide in adolescents. *Archives of General Psychiatry*, 60, 978–82.

Oliver, R.G. and Hetzel, B.S. (1972). Rise and fall of suicide rates in Australia: relation to sedative availability. *Medical Journal of Australia*, 2, 919–23.

Phillips, M.R., Li, X., and Zhang, Y. (2002*a*). Suicide rates in China, 1995–99. *Lancet*, 359, 835–40.

Phillips, M.R., Yang, G., Zhang, Y., Wang, L., Ji, H., and Zhou, M. (2002*b*). Risk factors for suicide in China: a national case-control psychological autopsy study. *Lancet*, 360, 1728–36.

Platt, S. (1984). Unemployment and suicidal behaviour: a review of the literature. *Social Science and Medicine*, 19, 93–115.

Platt, S. and Hawton, K. (2000). Suicidal behaviour and the labour market. In *The international handbook of suicide and attempted suicide*, (ed. K. Hawton and K. van Heeringen), pp. 309–383. Wiley, Chichester.

Proudfoot, J., Guest, G., Carson, J. *et al.* (1997). Effect of cognitive behavioural training on job-finding among long-term unemployed people. *Lancet*, 350, 96–100.

Qin, P., Agerbo, E., Westergard-Nielsen, N., Eriksson, T., and Mortensen, P.B. (2000). Gender differences in risk factors for suicide in Denmark. *British Journal of Psychiatry*, 177, 546–50.

Rose, G. (1992). *The strategy of preventive medicine*. Oxford University Press, London.

Sainsbury, P. (1955). *Suicide in London*. Chapman & Hall. Maudsley Monographs, London.

Sainsbury, P. (1983). Validity and reliability of trends in suicide statistics. *World Health Statistics Quarterly*, 36, 339–49.

Sainsbury, P., Jenkins, J., and Levey, A. (1979). The social correlates of suicide in Europe. In *The suicide syndrome*, (ed. R.D.T. Farmer and S.R. Hirsch), pp. 38–53. Cambridge University Press, London.

Saunderson, T.R. and Langford, I.H. (1996). A study of the geographical distribution of suicide rates in England & Wales 1989–92 using empirical Bayes estimates. *Social Science and Medicine*, 43, 489–502.

Schmidtke, A., Bille-Brahe, U., De Leo, D., Kerkhof, A., Bjerke, T., Crepet, P., *et al.* (1996). Attempted suicide in Europe: rates, trends, suicide attempters during the period 1989–1992. Results of the WHO/EURO Multicentre Study on Parasuicide. *Acta Psychiatrica Scandinavica*, 93, 337–8.

Skegg, K. and Cox, B. (1991). Suicide in New Zealand 1957–1986: the influence of age, period and birth-cohort. *Australian and New Zealand Journal of Psychiatry*, 25, 181–90.

Skog, O.J. (1993). Alcohol and suicide in Denmark 1911–24 – experiences from a 'natural experiment'. *Addiction*, 88, 1189–93.

Snowdon, J. and Hunt, G.E. (2002). Age, period and cohort effects on suicide rates in Australia, 1919–1999. *Acta Psychiatrica Scandinavica*, 105, 265–70.

Stack, S. (1983). The effect of religious commitment on suicide: a cross-national analysis. *Journal of Health and Social Behaviour*, 24, 362–74.

Swinscow, D. (1951). Some suicide statistics. *British Medical Journal*, (i), 1417–22.

US Department of Health and Human Services (2001). *National Strategy for Suicide Prevention: goal and objectives for action: summary*. USDHHS, Rockville, Maryland.

Wasserman, D. and Varnik, A. (1998). Suicide-preventive effects of perestroika in the former USSR: the role of alcohol restriction. *Acta Psychiatrica Scandinavica Supplement*, 394, 1–4.

Webb, D., Glass, G., Metha, A., and Cobb, C. (2002). Economic correlates of suicide in the United States (1929–1992): a time series analysis. *Archives of Suicide Research*, 6, 93–101.

Weyerer, S. and Wiedenmann, A. (1995). Economic factors and the rates of suicide in Germany between 1881 and 1989. *Psychological Reports*, 76, 1331–41.

Whitley, E., Gunnell, D., Dorling, D., and Davey Smith, G. (1999). Ecological study of social fragmentation, poverty, and suicide. *British Medical Journal*, 319, 1034–7.

World Health Organisation (2002). *The World Health Report 2002. Reducing risks, promoting healthy life*. WHO, Geneva

Yip, P.S., Callanan, C., and Yuen, H.P. (2000). Urban/rural and gender differentials in suicide rates: East and West. *Journal of Affective Disorders*, 57, 99–106.

Zonda, T., Rihmer, Z., and Lester, D. (1992). Social correlates of deviant behaviour in Hungary. *European Journal of Psychiatry*, 6, 236–8.

4

Contextual effects in suicidal behaviour: evidence, explanation, and implications

Stephen Platt, Stephen Davis, Michael Sharpe, and Fiona O'May

Introduction

This chapter argues for the importance of a contextual perspective on suicidal behaviour, citing recent developments in epidemiological theory and evidence from empirical investigations. A qualitative study of repeat deliberate self-harm, conducted by the authors, illustrates how personal disadvantage, adverse early life experiences, and processes of social exclusion combine with an impoverished local socio-economic and cultural context to increase the risk of self-harmful behaviour. These findings challenge accepted wisdom about the design of interventions to reduce repeat deliberate self-harm. Instead of reliance on medical, hospital-based treatments, we suggest a mixture of public policy and health-service interventions targeted at the more fundamental (or 'upstream') determinants of deliberate self-harm.

Contextual effects on health

A key feature of recent developments in epidemiology has been the loss of a contextual perspective and a shift in the level of analysis from the population to the individual (Pearce 1996; Diez-Roux 1998). While the individual risk factor approach has been associated with many notable advances in scientific knowledge (e.g. the relationship between cigarette smoking and lung cancer), concern has been rising about the limitations of an exclusive focus upon individuals and more proximal ('downstream') influences on health. Pearce and McKinlay argue for a 'back-to-the-future approach', whereby epidemiology will refocus on 'the major ['upstream'] determinants of health at the population level . . . , including history, culture and the role of socioeconomic factors . . .' (Pearce and McKinlay 1998, p. 644). An 'ecosocial' epidemiological framework (Krieger

1994; Susser and Susser 1996) integrates population-level thinking, and analyses health determinants and outcomes at different levels, in particular paying attention to the linkages between individuals and the social structures (groups, localities, organizations, etc.) in which they are embedded. Individual-level health outcomes cannot be adequately studied by reference to the characteristics of individuals alone. It is also necessary to examine the characteristics of the social groups to which they belong, or the neighbourhoods where they live (Kawachi and Berkman 2003), and to acknowledge the interaction between individuals and contexts (Diez-Roux 2003; Macintyre and Ellaway 2003).

The study of the effects of collective or group characteristics on individual-level outcomes is known as contextual analysis (Iversen 1991) or multilevel analysis (Hox and Kreft 1994). 'Contextual effects' is the term used to describe variation in health outcomes between groups or localities which can be explained in terms of the characteristics (e.g. cultural, economic, social) of those aggregate-level units. 'Compositional effects', on the other hand, refer to variation in health outcomes between groups or localities that can be explained in terms of the characteristics (e.g. social, psychological, genetic) of individuals who are members of those groups or live in those localities. Empirical studies of the presence and strength of contextual effects have become increasingly common with the advent of powerful statistical techniques (Duncan *et al.* 1998). Contextual analysis combines aggregate-level and individual-level variables into a single hierarchical regression analysis. Within epidemiology, the potential importance of aggregate-level variables in understanding health inequalities has been highlighted (Macintyre *et al.* 1993). A critical review of multilevel analyses of neighbourhood socio-economic context and health outcomes (mortality, infant and child morbidity, adult chronic disease, mental health, and health behaviours) synthesized findings from 25 studies (Pickett and Pearl 2001). Although all but two of the studies reported a statistically significant association between at least one measure of the social environment and a health outcome (contextual effect), after adjusting for individual-level socio-economic status (compositional effect), 'contextual effects were generally modest and much smaller than compositional effects' (Pickett and Pearl 2001; p. 111).

Evidence of contextual effects for suicidal behaviour

Ever since Durhkeim's seminal study (Durkheim 1952 [1897]), sociologists have been conducting aggregate-level analyses of suicide, examining the relationship between suicide rates and a wide range of social variables, both longitudinally and cross-sectionally, and between and within countries.

However, even when these studies report a positive aggregate-level association (which is by no means always the case—for reviews of the evidence on suicide and unemployment, see Platt 1984; Platt and Hawton 2000), they are open to the criticism of model mis-specification: the observed contextual effect may arise because of the omission of individual-level variables related to the outcome and to the aggregate characteristic which is being studied (Diez-Roux 1998). The well-known ecological fallacy (Robinson 1950) alerts us to the danger of using aggregate-level data (e.g. a correlation between the un-employment rate and the suicide rate) to infer relationships at the individual level (e.g. the likelihood that an unemployed person will commit suicide). Nevertheless, even when ecological confounding is controlled for, it is still possible that the prevalence of a risk factor in the population will modify the strength of individual risk associated with that risk factor at the individual level. Ecological effect modification (Greenland and Morgenstern 1989) as-sumes that relative risks may not be stable or constant across the population.

There is some evidence to support the existence of such an effect in the epidemiological literature on suicide and deliberate self-harm. A series of elegant studies by Neeleman and colleagues has made an important contribu-tion to the literature. An ecological study of associations between suicide rates and an index of religiosity in 26 European and American countries, adjusted for socio-economic variation, examined the effect of stratification according to levels of religiosity (Neeleman and Lewis 1999). The association between suicide rates and religiosity was weaker for men than for women and dis-appeared altogether after adjustment for confounding. After stratification according to levels of exposure to national levels of religiosity, contrasting patterns were uncovered: negative associations in the least religious nations and positive (though not significant) associations in the more religious na-tions. The authors conclude that 'the prevalence of religiosity modifies the strength of its own ecological association with male . . . suicide rates' (Neele-man and Lewis 1999, p. 208). In a study of the ecological association between religiousness and suicide rates in 11 Dutch provinces, Neeleman (1998) showed that orthodox beliefs and religious affiliation were the most powerful predictors of lower acceptance of suicide among individuals and of lower suicide rates in provinces. The aggregate-level association between religious-ness and suicide rates was best represented by a curvilinear regression line: '[T]he most plausible explanation . . . is that the protection afforded by given individual levels of religiousness varies with the regional prevalence of reli-giousness' (Neeleman 1998, p. 470). In a third study, Neeleman and Wessely (1999) undertook a small area analysis of ethnic minority suicide in south London. While high ethnic density was found to be positively (but weakly) associated with the suicide rate at the ecological (local area) level, individual members of ethnic minorities were at relatively low risk of suicide when living in areas that had the highest ecological risk. Adjusted for socio-economic deprivation, age and gender, ethnic minority suicide rates were lower in areas where there was a proportionately larger minority population.

Contextual effects for suicidal behaviour have also been explored in studies by Kreitman and colleagues in Edinburgh. Platt and Kreitman (1985) showed that the rate of unemployment in small areas (city wards) in Edinburgh was significantly and positively associated with the rate of parasuicide (non-fatal deliberate self-harm) among both employed and employed persons, and negatively associated with the relative risk of parasuicide among the unemployed compared to the employed. This finding suggests that the psychological impact of being unemployed is moderated by the prevailing level of unemployment in the local area: unemployment is a stronger risk factor for parasuicide when it is more uncommon. A second study (Platt 1985) sought to examine the evidence for a 'subculture of parasuicide' in small areas ('wards') in Edinburgh characterized by high rates of parasuicide. Buglass *et al.* (1970) had sought to determine whether the consistent pattern of differential parasuicide rates within the city could be accounted for in terms of differences in the composition (individual risk factors) of the population living in the different wards. Although the variance of parasuicide mortality ratios was reduced following simultaneous standardization on six socio-demographic factors, a statistically significant difference in parasuicide rates remained. It was subsequently hypothesized (Kreitman 1977, pp. 63–4) that geographical areas with high parasuicide rates are characterized by a distinctive subculture which is expected to facilitate suicidal behaviour. Platt's empirical test of this hypothesis demonstrated that areas of Edinburgh with high rates of parasuicide do, indeed, have a meaning system which is distinctive from that found in areas with low rates of parasuicide. However, not all differences between area types were in the expected direction. The 'subculture of parasuicide' remains speculative rather than proven.

The social context of deliberate self-harm: an empirical investigation

In their plea for a rediscovery of the population perspective in epidemiological research, Pearce and McKinlay (1998) call for the development of 'new appropriate methods', including 'rigorous qualitative approaches' as well as multi-level modelling and geographic information systems. We have undertaken an empirical study which seeks to contribute to the understanding of contextual effects in suicidal behaviour, using a wholly qualitative method-ology to explore how individual vulnerabilities, limited family resources, and precarious local social and cultural structures ('context') interact within biography to 'produce' self-harmful behaviour.

Methods used in the study

Sample recruitment

Ethical approval for the study was obtained from the health board's Local Research Ethics Committee. Respondents were recruited from a hospital toxi-cology ward following an act of repeat deliberate self-harm (DSH, defined as 'a non-fatal act in which a person causes self-injury or ingests a substance in excess of any prescribed or generally recognized therapeutic dosage'). Patients were included if they were resident within a designated, economically deprived area of Edinburgh (hereafter referred to as Eastcraig) and had experienced at least one previous act of deliberate self-harm. Potential respondents were excluded if they had taken an overdose which was assessed by clinicians to be 'recreational' rather than with the intent of self-harm, or they were aged under 16 years of age, or they were judged by the assessing clinician to be actively psychotic, or if language or cognitive impairment limited communication.

At the time of the patient interview, respondents were also asked for permission to contact and interview the doctor or nurse who assessed them, a significant other of their choosing, and the community professional most involved with their case (as identified by the patient). All patient interviews took place within 2 weeks of the episode of self-harm. The majority of patient interviews took place in the hospital ward and interviews with significant others were conducted at their homes.

Methods of data collection

Two data collection methods were used. First, secondary data sources were reviewed in order to build up a profile of the local community which would facilitate a contextualized understanding of interview data. The information captured from these sources included: demographics, labour market condi-tions, housing, morbidity and mortality rates, and information about local health and social services. Secondly, interviews were conducted with respond-ents who had committed an act of deliberate self-harm and, where consent was obtained, with significant others, and community and hospital professionals.

Response rates

During the recruitment period 142 people were admitted to the toxicology ward. Of these, 77 met the study criteria and 50 agreed to take part in the study

(16 were discharged before they could be contacted and did not respond to the postal invitation, and 11 refused). The non-contact rate was 21% (16/77) and the refusal rate was 18% (11/61).

In more than half the sample ($n = 27$) it was not possible to obtain consent to approach a significant other. For the remainder, 17 interviews were obtained with the 23 named significant others. The relationships of the significant others to the patients were as follows: father (1), mother/step-mother (5), daughter (2), spouse/partner (3 male, 2 female), brother (2), cousin (2 male), ex-fiancée (1), friend (5 female).

Data presentation

Findings are presented under three inter-related headings: *people, context,* and *people in context.* We concentrate on the accounts of those who had self-harmed and their significant others. The health professionals' data are only used to provide demographic and psychiatric diagnostic descriptions of the research sample. The interview extracts used are verbatim quotations. In order to aid ease of understanding these have been transcribed using standard English and not the Scottish vernacular. Each extract is followed by a code which consists of one/two letter(s) and a number. The letter 'R' indicates that the extract comes from a respondent who has self-harmed, while 'SO' denotes that the material is from an interview with a significant other. The number corresponds to the anonymous respondent ID.

People

The median age of respondents was 34 years, with approximately equal numbers of males and females (Table 4.1). Fourteen respondents were married or cohabiting with a partner, while 33 were single, divorced, separated, or widowed (the marital status of three was unknown). Twenty-three respondents

Table 4.1 Sample of deliberate self-harm respondents by gender and age groups

Age (years)	Male (*N*)	Female (*N*)
18–29	6	9
30–39	8	11
40–49	5	5
50–59	5	0
60+	0	1
Total	24	26

were living alone. At the time of the act of self-harm only four respondents were employed (2 male, 2 female), 15 were economically active but unemployed (9 male, 6 female), 29 were claiming either disability or long-term sickness benefit (12 male, 17 female) and two were retired (1 male, 1 female).

Respondents were given a psychiatric diagnosis by the assessing psychiatrist or specialist nurse at the time of hospital admission (Table 4.2). The most frequent diagnoses were substance misuse and adjustment disorder. Only five respondents were diagnosed with a depressive disorder, and in no case was this the sole diagnosis. Eighteen respondents also received additional medical diagnoses, the most common being back pain and arthritis.

Context

In 1998 the population of Eastcraig was estimated at around 16 000, just under 4% of the population of the city of Edinburgh. Twenty-five per cent were aged under 16 years (compared to 17% in the city) and 11% were aged 65+ years (15% in the city). Eastcraig contained an over-representation of households living in public rented dwellings (58%), and an under-representation of owner-occupied dwellings (28%), compared to the city as a whole (16% and 70%, respectively, in 1998). The level of educational qualification achieved by pupils attending local schools was markedly lower than in the city as a whole.

The official unemployment rate was twice as high in Eastcraig (12% in 1998/99) as in the city as a whole (6%), with a larger proportion of the unemployed having been out of work for at least a year (24% versus 18%). Approximately 22% of the working-age population considered themselves to be economically inactive. In 1999, 22% of 579 households reported a net income of less than £300 per month. It was estimated that at least 70% of Eastcraig's working households earned below the city average wage and nearly a quarter of

Table 4.2 Main psychiatric diagnosis recorded by assessing psychiatrists

Primary psychiatric diagnosis	All patients
Depressive disorder	5
Alcohol dependence	21
Drug misuse or dependence	12
Adjustment disorder	7
Personality disorder only	3
No diagnosis	2
Total	50

There was considerable co-morbidity.

households (23%) had no bank or building society account (compared to 12% in Scotland as a whole). The prevalence of school-based poverty indicators (e.g. receipt of free school meals, receipt of clothing grant) was two to three times higher in Eastcraig than in the city as a whole. In 1997 the total standardized mortality ratio (SMR) for Eastcraig was 115 compared to 92 in the whole of the city (Scotland = 100). The area is served by two health centres where free access to primary care services is available, and by a limited range of shops and other retail outlets.

Overall, Eastcraig is characterized by high levels of socio-economic deprivation and environmental degradation, and has a poor health record. The area is currently undergoing economic regeneration.

People in context

In this section we present data from interviews with people who had self-harmed and their significant others. Findings are presented under five broad headings: childhood experiences; adult relationships; employment, income and poverty; health; and the local environment.

Childhood experiences

A significant number of both respondent and significant other accounts related to early family experiences. These were focused on relationships and dynamics rather than on descriptions of past poverty or material disadvantage. Some accounts highlighted the existence of inter-generational transmission of poor parenting. In the extract below a respondent points to her own parents' lack of parenting skills, which she believed related in part to her own mother's upbringing.

> You know my mum and dad did not do anything cruel to me or batter me or . . . they gave me quite a good childhood, but there was no support there, when things weren't funny. I adore my mother she, she just did not know any better, she came out of an orphanage, she never got taught right, well she got taught right but she never got taught how to bring kids up. And my dad was always like, he should've known better, but he was just a dad that went to the pub and worked, know what I mean. (R20)

Many respondents reported alcohol-related problems in their childhood. Some referred to what might be termed 'family dynamics' (i.e. difficult relationships between parents or between siblings), others to abuse by alcoholic parents. Some respondents disclosed protracted sexual abuse and described the ways that this led them to engage in other self-damaging and negative behaviours (examples included criminal activities, prostitution, and early pregnancy).

> I got a year and 6 weeks when I was 14 going on 15, because they said I was unruly . . . well my dad was abusing me so I was running away from my house all the time and getting myself into trouble. (R44)

It was not uncommon for these kinds of experiences to be followed by family breakdown. Many respondents reported living with one birth parent (usually the mother) and one or more step-parents. Several other respondents had grown up in local authority care or spent periods of time in criminal justice institutions. In the following extract a 36-year-old man describes his perception of how growing up in care affected his ability to develop long-term friendships and confiding relationships.

> I've never been one for trusting friends, I was brought up in care and I think that's probably what done that. Hardly trust myself never mind anybody else, I've been let down so many times. (R04)

Adult relationships

The data relating to current family structure and networks present a complex picture. A combination of relatively large families and multiple (normally sequential) sexual relationships often led to multi-faceted and changing family dynamics. At the same time there is evidence to suggest that some of the types of problems experienced in respondents' own childhoods were recurring in the families that they were creating.

Relationship problems associated with alcohol and drug use and/or violence were commonly cited.

> [My mother and mother-in-law are] both alcoholics . . . They both give me and my wife grief, and my wife's brother and all, he's give us grief. . . . Well it's a bit stupid really, it's with them being alcoholics the drink goes for them when they drink . . . they just go crazy when they start drinking, they start abusing us and things like that. (R27)

Other respondents (mainly, although not exclusively, women) described the way that physical violence (often associated with alcohol or drug use) could lead to withdrawal from previous friendships or a distancing from other family members. A woman described how she tolerated her partner's violence because he accepted her addiction to alcohol. The key point which respondents repeatedly made was that drug and alcohol use and/or repeated acts of violence had extremely detrimental effects on the development of close confiding relationships.

> Interviewer: 'How were the people that you knew in the area, were they able to kind of support you while your ex-husband was getting involved?'
> Respondent: 'They don't want to get involved. I wasn't even allowed my own family to visit me whilst I was with him, that's how bad he was.' (R46)

The interviews with significant others highlighted a further dimension to these relationships, namely the stresses involved in trying to support individuals with multiple difficulties over long periods of time. Several reported the frustration that resulted and the ways that they sometimes withdrew support.

It is also worth bearing in mind that significant others (e.g. siblings) had often themselves either experienced similar childhoods or been involved in the self-harmer's upbringing (e.g. parents, aunts, or uncles). Many had also themselves experienced alcohol or drug problems.

> She's not got anyone to talk to, when she's at, when she's feeling down, because I mean her trying to come and talk to me about it she knows that I would just, well usually I lose the head at her (get angry), saying to her, well mum why are you feeling like this, you were doing good, or if she's had a drink, I hate her having a drink, I mean I do lose the rag at her for, for drinking, because simply for the fact I know she's gone to go away and do something crazy to herself, so I know that I, I've been a big cause of her problems in her life, because I used to be quite violent em, towards her. (SO49)

Still other respondents highlighted the effect of insecure on–off interpersonal relationships (both with sexual partners and parents and children). In these descriptions respondents highlighted the emotional roller-coaster associated with repeated separation and reconciliation and/or multiple short- to medium-term sexual relationships. Such accounts highlighted the ways in which, over time, people became wary of sharing their feelings and/or becoming too reliant (emotionally or financially) upon a partner.

> She is seeing someone at the moment, but again it's nothing sort of solid. She says it's just a casual sex thing, which again mucks up her head because she ends up going head-over-heels in love with people. She doesn't seem to have long-term relationships, she only seems to have short ones, then she gets really hurt. Most of the people she seems to meet, she meets when she is drunk and they are only looking for a fling. (SO44)

Several female respondents commented on the importance of maintaining their tenancy in their own names so as to protect themselves and their children from homelessness during difficult periods in their relationships.

Descriptions of interpersonal and family relationships also suggested that some respondents perceived themselves to have a major caring responsibility. At one level this related to the often complex structure of families which provided opportunities or demands for caring. At another level, however, many respondents described themselves as being perceived by other family members as good carers.

In some interviews respondents described caring as being stressful and detrimental to their sense of well-being. Elsewhere, however, caring responsibilities were cited as providing a sense of purpose and life satisfaction. Several mothers commented that, without their childcare duties, they would feel far worse. One respondent made an explicit link between her caring behaviours and coping with her own problems.

> I'm used to always having somebody about me. And always having somebody with a problem. It's like, I can shut my own problems off if I'm dealing with somebody else's.

Well as Michael says he's nineteen, as long as he can remember I've always dealt with somebody else's kids or whatever. (R40)

Employment, income, and wealth

All four respondents in paid employment were working in low-skilled service-sector jobs. Very few unemployed respondents indicated that they were actively seeking work and many described themselves as being unfit for work, owing to reported illness and/or drug or alcohol dependence. Despite the fact that the majority of respondents were in receipt of benefits, poverty was not much mentioned as an explicit source of stress or anxiety. At the same time, respondents' descriptions of daily life pointed to difficulties in making ends meet and tensions caused through limited income. A lack of money, in combination with tobacco, alcohol, or drug use, resulted in some respondents not eating properly or cutting back on heating. Other respondents explicitly linked their financial difficulties to problematic partner/family relationships. These situations were particularly marked in relation to abusive partners and often linked to housing problems.

> I'm with a housing association and if you damage it, you've got to repair it. So he's defaced like nearly every one of my doors. So I can't get away. . . . because I only had to repair, (my son) had accidentally pushed the living room door into the cupboard door. There was no stoppers or anything. . . . And he defaced, near enough every door he broke. And he smashed the window and wrote in blood 'cow' on my wall. He's wrote 'slut' on my wall, with a knife engraved. . . . They want four hundred and eight pounds because he's caused that much damage. . . . All these housing associations are funny . . . They won't rehouse you if you've got damage to property. No matter how, you know, it was caused. (R39)

Some respondents appeared to have had periods when they had run up considerable debts, either through the use of store cards or not paying their rent. Several were currently being pursued through the courts to recover outstanding debts.

Physical and mental health

Many respondents described themselves as being 'depressed', although this description was often at variance with the clinical diagnosis made by psychiatrists at the time of hospital admission (Table 4.2). Respondents' most common explanations for their 'depression' were continuing and chronic stressors. The directional relationships between alcohol and drug abuse, difficult life circumstances, and 'depression' were commonly unclear, even to the respondents themselves.

> Interviewer: . . . is the depression because of the alcohol or is the depression because of the things outside of your life?

Respondent: Well the two, the two of them, the drinks not helping . . . It's not helping, I think it's helping and it's helping me at the time. . . . But I've still got my problems in the morning. (R11)

Well if you're from an area like Eastcraig everyone's in the same boat, you know, you aren't working and everything, so you're on benefit. They've got used to certain things to get money, they end up depressed, drinking alcohol, end up in fights you know, it just, it does that, it does that to you if you're on the sick through no fault of your own, and I mean, all your dreams and wishes are taken away from you, it can be very, very depressing you know. You end up just not realising you're going into a depression and getting further and further in, with this depression you just keep thinking constantly all the time, I just think I deserve better than this. (R07)

Several respondents reported that they were suffering ongoing medical problems. In some cases these were cited as reasons for not being able to work. On other occasions it appeared that these problems were related to long-term alcohol or drug use. What these respondents shared was the view that their physical health constituted yet another source of difficulty which they faced on a daily basis.

And no amount of tablets will take away that pain [alcohol-related pancreatitis] you know, I've got to get in touch with the doctor and that's when I end up in the hospital you know. You know and you feel sore all over you know, and then my legs sometimes I get up to walk and it's as though my legs have went numb and you know that's it you just don't realise you know. I just take it obviously day, day by day really. (R22)

The local environment

Comments from respondents about the local area concerned both the physical fabric and the socio-cultural environment. In relation to both aspects of the environment, respondents pointed out that there were differences between various sub-areas. Accommodation, for example, ranged from newly built semi-detached houses to 1970s high-rise tower blocks. Not surprisingly, more physical problems were cited in relation to older buildings. Similarly, distinctions were drawn between 'good' and 'bad' areas, in terms of levels of drug use, vandalism, 'joy-riding', and violence. In relation to the worst areas, several people described the environment through the use of analogies with well-known violent or war zone areas.

It's like the Bronx . . . They've spent a hell of lot of money on improve all em, yes building a couple houses, oh yes, excellent they've build a couple of houses. It still doesn't eliminate the problem. (R09)

It's like Vietnam, I swear to God that's what it's like, I do not want my bairn (child) being brought up in any place like that. (R03)

The most strongly expressed views regarding causes of difficulties within the local area were related to problems with drugs and alcohol. These problems in turn were often seen as arising from a combination of availability, boredom, and the socialization of people into negative health-damaging behaviours. Other respondents pointed to general antisocial behaviour and crime, ranging from noise, graffiti, and smashed windows to burglary and murder. There was general anxiety about possible repercussions if complaints were made to statutory agencies about these problems.

> I've never seen so many drugs in my life, I didn't know what dihydrocodeine or methadone was before I moved up here . . . This area, I think you'd find some of it's just abusing drugs in every single stair. In this area, honestly, its that bad around here . . . You see the people standing down the shopping centre waiting to buy tablets. (R31)
>
> The stair [block of flats] that she's [self-harmer] is in, it's, well it's like this block, but it's full of junkies (drug addicts), and you are getting people actually doing human toilet in the stair like . . . Well, basically she's stuck right in the heart of Eastcraig and it's, she's surrounded by junkies and dealers. (SO49)
>
> It's all drink from morning to night, drink. You know, everywhere you go, you cannot get away from it. See, right now, when people say they need help from alcohol and that, I know exactly what they mean. They need to get out the environment. (R44)
>
> They play the music loud at night and that when the bairns [children] are in bed, and just the bairns running up and down the balcony all the time. It's not an environment that I want to bring my bairn up in. (R47)
>
> Because I had problems with, there's a school nearby and kids are just throwing bricks through your window . . . Last year . . . I had . . . three bricks through my window so, don't know why but they just do it, just for, just for a laugh . . . but for me it's no laugh. (R19)

The relevance of the findings to understanding self-harm

It has been argued that much of the previous research that has attempted to understand the social causation of health and illness has only achieved a charting of (typically individual) risk factors (Frohlich *et al.* 2001). This criticism could certainly be applied to the literature on deliberate self-harm. Questions concerning how risks are created and maintained, and the determination of which social processes create potentially health-damaging social environments, remain unanswered. In their contribution to the debate on social context, Frohlich and co-workers argue that it is necessary to gain a better understanding of the relationships between 'agency (the ability for people to deploy a range of causal powers), practices (the activities that make and transform the world we live in) and social structure (the rules and resources within society)' (Frohlich *et al.* 2001, p. 781).

We have attempted to apply this perspective to deliberate self-harm by examining the lived experiences of a group of repeat self-harmers. Their accounts confirm the importance of linking agency and practice, with an additional focus upon the role of structured social space (for an alternative perspective on agency and deliberate self-harm, based on data from the same study, see Redley 2003). Respondents' accounts documented perceptions of key influences across the lifecourse and the ways that these contributed to their current life circumstances and their decisions to engage in acts of self-harm. Most respondents noted the importance of early life experiences. However, the emphasis was not on material disadvantage (although this seemed to exist in many cases) but rather on damaging familial relationships. Violence, sexual abuse, and difficulties related to drug and alcohol use were commonly reported. In turn, these difficulties were cited as resulting from cultural patterns of behaviour and/or their parents' own problematic childhoods.

Respondents' accounts also highlighted the need to understand the pathways of inter-generational transmission of norms, values, and patterns of behaviour. The family is one of the primary locations for socialization, and it seems clear that respondents learnt what it means to live in a family and what were 'appropriate' roles for men, women, and children during early childhood. They also commonly adopted ways of using or abusing various substances (illicit drugs, alcohol, tobacco) and attitudes toward violence. In adult life the local environment then provided respondents with cultural cues concerning appropriate values and behaviours. It supplied people with whom respondents interacted and a socio-cultural background against which to understand and interpret the appropriateness of social actions. Respondents met partners and developed families with individuals who often shared similar early life experiences. They also made sense of actions and behaviours (their own and others) against the wider norms and values of their community.

We are not suggesting that local residents or respondents formed part of an under-class or counter-culture which stood in opposition to mainstream social values, in the ways outlined by Murray (1990). Rather, we identify a long-term process of social exclusion (Walker and Walker 1997), illustrated by the relative isolation of the community and the development of a parochial and inward looking subculture. Respondents often aspired toward supportive, non-violent interpersonal relationships and the creation of nuclear families. It was also common for them to recognize the impact of drug and alcohol abuse on the community and to express a desire for their social situations to be different. However, cumulative social disadvantage appears to have restricted horizons and perceived opportunities: respondents spent most of their time interacting with people living nearby—they did not very often travel outside of their immediate locality nor did they make use of the city's wider resources. These findings underline the complexity of the relationships between agency, practice, and social structure. People make choices but what they see as 'valid' or 'good' choices are shaped by personal history/biography and socio-economic and socio-historic context. Respondents' accounts document inter-relation-ships between various life domains (e.g. family and education, family and criminal activity) but also point to ways in which their choices were shaped by cultural contexts and material resources.

Implications for practice and prevention

The volume of the repetition of deliberate self-harm has been highlighted as a massive economic burden for families, communities, and societies, and rep-resents a major risk factor for completed suicide. One-third to half the patients admitted to hospital following an episode of deliberate self-harm will already have a history of previous self-harm (Kreitman and Casey 1988; Platt *et al.* 1988; Bille-Brahe *et al.* 1997; Sakinofsky 2000), while 6–30% (median 16%) will harm themselves within a year (NHS Centre for Reviews and Dissemin-ation 1998). About 1% of patients referred to general hospitals in the UK for deliberate self-harm commit suicide within a year of the self-harm episode (a risk which is approximately 100 times that of the general population) (Greer and Bagley 1971; Hawton and Fagg 1988), and 2–13% (median 3%) within 5–10 years (NHS Centre for Reviews and Dissemination 1998). Based on evidence from studies of psychiatric populations, the best predictor of eventual suicide is a history of deliberate self-harm, with 'grand repeaters' (i.e. those having multiple repeated episodes of self-harm) constituting a particularly vulnerable subgroup (Hawton and Fagg 1988). Between 40% and 50% of those who commit suicide have a history of deliberate self-harm (Ovenstone and Kreitman 1974; Hawton and Fagg 1988).

What is the health service to do to help those who engage in this behaviour? A range of hospital-based medical and psychosocial interventions to reduce repeat deliberate self-harm has been evaluated by means of randomized controlled trials. Recent systematic reviews (van der Sande *et al.* 1997; Hawton *et al.* 1998; NHS Centre for Reviews and Dissemination 1998) are unanimous in concluding that very few of these have been shown to be consistently effective. One response to this failure has been to urge larger trials, irrespective of the limited evidence of success so far and poor patient adherence to outpatient aftercare programmes (van der Sande *et al.* 1997). However, an alternative approach has been advocated by Hawton *et al.* (1998), who argue for the 'need for development of further treatment approaches informed by current knowledge about the psychosocial and biological characteristics of these patients and the socioeconomic and sociocultural context of the beha-viour' (Hawton *et al.* 1998, p. 446).

The findings of the study reported in this chapter support this conclusion, confirming that a reconsideration of the nature of interventions designed to reduce repetition of deliberate self-harm is necessary. Indeed, our most challenging recommendation is that the quest for exclusively medical and psychosocial hospital-based treatments aimed at reducing deliberate self-harm as a primary objective should be abandoned. Instead, we suggest a mixture of public policy and practice (including health service) interventions targeted at the more fundamental 'upstream' determinants (Pearce and McKinlay 1998) of deliberate self-harm, in particular pervasive forces of social exclusion.

Public policy instruments should be used at both national and local levels. Government departments and associated agencies need to consider how to enhance opportunities for developing lifeskills, achieving educational qualifications, obtaining suitable employment, undertaking meaningful activity, and participating in community life among those who have hitherto lacked such opportunities. Consideration should also be given to changes in local government housing policy in order to prevent the concentration of vulnerable individuals in localities that offer easy access to drugs and alcohol and (albeit inadvertently) nurture conditions which enhance violence and hopelessness.

Service interventions targeted at both individuals and groups should have the following characteristics: based in the community (not in hospital); delivered through co-ordinated and integrated inter-sectoral partnerships (the health service working in effective collaboration with other public sector and voluntary organizations); and building on those aspects of existing services that are seen as positive, i.e. teaching life and parenting skills (currently done in a limited way by a variety of community agencies) and providing long-term, continuing supportive contact or mentoring (currently offered mostly by GPs but limited by their biomedical role).

Conclusion

Our data suggest that DSH is only one among several coping strategies employed by persons living in the context of social disadvantage. We further propose that it is unhelpful to separate DSH from these other coping responses, particularly illicit drug use and alcohol abuse. Rather, we argue that it is necessary to appreciate the complex and reciprocal inter-relationships between different coping behaviours in specific social contexts if we are to devise effective primary or secondary prevention interventions.

Acknowledgements

The fieldwork for the study reported in this chapter was conducted by Dr Marcus Redley. The study was funded by the Chief Scientist Office (CSO) of the Scottish Executive Health Department. The Research Unit in

Health, Behaviour and Change is funded by CSO. However, the opinions expressed in this paper are those of the authors, not of the CSO.

References

Bille-Brahe, U., Kerkhof, A., DeLeo, D., Schmidtke, A., Crepet, P., Lonnqvist, J., *et al.* (1997). A repetition-prediction study of European parasuicide populations: a summary of the first report from Part II of the WHO/EURO Multicentre Study on parasuicide in co-operation with the EC Concerted Action on Attempted Suicide. *Acta Psychiatrica Scandinavica*, **95**, 81–6.

Buglass, D., Dugard, P., and Kreitman, N. (1970). Multiple standardisation of parasuicide ('attempted suicide') rates in Edinburgh. *British Journal of Preventive and Social Medicine*, **12**, 241–53.

Diez-Roux, A.V. (1998). Bringing context back into epidemiology: variables and fallacies in multilevel analysis. *American Journal of Public Health*, **88**, 216–22.

Diez-Roux, A.V. (2003). The examination of neighbourhood effects on health: conceptual and methodological issues related to the presence of multiple levels of organization. In *Neighborhoods and health*, (ed. I. Kawachi and L.F. Berkman), pp. 45–64. Oxford University Press, Oxford.

Duncan, C., Jones, K., and Moon, G. (1998). Context, composition and heterogeneity: using multilevel models in health research. *Social Science and Medicine*, **46**, 97–117.

Durkhiem, E. (1952 [1897]). *Suicide. A study in sociology*. Routledge and Kegan Paul, London.

Frohlich, K.L., Corin, E., and Potvin, L. (2001). A theoretical proposal for the relationship between context and disease. *Sociology of Health and Illness*, **23**, 776–97.

Greenland, S. and Morgenstern, H. (1989). Ecological bias, confounding and effect modification. *International Journal of Epidemiology*, **18**, 269–74.

Greer, S. and Bagley, C. (1971). Effect of psychiatric intervention in attempted suicide: a controlled study. *British Medical Journal*, **1**, 168–74.

Hawton, K. and Fagg, J. (1988). Suicide, and other causes of death, following attempted suicide. *British Journal of Psychiatry*, **152**, 359–66.

Hawton, K., Arensman, E., Townsend, E., Bremner, S., Feldman, E., Goldney, R., *et al.* (1998). Deliberate self harm: systematic review of efficacy of psychosocial and pharmacological treatments in preventing repetition. *British Medical Journal*, **317**, 441–7.

Hox, J. and Kreft, I. (1994). Multilevel analysis methods. *Sociological Methods and Research*, **22**, 282–99.

Iversen, G. (1991). *Contextual analysis*. Sage Publications, Newbury Park, California.

Krieger, N. (1994). Epidemiology and the web of causation: has anyone seen the spider? *Social Science and Medicine*, **39**, 887–903.

Krietman, N. (ed.) (1977). *Parasuicide*. John Wiley, London.

Kreitman, N. and Casey, P. (1988). Repetition of parasuicide: an epidemiological and clinical study. *British Journal of Psychiatry*, **153**, 792–800.

Macintyre, S. and Ellaway, A. (2003). Neighborhoods and health: an overview. In *Neighborhoods and health*, (ed. I. Kawachi and L.F. Berkman), pp. 20–42. Oxford University Press, Oxford.

Macintrye, S., Maciver, S., and Sooman, A. (1993). Area, class and health: should we be focusing on places or people? *Journal of Social Policy*, 22, 213–34.

Murray, C. (1990). *The emerging British underclass*. Institute of Economic Affairs, London.

Neeleman, J. (1998). Regional suicide rates in the Netherlands: does religion still play a role? *International Journal of Epidemiology*, 27, 466–72.

Neeleman, J. and Lewis, G. (1999). Suicide, religion, and socioeconomic conditions. An ecological study in 26 countries, 1990. *Journal of Epidemiology and Community Health*, 53, 204–10.

Neeleman, J. and Wessely, S. (1999). Ethnic minority suicide: a small area geographical study in south London. *Psychological Medicine*, 29, 429–36.

NHS Centre for Reviews and Dissemination (1998). Deliberate self-harm. *Effective Health Care*, 4 (6), 1–12.

Ovenstone, I. and Kreitman, N. (1974). Two syndromes of suicide. *British Journal of Psychiatry*, 124, 336–45.

Pearce, N. (1996). Traditional epidemiology, modern epidemiology, and public health. *American Journal of Public Health*, 86, 678–83.

Pearce, N. and McKinlay, J.B. (1998). Back to the future in epidemiology and public health: response to Dr Gori. *Journal of Clinical Epidemiology*, 51, 634–6.

Pickett, K.E. and Pearl, M. (2001). Multilevel analyses of neighbourhood socioeconomic context and health outcomes: a critical review. *Journal of Epidemiology and Community Health*, 55, 111–22.

Platt, S. (1984). Unemployment and suicidal behaviour: a review of the literature. *Social Science and Medicine*, 19, 93–115.

Platt, S. (1985). A subculture of parasuicide? *Human Relations*, 38, 257–97.

Platt, S. and Hawton, K. (2000). Suicidal behaviour and the labour market. In *The international handbook of suicide and attempted suicide*, (ed. K. Hawton and K. van Heeringen), pp. 309–84. John Wiley and Sons, Chichester.

Platt, S. and Kreitman, N. (1985). Parasuicide and unemployment among men in Edinburgh 1968–82. *Psychological Medicine*, 15, 113–23.

Platt, S., Hawton, K., Kreitman, N., Fagg, J. and Foster, J. (1988). Recent clinical and epidemiological trends in Edinburgh and Oxford: a tale of two cities. *Psychological Medicine*, 18, 405–18.

Redley, M. (2003). Towards a new perspective on deliberate self-harm in an area of multiple deprivation. *Sociology of Health and Illness*, 25 (4), 348–73.

Robinson, W. (1950). Ecological correlations and the behaviour of individuals. *American Sociological Review*, 15, 351–7.

Sakinofsky, I. (2000). Repetition of suicidal behaviour. In *The international handbook of suicide and attempted suicide*, (ed. K. Hawton and K. van Heeringen), pp. 385–404. John Wiley and Sons, Chichester.

Susser, M. and Susser, E. (1996). Choosing a future for epidemiology. II From black box to Chinese boxes and eco-epidemiology. *American Journal of Public Health*, 86, 674–7.

Van der Sande, R., Buskens, E., Allart, E., van der Graaf, Y., and van Engeland, H. (1997). Psychosocial intervention following suicide attempt: a systematic review of treatment interventions. *Acta Psychiatrica Scandinavica*, 96, 43–50.

Walker, A. and Walker, C. (1997) *Britain divided: the growth of social exclusion in the 1980s and 1990s*. CPAG, London.

5

Psychology and suicidal behaviour: elaborating the entrapment model

J. Mark G. Williams, Catherine Crane,
Thorsten Barnhofer, and Danielle Duggan

Introduction and background

Early cognitive accounts of suicidal behaviour were developed from cognitive theories of depression. Suicidal patients were assumed to share depressed patients' high frequency of negative thinking, compounded by logical errors (e.g. overgeneralization, catastrophization, black and white thinking), and a tendency for long-term schemas or belief structures to be activated by current life events. In addition to sharing the general cognitive characteristics of depression, Beck showed that suicidality was particularly closely associated with hopelessness for the future and an imbalance between reasons for living and reasons for dying. Further research emphasized the widespread impairments in interpersonal problem solving in suicidal patients, findings that led to the development of brief problem-solving therapies. Indeed, of all the psychological variables that are studied in suicidal patients, it is those of depression, hopelessness, and problem solving that have become a recurrent theme.

This emergence of cognitive theories of suicidality from theories of depression is justified by the fact that suicidality seems very often to represent a complication of depression. Suicidal ideation arises initially as a symptom of depression, especially if there are reasons for a person to feel hopeless about the future. Studies of major depression in clinical populations show rates of suicidal ideation in excess of 50%. However, the majority of individuals who experience suicidal ideation do not make a suicide attempt (Kessler *et al.* 1999). Thus it may be less important to explain how suicidal ideation arises in the first place, than to explain why it is maintained and exacerbated to the point where an individual gets more and more caught in the fantasy of dying and how to bring it about.

In our previous work, we have suggested that suicidal ideation and behaviour arise from feelings of entrapment, that there is no escape (arrested flight), and that this represents a particular pattern of information processing about the self and the world (Williams 2001). When someone feels suicidal, the ideation may last only a short while if they can think of other, alternative ways to solve their problems. Impairments in problem-solving reduce this capacity. Even if no solution suggests itself, suicidal feelings may abate if the person feels he or she has something to look forward to in the future, some important reasons for living, despite the way they feel at the moment. Hopelessness about the future takes away these possibilities. It is not hard to see why the combination of poor problem-solving and hopelessness has become the main object of study for suicidologists interested in psychological processes; these processes are the most likely to make a person feel completely trapped and helpless about ever escaping from current difficulties.

In this chapter we shall review and update some of our recent research on the psychological processes underlying suicidal behaviour. First, we shall define 'entrapment' and say how different aspects of the way people process information about themselves and their world contribute to difficulties they have with solving current problems and in remaining hopeful for the future. We shall then discuss the arrested flight model of suicidal behaviour (Williams 2001), outline what we see as potential problems for this model as it stands (particularly the state/trait issue), and how we might begin to understand how to resolve these problems. In particular, we shall outline how differential activation theory, a model that has proved extremely important in related research with relapse in major depression, may explain how some individuals continue to be vulnerable to further suicidal behaviour, even when they appear to have recovered from the immediate suicidal crisis.

Defining entrapment

Entrapment can be defined as the inability (or perceived inability) to get away from an aversive environment after one has suffered a defeat, loss, or humiliation. The idea arises from evolutionary psychologists' attempts to explain the origins of depression (Gilbert and Allan 1998). In the animal world, very often an animal that loses an encounter with a more powerful rival suffers little ill effect if it can get away. Its social repertoire remains intact, and few differences are observed. By contrast, if the animal that has been defeated cannot escape, the combination of the high motivation to get away, plus the inability to do so, produces a very different outcome. Its behaviour becomes very submissive. The submissiveness of the loser usually succeeds in the winner ending the attack. Indeed, evolutionary psychologists observe that the survival function of such 'loser behaviour' is to allow the winner to get on with the business of being the boss, choosing mates, etc., without the fear of being continually challenged by the loser (see Gilbert and Allan 1998).

It is a short step, from these observations, to the hypothesis that humans may retain some of these evolutionarily primitive brain systems, and that humiliations, losses, and rejections may trigger such 'scripts' in situations where escape is not possible. In fact, George Brown, who published some of the most influential early work on how negative life events trigger depression, has now returned to some of his earlier data and shown that if these events were characterized by humiliation and entrapment (as judged by raters who are blind to other details of the person), then these events are much more likely than loss events to be associated with the onset of depression (in both community and clinical samples, see Fig. 5.1) (Brown *et al.* 1995). From such observations, we suggest, first, that it is particularly when such defeats, humiliations, and entrapments occur that the risk of suicidal behaviour will be increased. This will occur across different diagnoses, and may be especially relevant in situations where the symptoms of a mental health problem (as, for example, auditory hallucinations in schizophrenia) are themselves a source of humiliation and entrapment for the person (see Drake and Cotton 1986; Iqbal *et al.* 2000).

Secondly, however, people vary in how much they will see the same event as humiliating and entrapping. Gilbert and Allan (1998) have devised a

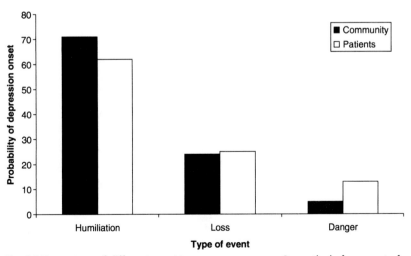

Fig. 5.1 Percentage of different event types among women 6 months before onset of depression (from Brown *et al.* (1995). *Psychological Medicine,* **25**, 7–21).

questionnaire measure of perceived defeat and entrapment, both entrapment by internal events such as one's thoughts and feelings, and by external circumstances (see Table 5.1). They find that these measures (especially defeat and external entrapment) predict levels of depression and hopelessness in both student and clinical samples. Their major contribution is to confirm that people vary in their general tendency to see events though the lenses of defeat and entrapment. These individual differences in processing information influence the likelihood that helplessness scripts will be activated in response to humiliating or defeating events, and thus influence the levels of depression that result.

However, these data raise a number of questions. First, depression, hopelessness, and suicidal feelings sometimes arise a considerable time after the occurrence of a defeating or humiliating event. We need to understand what it is that allows such events to affect behaviour despite the fact that the actual event is not a present reality in the person's world. Secondly, some individuals experience an enormous amount of adversity but do not become suicidal. We need to understand this resilience. Thirdly, we know that after a first episode of depression, subsequent episodes are more easily triggered, a process referred to as 'kindling' (e.g. Post 1992; Segal *et al.* 1996). Can suicidal ideation and behaviour, like depression, become more easily triggered over time (e.g. Joiner and Rudd 2000)? If this is the case, we need to explain the mechanisms underlying 'kindling' of suicidal behaviour and its relationship to depression. Our research is examining the possibility that the way individuals process information about themselves and the world helps to determine the lag between event and reaction, individual differences in response to events, and the cumulative effect of previous history on current vulnerability to suicidal behaviour.

The arrested flight ('cry of pain') model

The arrested flight model has three components: sensitivity to cues in the environment that signal defeat or humiliation and give rise to an overwhelming feeling of *needing to escape*; a sense of being *unable to escape*; and the sense that *this state of affairs will continue indefinitely* (that there will be no rescue).

Table 5.1 Items from the External Entrapment Scale (Gilbert and Allan 1998)

I am in a relationship I can't get out of
I have a strong desire to escape from things in my life
I often have the feeling that I would just like to run away
I feel trapped by other people

The first component, sensitivity to cues signalling defeat, suggests that, in addition to exposure to actual events (of the type described by Brown *et al.* 1995), some people become sensitized to these themes. As a result they are prone to interpret even relatively neutral events as representing humiliation or defeat, at least when they get into particular moods. A glance from a workmate that is not a smile, may, for some, constitute a rejection. Overhearing a colleague being praised for good work is seen as a defeat ('Why not me? Because I'm no good'). A lower than expected grade on a test is seen as a shameful failure. The fact that such sensitivities give rise to feelings of needing to escape is apparent in the reasons that attempted suicide patients give for their actions, in which escape motivations predominate.

The second component, being unable to escape, arises from deficits in interpersonal problem solving. Our research has found that such problem-solving difficulties are closely associated with the tendency to retrieve personal memories from the past in an overgeneral way. Current theories of autobiographical memory acknowledge that our personal memories tend to be hierarchically organized (Conway and Pleydell-Pearce 2000), with general event summaries (e.g. 'meetings at work') helping us, normally, to come up with a memory record of a specific event we need to call to mind (e.g. 'our meeting last Tuesday'). The memory records of specific events will usually provide the detailed information required to guide ongoing behaviour (e.g. 'we decided not to meet again!'), but general event summaries are necessary to enable us to navigate through the memory hierarchy.

It has been known for some time that when attempting to retrieve memories of specific events, suicidal patients, like those with depression, appear to get stuck at the general event summary level (e.g. Williams and Broadbent 1986). For example a depressed or suicidal patient given the cue word '*sorry*' and asked to retrieve a specific event memory might respond '*I feel sorry for all the times I have hurt my family*'. One reason for this overgenerality may be that the recollection of specific details of events has become associated with strong and aversive affect. Indeed, there is now a great deal of evidence that overgeneral recall occurs in those groups (from both clinical and community populations) that have suffered adversity or abuse, particularly sexual abuse or war trauma (see Henderson *et al.* 2002, for an example of this research). While overgenerality may initially be protective, helping individuals to avoid traumatic memories, there is increasing evidence to suggest that it also contributes significantly to the deficits in problem solving seen in suicidal patients.

For example, Pollock and Williams (2001) examined autobiographical memory specificity and problem-solving performance in a group of patients who had very recently attempted suicide. They found a highly significant association between overgenerality of memory and the severity of the problem-solving deficits observed. Other studies (e.g. Evans *et al.* 1992; Sidley *et al.* 1999) have identified a similar association, with those patients who have most difficulties in navigating through their own personal memory system (so having fewer specific memories on which to draw), also having most difficulty in coming up with solutions to current problems. This, and other research, such as the work of Hutchings *et al.* (1998), who identified the same relationship in a study of memory and real-life problem-solving behaviour (treatment compliance), demonstrates that overgeneral memory is fundamentally entrapping. This may help us to answer the question of why trauma, which is associated with increases in overgeneral memory, has such long-lasting effects.

The third aspect of the arrested flight model is the tendency to project such entrapment into the future—hopelessness. We have examined whether hopelessness is mostly the anticipation of a negative future, or the lack of being able to think of a positive future (MacLeod *et al.* 1993). Using a fluency test, participants are asked to think of as many good events (or, in counterbalanced order, as many bad events) that might occur in the future (e.g. next week, month, year, or 5–10 years), we have found that greater hopelessness is a function of lack of positive future, not an excess of negative future. This original work has now been replicated by MacLeod in several studies (MacLeod *et al.* 1997*a, b*), and by O'Connor and colleagues (O'Connor *et al.* 2000).

The arrested flight model of suicidal behaviour has recently received further empirical support. O'Connor (2003) compared suicidal patients and hospital controls on measures of perceived stress, perceived opportunity for escape from most stressful recent experience, feelings of defeat, and level of social support (opportunity for rescue). Parasuicide patients were found to be more depressed, anxious, and hopeless, and to have higher levels of stress than hospital controls. Importantly, they also reported significantly higher levels of defeat, lower levels of escapability, and lower levels of social support. Logistic regression correctly assigned 90% of participants to the parasuicide or control group, with levels of social support, feelings of defeat, and the interaction between social support and defeat, being significant predictors of group membership. High levels of social support were protective. Individuals who reported high levels of inescapability nevertheless fell into the control, rather than parasuicide, group, if they had social support. These findings indicate that defeat and entrapment are likely to be key contributory factors in understanding suicidal behaviour, with perceived opportunity for rescue playing a mediating role.

Trait versus state

The arrested flight model, like other theories of suicidal behaviour, includes a number of explanatory variables. But all models of such behaviour, no matter how elegant, have in the end to answer the question: which variables contribute to long-term vulnerability (a trait) and which represent short-term precipitating factors. Of course, it is possible that the variables that appear to be short-term precipitating factors may turn out to be reactions to the mood disturbance of the suicidal crisis, rather than causes. There is an extra complexity in the case of suicidal behaviour. Although it is episodic, occurring most often when a person is in an episode of depression and not when they are in remission, not all people who suffer from recurrent depression become suicidal, and some suicidal behaviour occurs in individuals who are not clinically depressed. As Mann *et al.* (1999) point out, we need a model that helps us to determine who remains vulnerable, despite seeming to have recovered, and how this underlying vulnerability relates to the acute suicidal state.

In fact, when we look at the evidence on both hopelessness and problem solving, we see that they have *both* trait and state factors. Let us look at hopelessness first. Malone and colleagues examined which of their depressed patients (all with a diagnosis of major depression) had a history of suicidal behaviour (Malone *et al.* 2000). Even though the suicidal behaviour itself had occurred some time before, they found that the hopelessness levels were still significantly higher in those with such a history. Data from other studies support this conclusion, hopelessness remains higher between episodes of deliberate self-harm, and thus it seems to represent a vulnerability to suicidal ideation and behaviour (Young *et al.* 1996). On the other hand, Schotte *et al.* (1990) found clear evidence that hopelessness levels fall rapidly after the suicidal crisis is over (see Fig. 5.2). This is important, since most research studies test patients within a week of the DSH event, without being concerned how many days have elapsed. Clearly, it matters a great deal when people are tested. But for the present purposes, the important message is that hopelessness shows evidence of being state-like, as well as trait-like. It is higher than normal between episodes, but it rises still further in a crisis, falling again afterwards.

Are both trait and state levels related to the same underlying phenomena? The data suggest that they are. Both trait levels of hopelessness and the higher state levels that occur in the midst of a crisis appear to be closely related to the inability to imagine positive events in the future. This 'dysfluency' for positive events is itself related to reduced levels of positive mood, which, of course, can vary over time. What emerges is a picture in which low levels of positive affect

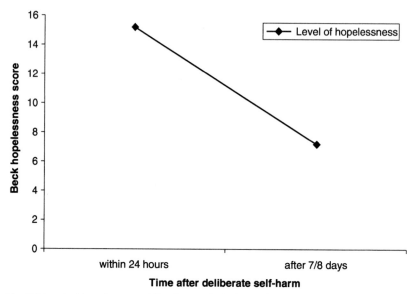

Fig. 5.2 Level of hopelessness shifts down relatively rapidly in the week after deliberate self-harm (data from Schotte *et al.* 1990).

and an absence of positive thoughts about the future are very closely connected. While it is feelings of depression that may be most associated with a sense of defeat and the urge to escape, it is positive cognitions that provide resilience and protect the individual from harming him or herself. Positive mood tends to be fairly low even in between episodes, but further reductions in positive mood that occur at difficult times compound existing problems that a vulnerable person has when he or she tries to generate thoughts of a positive future. This causes hopelessness to rise, bringing with it any other moods and thoughts that have become associated with hopelessness in the past. It is the nature of this association that we will turn to in a moment. But before we do, let us see if problem solving also has this feature of being both a trait and a state phenomenon.

Figure 5.3 (left-hand graph) shows the changes that occur in patients' scores on the Means Ends Problem Solving task (MEPS—a standardized problem-solving task) in the immediate aftermath of a suicidal crisis (data from Schotte *et al.*, 1990). It is clear that problem-solving abilities recover quite quickly. However, Pollock and Williams (2004) followed people up after a suicidal crisis from their first week following the crisis to 6 weeks later, during which time their mood disturbance improved significantly. These data are shown in the right-hand graph of Fig. 5.3. As can be seen, despite the mood change, the

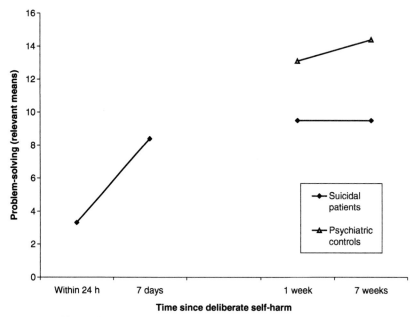

Fig. 5.3 Problem-solving (number of relevant means) improves in the week following deliberate self-harm (data on the left; Schotte *et al.* 1990), but stabilizes over the next few weeks to a level that remains more impaired than in psychiatric patients (matched control) (data on the right; Pollock and Williams 2004).

problem-solving performance remained impaired. These data confirm that there are trait elements as well as state elements to problem solving.

So *both* hopelessness and problem solving act as *both* trait and state factors. If we want to understand the interaction of trait and state aspects of these variables, we need a model of what is going on at this interface. We need to understand differential activation.

Differential activation

For some years, psychologists have studied what is known as 'context-dependent memory'—the phenomenon by which a person recalls information better if they are recalling it in the context in which they learned, or first thought of it. A striking example of this comes from a study of divers in the North Sea. If divers learn a list on the shore, they find that when underwater they cannot recall the list so well. They have to return to shore if they wish to recall the list fully. But a similar thing happens if they learn a list underwater. In this case they cannot recall it so well on shore, and have to return underwater to remember it well (Godden and Baddeley 1975).

Further research shows that a negative or positive mood can act like the water, or the shore, providing a context for learning. As a result, returning to a certain mood makes more accessible whatever has been laid down in memory when this mood has been active in the past. Returning to that mood can reinstate the whole context of whatever was going on: thinking patterns, bodily sensations, attentional biases and sensitivities, and so on.

What implications does this have for understanding suicidal thoughts and behaviour? It suggests that we need to look at what patterns have become associated together with different moods throughout the learning history of any individual. Figure 5.4a shows some of the elements that can be activated when someone feels depressed. These elements may initially occur together in fairly loose association the first time a person feels down, perhaps during adolescence, even if, at this time, the criteria for major depression are not met. If the depression occurs again, however, the pattern starts to become established and learned associations build up between the moods, the thinking and the bodily sensations (for example between feelings of hopelessness, entrapment, agitation, and suicidal ideation). From then on these patterns may be reactivated whenever mood is low.

Even when the mood normalizes between episodes, the associations are still there: they remain latent even when the person is not currently depressed and can be more and more easily activated by depression as well as by other moods that may have become associated with the entrapment processing pattern in the past. This is the same process we see in context-dependent memory: the learned material is still present, but not sufficiently activated to be conscious. It is the reinstatement of the context (in this case low mood) that reassembles the patterns, suddenly making accessible negative self-talk, low self-esteem, sluggish or agitated bodily states, hopelessness, and so on (see Fig. 5.4b). If suicidal ideation has occurred during one episode of depression, it is likely to be reactivated, along with these other features of depressive thinking, on subsequent occasions. For some people, suicidal ideation has never become a part of what they experience when depressed. As a result suicidal ideation has never been linked to the rest of the pattern, so reactivation of depressed mood will not tend to activate suicidal ideation or behaviour. This is, of course, unless a severely humiliating and entrapping life event occurs, in which case suicidal thoughts might be introduced into the pattern. Once introduced, other elements of the pattern (e.g. depression, anger, bodily sluggishness) would gain the capacity to reactivate this suicidal ideation.

In some cases, the depression and associated suicidal ideation will be severe enough, even on a first episode, to produce attempts to commit suicide that are highly lethal. In other cases, suicidal behaviour will occur only following

(a)

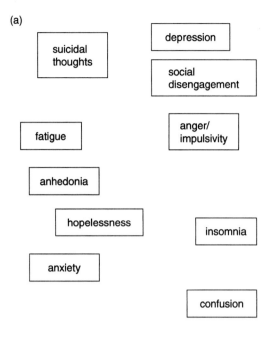

(b)

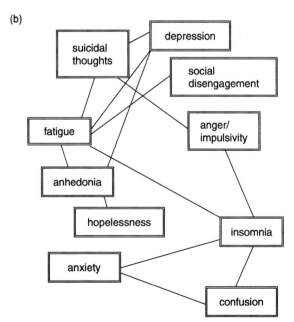

Fig. 5.4 Symptoms of depression co-occur (a) and, if activated repeatedly, form associations (b) that will share some characteristics between people, but have some features that are unique to each person.

repeated episodes of reactivation of suicide ideation. During such repeated activation suicidal ideas may become elaborated and other negative moods (such as anger) may become associated with the suicidal ideation. These negative moods will then gain the potential to elicit the holistic 'entrapment' schema (and suicidal behaviour), even in the absence of depression. This is how co-morbidity comes to be able to predict suicidal behaviour more clearly than a single diagnosis alone; it offers many more moods, thoughts, and contexts (including body sensations) to which suicidal ideation can become associated. Each of these may act as a trigger for reinstating the suicidal pattern of processing at a later date; for example, the start of another episode of major depression (Yen *et al.* 2003).

Between episodes, someone who is vulnerable to further suicidal behaviour will not be easily distinguishable from someone who has been suicidal but found a way of allowing their mood to vary without activating other moods and the suicide 'mode' or pattern. The question is, if some (previously) suicidal people carry around with them a pattern of processing which is latent, but which may be activated by a range of moods, how can we tell who has really recovered, and who remains vulnerable? We could wait until mood is disturbed by a life event, and hope to be there soon enough to monitor changes in the dysfunctional and self-critical patterns of thinking that may be activated. But the alternative is to invite people, in the clinical laboratory, to experience a small amount of sad mood, and to monitor closely what changes this mood brings about under these controlled conditions. This 'mood challenge' paradigm has been used to help understand relapse and recurrence in major depression and, although suicidal behaviour is different in many ways from depression, we may learn a lot about suicidal thinking from this aspect of research on recurrence.

Segal and colleagues conducted a study in which depressed patients were assessed after recovery from depression (Segal *et al.* 1999). They had been treated either with antidepressant medication or by cognitive therapy, and both groups had achieved remission. The researchers wanted to predict who was more vulnerable to future depression. It is well known that the number of previous episodes is the biggest predictor of future episodes, but at the time of potential recurrence, this historical variable needs a proximal (immediate) psychobiological process by which this risk is translated into a current downturn in mood. Segal and colleagues wished to test the hypothesis that, at times of incipient relapse or recurrence, it is the strength of the activation process (how easily negative thoughts and dysfunctional attitudes can be recruited by small changes in mood) that determines whether a person slides down into another episode.

They gave their patients the Dysfunctional Attitudes Scale (DAS) (Table 5.2). In previous studies it has been established that scores on this measure are higher in patients who are currently depressed, but return to normal, or near normal, when depression has remitted (not unlike hopelessness in the case of the suicidal patient). Segal and colleagues gave the recovered patients a Mood Induction Procedure, inviting them to listen to some sad music and to think of a sad memory. They then measured the DAS again, and found that the scores had risen in response to the mood induction, in some people much more than others. In some patients mood shifted a lot, yet this DAS score shifted only a little. For others, small amounts of mood shift had activated large shifts in dysfunctional attitudes. Thirty of these patients were followed up between 13 and 48 months later. The authors found that the DAS levels *after* the mood activation procedure significantly predicted recurrence of depression, even after taking into account the patients' pre-activation DAS scores.

Two recent studies indicate that differential activation may be very relevant to understanding what is happening when an individual slips into a suicidal crisis. The first, by Goldstein and Willner (2002), showed that feelings of defeat and entrapment (like dysfunctional attitudes), can be reactivated by a mood induction, particularly in individuals who have higher baseline levels of depression. The second study, by Williams and colleagues (2005), compared individuals who, although not currently depressed, had a history of depression either with or without suicidal ideation. Rather than using a negative mood induction, individuals were asked to indicate how much they experienced a range of thoughts and feelings when their mood was somewhat lower than normal (using a standardized questionnaire, the Leiden Index of Depression Sensitivity (LEIDS); Van der Does 2002). Individuals who had been suicidal during previous episodes of depression endorsed the LEIDS items measuring hopelessness and suicidal ideation much more strongly than those who had a history of depression without suicidal ideation. In contrast, the two groups did not differ on other items, such as those measuring aggression and harm avoidance. These studies provide preliminary evidence that feelings of defeat and entrapment can be reactivated by negative mood,

Table 5.2 Sample items from the Dysfunctional Attitudes Scale

I cannot find happiness without being loved by another person
People who have the marks of success/good looks/fame/wealth are bound to be happier than people who do not
I should be happy all the time
Turning to someone else for help or advice is an admission of weakness

and that, in those with a history of suicidal ideation or behaviour, depressed mood more readily reinstates hopelessness and suicidal ideation.

What it is that is activated?

We have seen that, in depression, recurrence is more likely if a person reacts to small amounts of mood change with large amounts of negative thinking. Other research on depression suggests that this is not the whole story. For sad mood not only activates certain themes, but also activates certain processes. These processes may turn out to be as, or more, pernicious than the negative themes. The most pernicious of all is rumination, and it is one of the most difficult for people to deal with because it feels as if it should be helping. Rumination, in this context, can be defined as the tendency to react to depression by trying to 'figure things out' or contemplate the 'why' of things. Susan Nolen-Hoeksema shows how such rumination makes people vulnerable to depression because, as soon as they feel a little bit sad, they do something which focuses more and more on their symptoms and on what might be causing themselves to be sad (Nolen-Hoeksema 1991). If they cannot see a cause, they continue to brood on their sadness, and to think of things that might be causing the sadness. They are effectively putting themselves through a mood induction procedure, but this time not in the relative safety of the laboratory. Sometimes they go away by themselves to try and figure things out: 'What's going wrong with me?', 'Where will this all lead?', 'Why am I like this?'. If asked, they say that this ruminative thinking will help them solve their problems, but the evidence from experiments is that just the opposite happens: problem solving is reduced when rumination takes hold.

Could it be, then, that when mood acts like a context reactivating negative themes, it also reactivates ruminative processes, that carry on without further prompting from mood? As a result of this ruminative self-focus, the person can become depressed about being depressed: they feel guilt about having no energy, or they feel bad about focusing on themselves so much, but these bad feelings simply cause them to ruminate even more, creating a vicious circle.

This may, at last, help us understand the processes by which someone can be depressed or suicidal even when the event that initially triggered feelings of humiliation or entrapment took place some months or years before. The event may have started a process, allowing suicidal ideation to become associated with low mood. Over many iterations of the mood/thinking/rumination cycle, these associations become a pattern that takes on a life of its own, able to be reactivated by even relatively small shifts in mood. An example of this sensitization comes from a study by Joiner and Rudd (2000). They found that distressed individuals who had made several previous suicide attempts showed a much weaker relationship between the severity of current suicidal ideation and the presence of negative life events than those who had only thought about suicide or harmed themselves on a single occasion, a pattern that is consistent with sensitization or kindling of suicidal ideation and behaviour.

The fact that mood is able to activate both negative themes, and a negative process is critical to understanding what occurs in a suicidal crisis. The rumination feeds on itself, adding to and exacerbating even the worst situations. Additionally, in terms of the models of suicidal behaviour with which we are familiar, rumination also affects problem solving. How does it do this?

Watkins and colleagues experimentally manipulated how much people ruminated, asking them either to ruminate for 8 min, or to fill their minds with unrelated material for 8 min (Watkins *et al.* 2000). They found an increase in overgeneral memory following rumination, and a decrease in overgeneral memories following distraction. These data suggest that if ruminative processes are reactivated, they set off increased overgeneral memory, which, as discussed, is known to impair problem solving in suicidal patients (Pollock and Williams 2001).

Clinical implications

It is common for clinicians to ask their suicidal patients about what events happened that might have precipitated the suicidal behaviour. It is not always apparent why this or that particular event was important in the causal chain, however. Our approach suggests that certain key events can be humiliating, defeating, and entrapping (or seen by the person to be such), and it is these themes, and how they may be reactivated, that need to be the focus of enquiry. But we have also noted that the effects of these events may not be immediate. The moods, thoughts, and body sensations associated with them may take time to incubate. Associations are built up not only by the constant reminders of such events that often occur, but by any downturn in mood. The differential activation model says that people differ, one from the other, in the *ease with which* small changes in mood can reactivate particular constellations of self-referent, negative thoughts, and in the *particular content* of these patterns of thinking (an overwhelming sense of needing to escape, entrapment, and no rescue).

The implication of this is that our treatments need to consider the combined effect of mood on a cognitive system that is vulnerable, and the way that it has built up a pattern of association between depressed mood, inhibition of positive mood, negative thinking, and rumination. Problem-solving approaches may not be as powerful as they might be because we have not been clear enough about how such deficits arise and are maintained. If it is true that problem solving becomes more and more difficult as rumination increases, and that this is because it increases overgeneral memory, then these processes need to be made explicit in treatment. And if hopelessness increases as the increased inhibition of positive mood reduces access to positive future events, then treatment approaches need to focus on increasing accessibility of specific future events, starting with the next 24 hours and the next week.

Patients need to know the extent to which these cognitive mechanisms (poor positive fluency and overgeneral memory) can affect their own suicide-related thinking patterns, how these may have become established over their lifetime, and how, despite their best efforts, this pattern may escalate, once it has been activated. Suicide ideation and planning may have first entered their lives as a mere co-occurring feature of depression, but are now maintained and exacerbated. Why? Because the capacity to switch them off has diminished. There are too few positive future scenarios which would naturally stop the suicidal rumination in its tracks. There are too few specific memories of past coping behaviour to help generate alternative solutions to current problems. Suicidal ideation gets rapidly out of control because there is nothing to stop it doing so.

Our treatments will not have sufficient power to reduce suicide urges unless they enable the person to see how best they can deal with these patterns of cognitive reactivity, allowing moods to come and go without bringing about such catastrophic changes in both the cognitive themes and in the cognitive processes. Our research is therefore examining how a mindfulness-based cognitive therapy (MBCT) approach may help. MBCT was developed to address the issue of recurrence and relapse in chronic and recurrent depression. It is based on the observation referred to earlier, that once a person has recovered from an episode of depression, a relatively small amount of negative mood can trigger a large number of negative thoughts (e.g. 'I am a failure', 'I am weak', 'I am worthless') together with bodily sensations (e.g. weakness or fatigue or unexplained pain). Both the negative thoughts and the fatigue often seem out of proportion to the situation. Patients who believed they had recovered may find themselves feeling 'back to square one', and end up inside the types of rumination loops described earlier.

Based on Jon Kabat-Zinn's Stress Reduction program at the University of Massachusetts Medical Center (Kabat-Zinn 1991), MBCT includes simple breathing meditations and yoga stretches to help participants become more aware of the present moment, including getting in touch with moment-to-moment changes in the mind and the body. In eight weekly classes (the atmosphere is that of a class, rather than a therapy group), and by listening to tapes at home during the week, class participants learn the practice of mindfulness meditation. MBCT also includes basic education about depression, and several exercises from cognitive therapy that show the links between thinking and feeling, and how participants can best look after themselves when depression threatens to overwhelm them.

Mindfulness-based cognitive therapy helps participants in the classes to see more clearly the patterns of the mind; and to learn how recognize when their mood is beginning to go down. It helps break the link between negative mood and the negative thinking that it would normally have triggered. Participants develop the capacity to allow distressing mood, thoughts, and sensations to come and go, without having to battle with them. They find that they can stay in touch with the present moment, without having to ruminate about the past, or worry about the future.

Preliminary evidence that mindfulness may have an important role to play in helping people with suicidal behaviour can be found, both in its use to treat borderline personality disorder patients who are chronically suicidal (Linehan *et al.* 1993; Williams and Swales 2005), and in the evidence that mindfulness-based cognitive therapy reduces overgenerality in memory (Williams *et al.* 2000). MBCT has been found to reduce relapse and recurrence in major depression (Teasdale *et al.* 2000; Segal *et al.* 2002; Ma and Teasdale 2004). The next stage in research is to examine whether it can also help people to recognize their patterns of suicidal reactivity earlier, and deal with them in a skilful way that does not simply exacerbate them.

References

Brown, G.W., Harris, T.O., and Hepworth, C. (1995). Loss, humiliation and entrapment among women developing depression: A patient and non-patient comparison. *Psychological Medicine*, 25, 7–21.

Conway, M.A. and Pleydell-Pearce, C.W. (2000). The construction of autobiographical memories in the self-memory system. *Psychological Review*, 107, 261–88.

Drake, R.E. and Cotton, P.G. (1986). Depression, hopelessness and suicide in chronic schizophrenia. *British Journal of Psychiatry*, 148, 554–9.

Evans, J., Williams, J.M.G., O'Loughlin, S., and Howells, K. (1992). Autobiographical memory and problem-solving strategies of parasuicide patients. *Psychological Medicine*, 22, 399–405.

Gilbert, P. and Allan, S. (1998). The role of defeat and entrapment (arrested flight) in depression: an exploration of an evolutionary view. *Psychological Medicine*, 28, 585–98.

Godden, D.R. and Baddeley, A.D. (1975). Context-dependent memory in two natural environments. *British Journal of Psychology*, 66, 325–31.

Goldstein, R.C. and Willner, P. (2002). Self-report measures of defeat and entrapment during a brief depressive mood induction. *Cognition and Emotion*, 16, 629–42.

Henderson, D., Hargreaves, I., Gregory, S., and Williams, J.M.G. (2002). Autobiographical memory and emotion in a non-clinical sample of women with and without a reported history of childhood sexual abuse. *British Journal of Clinical Psychology*, 41, 129–141.

Hutchings, J., Nash, S., Williams, J.M.G., and Nightingale, D. (1998). Parental autobiographical memory: Is this a helpful clinical measure in behavioural child management? *British Journal of Clinical Psychology*, 37, 303–12.

Iqbal, Z., Birchwood, M., Chadwick, P., and Trower, P. (2000). Cognitive approach to depression and suicidal thinking in psychosis. 2. Testing the validity of a social ranking model. *British Journal of Psychiatry*, 177, 522–8.

Joiner, T.E. and Rudd, M.D. (2000). Intensity and duration of suicidal crises vary as a function of previous suicide attempts and negative life events. *Journal of Consulting and Clinical Psychology*, 68, 909–16.

Kabat-Zinn, J. (1991) *Full catastrophe living*. Dell Publishing, New York.

Kessler, R.C., Borges, G., and Walters, E.E. (1999). Prevalence of and risk factors for lifetime suicide attempts in the national comorbidity survey. *Archives of General Psychiatry*, 56, 617–26.

Linehan, M.M., Heard, H.L., and Armstrong, H.E. (1993). Naturalistic follow-up of a behavioral treatment for chronically parasuicidal borderline patients. *Archives of General Psychiatry*, 50, 971–4.

Ma, S.H. and Teasdale, J.D. (2004). Mindfulness-based cognitive therapy for depression: Replication and exploration of differential relapse prevention effects. *Journal of Consulting and Clinical Psychology*, 72, 31–40.

MacLeod, A.K., Rose, G.S., and Williams, J.M.G. (1993). Components of hopelessness about the future in parasuicide. *Cognitive Therapy and Research*, 17, 441–55.

MacLeod, A.K., Pankhania, B., Lee, M., and Mitchell, D. (1997a). Parasuicide, depression and the anticipation of positive and negative future experiences. *Psychological Medicine*, 27, 973–7.

MacLeod, A.K., Tata, P., Kentish, J., and Jacobson, H. (1997b). Retrospective and prospective cognitions in anxiety and depression. *Cognition and Emotion*, 11, 467–79.

Malone, K.M., Oquendo, M.A., Haas, G.L., Ellis, S.P., Li, S.H., and Mann, J.J. (2000). Protective factors against suicidal acts in major depression: Reasons for living. *American Journal of Psychiatry*, 157, 1084–8.

Mann, J.J., Waternaux, C., Haas, G.L., and Malone, K.M. (1999). Toward a clinical model of suicidal behavior in psychiatric patients. *American Journal of Psychiatry*, 156, 181–9.

Nolen-Hoeksema, S. (1991). Responses to depression and their effects on the duration of depressive episodes. *Journal of Abnormal Psychology*, 100, 569–82.

O'Connor, R.C. (2003). Suicidal behaviour as a cry of pain: Test of a psychological model. *Archives of Suicide Research*, 7, 1–12.

O'Connor, R.C., Connery, H., and Cheyne, W. M. (2000). Hopelessness: the role of depression, future directed thinking and cognitive vulnerability. *Psychology, Health and Medicine*, 5, 155–61.

Pollock, L.R. and Williams, J.M.G. (2001). Effective problem solving in suicide attempters depends on specific autobiographical recall. *Suicide and Life-Threatening Behavior*, 31, 386–96.

Pollock, L.R. and Williams, J.M.G. (2004). Problem solving in suicide attempters. *Psychological Medicine*, 34, 163–7.

Post, R.M. (1992). Transduction of psychosocial stress into the neurobiology of recurrent affective-disorder. *American Journal of Psychiatry*, 149, 999–1010.

Schotte, D.E., Cools, J., and Payvar, S. (1990). Problem-solving deficits in suicidal patients—trait vulnerability or state phenomenon. *Journal of Consulting and Clinical Psychology*, 58, 562–4.

Segal, Z.V., Williams, J.M., Teasdale, J.D., and Gemar, M. (1996). A cognitive science perspective on kindling and episode sensitization in recurrent affective disorder. *Psychological Medicine*, 26, 371–80.

Segal, Z.V., Gemar, M., and Williams, S. (1999). Differential cognitive response to a mood challenge following successful cognitive therapy or pharmacotherapy for unipolar depression. *Journal of Abnormal Psychology*, 108, 3–10.

Segal, Z.V., Teasdale, J.D., Williams, J.M., and Gemar, M.C. (2002). The mindfulness-based cognitive therapy adherence scale: Inter-rater reliability, adherence to protocol and treatment distinctiveness. *Clinical Psychology and Psychotherapy*, 9, 131–8.

Sidley, G.L., Calam, R., Wells, A., Hughes, T., and Whitaker, K. (1999). The prediction of parasuicide repetition in a high-risk group. *British Journal of Clinical Psychology*, 38, 375–86.

Teasdale, J.D., Segal, Z.V., Williams, J.M.G., Ridgeway, V.A., Soulsby, J.M., and Lau, M.A. (2000). Prevention of relapse/recurrence in major depression by mindfulness-based cognitive therapy. *Journal of Consulting and Clinical Psychology*, 68, 615–23.

Van der Does, A.J.W. (2002). Cognitive vulnerability to depression: Validity of a new measure. *Journal of Affective Disorders*, 68, 137–8.

Watkins, E., Teasdale, J.D., and Williams, R.M. (2000). Decentring and distraction reduce overgeneral autobiographical memory in depression. *Psychological Medicine*, 30, 911–20.

Williams, J.M.G. (2001). *Suicide and attempted suicide.* Penguin, London.

Williams, J.M.G. and Broadbent, K. (1986). Autobiographical memory in suicide attempters. *Journal of Abnormal Psychology*, 95, 144–9.

Williams, J.M.G. and Swales, M. (2005). The use of mindfulness-based approaches for suicidal patients. *Archives of Suicide Research*, 8, 315–30.

Williams, J.M.G. and Van der Does, A.J.W., Barnhofer, T., Crane, C., and Segal, Z. S. (2005). Cognitive reactivity, suicidal ideation and future fluency: investigating a differential activation theory of suicidality, submitted.

Williams, J.M.G., Segal, Z.V., Teasdale, J.D., and Soulsby, J. (2000). Mindfulness-based cognitive therapy reduces overgeneral autobiographical memory in formerly depressed patients. *Journal of Abnormal Psychology*, 109, 150–5.

Yen, S., Shea, M.T., Pagano, M., Sanislow, C.A., Grilo, C.M., McGlashan, T.H. *et al.* (2003). Axis I and axis II disorders as predictors of prospective suicide attempts: Findings from the collaborative longitudinal personality disorders study. *Journal of Abnormal Psychology*, 112, 375–81.

Young, M.A., Fogg, L.F., Scheftner, W., Fawcett, J., Akiskal, H., and Maser, J. (1996). Stable trait components of hopelessness: Baseline and sensitivity to depression. *Journal of Abnormal Psychology*, 105, 155–65.

6

Psychobiological approaches to the predisposition to suicidal behaviour: implications for treatment and prevention

Kees van Heeringen

Introduction

Suicidal behaviour is strongly associated with psychiatric disorders. Over 90% of suicide completers and suicide attempters suffer from a diagnosable psychiatric illness (Beautrais *et al.* 1996; Cavanagh *et al.* 2003), and an increased risk of suicide is present in virtually all psychiatric disorders (Harris and Barraclough 1997), but particularly in mood disorders, alcohol dependence and schizophrenia. Personality disorders, including borderline and antisocial personality disorders, are also associated with an increased risk of non-fatal and fatal suicidal behaviour (Linehan *et al.* 2000). Attempted suicide patients with co-morbid axis I and axis II disorders show a higher rate of repetition suicide attempts, and may have a greater suicide risk than those without such a co-morbidity (Hawton *et al.* 2003).

Psychiatric diagnosis thus constitutes an important part of the assessment of the risk of suicidal behaviour in the individual patient. However, lack of specificity in terms of symptoms (e.g. suicidal ideation) and outcome (e.g. suicide) is a major drawback associated with the assignment of psychiatric diagnoses using diagnostic criteria such as those provided in the DSM classification system. Even in groups of psychiatric patients with the highest risk, such as discharged hospital populations, most patients never show suicidal behaviour. The inclusion of psychosocial characteristics, such as marital and employment status, financial situation, and social integration, may increase the accuracy of risk assessment, but these characteristics are similarly non-specific with regard to their association with suicidal behaviour.

It thus follows that the accuracy of assessing the risk of suicidal behaviour would increase substantially through the identification of characteristics that determine the specific suicidal reaction to particular circumstances. Evidence is accumulating that suicidal behaviour is indeed associated with a predisposition or diathesis; that is, a constitutional make-up that makes a person react in specific ways to extrinsic stimuli, thereby tending to make them more susceptible than normal to certain disorders (Mann 2003). From a psychiatric point of view several features have been suggested to be part of this diathesis, including aggression/impulsivity and pessimism (Mann 2003), and anxiety and hopelessness (Van Heeringen 2001).

In addition to the importance of identifying this diathesis for risk assessment, it may well be of crucial importance for risk reduction, including the risk of repetition following non-fatal suicidal behaviour. While there is no doubt about the strongly increased risk of repeated suicide attempts and completed suicide following deliberate self-harm, it is currently not clear how the risk of repetition can be diminished by treatment (Hawton *et al.* 1998). The description of the diathesis for suicidal behaviour in terms of targets for psychological and/or biological treatment may thus contribute to its prevention.

This chapter will describe a psychobiological approach to the study and treatment of the predisposition to suicidal behaviour. First, relevant findings from cognitive psychological and neuropsychological studies of suicidal behaviour, which follow logically from the previous chapter, will be reviewed. Secondly, recent insights in the neurobiology of suicidal behaviour will be addressed. The third part of this chapter will then describe the association between biological and psychological characteristics, following which implications for treatment and prevention will be discussed.

Cognitive psychological and neuropsychological aspects of the predisposition to suicidal behaviour

Knowledge about the state of mind of suicidal individuals remains limited. Although thoughts and attitudes around the time of a suicidal act may predict future suicidal behaviour (Beck *et al.* 1999), relatively little is known about the most basic aspects of cognitive processing in suicidal individuals. However, impaired cognitive functioning in psychiatric disorders for which suicide risk is elevated is now well documented (Mann *et al.* 1999), and insight into the cognitive characteristics of suicidal individuals is increasing (Williams and Pollock 2001; see also Chapter 5 of this book). It has thus become clear that three characteristics differentiate depressed individuals who are suicidal from depressed people who are not. These characteristics include:

(1) a sensitivity to particular life events reflecting signals of defeat, leading to involuntary hypersensitivity to stimuli signaling 'loser' status;

(2) 'no escape': the sense of being trapped, which is related to an insufficient capacity to solve problems, which arise from the confrontation with stimuli as described above;

(3) 'no rescue': the absence of rescue factors, mediated by deficient prospective cognitive processes and leading to feelings of hopelessness.

Although the involvement of these cognitive characteristics in the development of suicidal behaviour has been shown consistently, little is known about their neural basis (Van Heeringen and Marušič 2003).

The sensitivity to particular life events

With regard to the sensitivity to particular life events, early studies focused on the hypothesis that a generalized cognitive rigidity mediates the relationship between stressful life events and suicidal behaviour. However, more recent findings are consistent with the suggestion that, among depressed people, those who attempt suicide differ from those who do not on some, but not all, neuropsychological tests (King *et al.* 2000). Using a modified Stroop task, Becker *et al.* (1999) found that the level of suicidal ideation in depressed individuals correlates particularly with biases in selective attention. Another study could not demonstrate any difference in attention measures between suicide attempters and non-attempters in a group of depressed people (Keilp *et al.* 2001). Although clearly much more research is needed, these findings suggest a role of attentional biases in the development of suicidal ideation, but not suicidal behaviour, in people with depression.

Escape and problem solving

Williams and Pollock (2001) have argued convincingly with regard to the second characteristic, that the sense of being trapped is associated with trait-dependent deficiencies in problem-solving skills, which, in turn, appear to depend upon deficiencies in autobiographical memory (see also Chapter 5 of this book). Several studies have shown an association between attempted suicide and overgeneral autobiographical memory (Evans *et al.* 1992; Sidley *et al.* 1997). These studies indicate that overgeneral autobiographical recall (probably mediated by the frontal lobes of the brain) affects the occurrence of suicidal behaviour by its effects on the ability to recall specific memories among people who attempt suicide, which correlates positively with the effectiveness of the solutions suggested for solving hypothetical (social or interpersonal) problems.

Rescue and prospective cognition

With regard to the third cognitive psychological characteristic, the relatively new research approach addressing prospective cognition may well be useful. One study (Audenaert *et al.* 2002), but not another (McLeod *et al.* 1993), found differences between people who attempted suicide and a non-depressed control group, using a neutral fluency task. By using a modified fluency test, it was demonstrated recently that participants who had attempted suicide were less fluent in coming up with positive events that might happen in the future (Williams and Pollock 2001). Moreover, hopelessness, which is a core psycho-pathological characteristic in association with suicidal behaviour, was found to correlate significantly with the lack of generating future positive events and not with an excessive anticipation of negative things in the future.

It thus appears that the three core cognitive psychological characteristics of suicidal ideation and behaviour are associated with biases in neuropsychological functioning in terms of attention, memory, and fluency, respectively.

The neurobiology of the predisposition to suicidal behaviour

The involvement of at least three neurobiological systems in suicidal behaviour has been documented using a vast number of divergent research approaches. These include the serotonergic system, the noradrenergic system and the hypothalamic–pituitary–adrenal (HPA) axis. With regard to the dopaminergic system, there are too few studies to determine whether it is involved in suicidal behaviour (Mann 2003).

The role of serotonin in the predisposition to suicidal behaviour

Following the first report of the involvement of the serotonergic system in suicidal behaviour (Åsberg *et al.* 1976), the association between serotonergic dysfunction and suicidal behaviour has been studied and confirmed using a vast array of research approaches. The main findings from post-mortem, cerebrospinal fluid (CSF), challenge, and functional neuroimaging studies will be reviewed shortly here (for detailed overviews, including references, see Mann 2003; Van Heeringen 2003). *Post-mortem* studies have shown: (1) fewer presynaptic serotonin (5-HT) transporter sites in the (ventromedial) prefrontal cortex, hypothalamus, occipital cortex, and brainstem; and (2) an upregulation of postsynaptic 5-HT_{1a} and 5-HT_{2a} receptors in the prefrontal cortex of suicide victims. Post-mortem studies have also demonstrated relatively low concentrations of serotonin and 5-HIAA (5-hydroxyindoleacetic acid, the main metabolite of 5-HT) in the brainstem of suicide victims. Comparatively low concentrations of 5-HIAA have been found in the *cerebrospinal fluid* (CSF) of suicide attempters suffering from major depression, schizophrenia, and personality disorders, as compared to persons with the same diagnoses but no history of attempted suicide. CSF 5-HIAA concentrations correlate with the lethality of the suicide attempts, and low CSF 5-HIAA has been shown to predict future suicide attempts and completed suicide. Suicide attempters with major depression or a personality disorder have shown a blunted response to *challenge* of the serotonergic system by means of the 5-HT agonist fenfluramine. Again, the lethality of the suicide attempt correlated with the level of reduced response to this pharmacological stimulation.

Functional neuroimaging using positron emission tomography (PET) and fenfluramine challenge, measuring brain glucose utilization in high-lethality versus low-lethality suicide attempters, has shown relative hypometabolism in the ventral, medial, and lateral prefrontal cortex in high-lethality attempters compared with low-lethality attempters, the difference becoming more marked after fenfluramine administration (Oquendo *et al.* 2003). While controlling for age, lethality of the attempt appeared to be inversely correlated with metabolism in the ventromedial prefrontal cortex after fenfluramine challenge.

Using SPECT (single photon emission computed tomography) and the highly selective $[^{123}I]5$-I-R91150 radioligand, it could be demonstrated that the binding potential of 5-HT$_{2a}$ receptors in the (particularly dorsolateral) prefrontal cortex of attempted suicides was significantly lower than that of healthy controls (Audenaert *et al.* 2001). The decrease in binding potential was significantly less marked in patients who took overdoses than in those using more violent methods to attempt suicide.

The 5-HT$_2$ receptor was also studied by Meyer and colleagues (1999), with the $[^{18}F]$setoperone radioligand and PET. In short, they demonstrated that there was no significant difference in 5-HT$_2$ receptor binding between depressed patients without a history of suicidal behaviour in the past 5 years and healthy controls. A more recent PET study using the same ligand in a sample of depressed patients, without specification of the presence or absence of a history of suicidal behaviour, showed a significantly decreased 5-HT$_2$ receptor binding potential in depressed patients when compared to healthy controls (Yatham *et al.* 2000).

Noradrenaline and suicidal behaviour

A number of studies have indicated the involvement of a dysfunctional noradrenergic system in the development of suicidal behaviour, but, unlike the serotonin system, it is not clear to what extent this dysfunction relates to a trait-dependent predisposition.

Post-mortem studies of the noradrenergic system have revealed fewer noradrenergic neurons in the locus coeruleus of suicide victims, increased brainstem levels of tyrosine hydroxylase, and lower levels of postsynaptic adrenergic receptors in the cortex. A possible explanation for these findings is that they are associated with an increased stress response before suicide, resulting in an excessive release of noradrenaline, a secondary upregulation of tyrosine hydroxylase biosynthetic activity, and a downregulation of postsynaptic adrenergic receptors in the cortex (Mann 2002). In general, these findings, together with those from other studies, including challenging with the α_2-adrenergic agonist clonidine, suggest a state-dependent anxiety/agitation-related condition in which increased noradrenaline release leads to transmitter depletion.

Suicidal behaviour and the HPA axis

Most, but not all, studies indicate increased activity of the HPA axis in association with suicidal ideation and/or behaviour. Increased urinary cortisol secretion (Van Heeringen et al. 2000) has been demonstrated in attempted suicide patients, while elevated CSF levels of corticotrophin-releasing hormone (CRH; Arato et al. 1989) and reduced post-mortem CRH binding sites were found in suicide completers. Non-suppression of plasma cortisol levels after administration of dexamethasone was associated with a 14-fold increase in the likelihood of suicide during 15 years of follow-up (Coryell and Schlesser 2001).

The psychobiology of the predisposition to suicidal behaviour

While the cognitive psychological, neuropsychological, and neurobiological studies, as reviewed above, have contributed substantially to our insights into the predisposition to suicidal behaviour, much more can be learned from the study of the correlations between findings in these different research domains. This section will describe many examples of such correlations, using the three cognitive psychological characteristics of the predisposition to suicidal behaviour as a starting point.

The psychobiology of sensitivity to particular life events

As discussed above, sensitivity to certain life events as a predisposition to suicidal behaviour may be particularly involved in the development of suicidal ideation following exposure to psychosocial adversity. Research has indeed shown that social, and particularly interpersonal, stressors commonly precipitate suicidal behaviour From a personality-based point of view, temperamental dimensions such as 'reward dependence' (Cloninger 1994) or 'stability' (Engström *et al.* 1996) mediate sensitivity to interpersonal events. Attempted suicide patients show lower scores on reward dependence (i.e. the bias in reacting to actual rewards and thereafter in maintaining behaviour previously associated with rewards) than psychiatric controls without a history of suicidal behaviour. Lower scores on reward dependence reflect emotional distance or aloofness. These scores correlate negatively with urinary cortisol secretion, the latter reflecting HPA-axis activity (Van Heeringen *et al.* 2000). It thus appears that this component of the predisposition comprises an interrelated trait-dependent interpersonal sensitivity and activation of the HPA axis, possibly mediated by attentional biases.

It has been suggested that the frontotemporal 5-HT_{1a} system (in conjunction with the hippocampus) is involved in resilience in the face of psychosocial stressors (Deakin 1996). The recent finding of a significant correlation between reward dependence scores and regional cerebral blood flow, particularly in the parahippocampal, temporal, and frontal cortices (Sugiori *et al.* 2000), is noteworthy in this regard. It thus appears that these regions are indeed involved in this component of the predisposition to suicidal behaviour.

The possibly interrelated roles of noradrenaline and attentional biases within this psychobiological constellation clearly need further investigation. However, in this respect it is important to point at the suggested modulatory role of noradrenaline in attentional processes (see, for example, Kodama *et al.* 2002) and reward dependence (Cloninger *et al.* 1993).

There are several additional issues related to this component of the predisposition to suicidality, which are worth noting because of their potential relevance for the development, treatment, and further study of suicidal behaviour. A role of the neuropeptides oxytocin and vasopressin has been suggested in the modulation of reward dependence (Cloninger 1994) and in the attenuation of psychosocial stress (see, for example, Carter 1998). It was shown recently that social support and (intra-nasally administered) oxytocin interact to suppress cortisol and subjective responses to psychosocial stress (Heinrichs *et al.* 2003). One study (Inder *et al.* 1997), but not another (Brunner *et al.* 2002), found increased plasma and/or CSF levels of arginine vasopressin (AVP) in depressed suicide attempters, while both studies demonstrated a correlation between AVP and cortisol concentrations. Further study is needed to explore whether the demonstrated association between comparatively low scores on reward dependence among attempted suicide patients, which may become manifest as aloofness, and increased cortisol secretion (see above) is mediated by a lack of social support, increased levels of AVP, and decreased levels of oxytocin. This may well have consequences for treatment, as the administration of oxytocin may attenuate the impact of psychosocial stress, and thus prevent the increase in production of cortisol. Later in this chapter it will be shown that such a reduction of cortisol secretion may well be important in the prevention of the development of feelings of hopelessness.

The psychobiology of 'no escape'

From neuropsychological and psychobiological points of view, little is known about the mechanisms that may be involved. Keilp and colleages (2001) studied memory functions in depressed suicide attempters, and found that high-lethality attempters performed worse on memory tasks than both depressed non-attempters and low-lethality attempters.

As described above, autobiographical memory characteristics are thought to play a crucial role in the development of this component of the diathesis. The definition of a diathesis or predisposition in terms of memory (and learning) is a major characteristic of Cloninger's psychobiological model of personality (Cloninger et al. 1993). This model is based on the constructs of temperament and character that are involved in perceptual processes and the development of concepts, respectively. During the process of determining the significance and salience of perceived stressors, human beings convert sensory inputs (i.e. percepts) into abstract symbols (i.e. concepts). Stimulus–response characteristics thus depend on the conceptual significance and salience of perceived stimuli.

The involved perceptual and conceptual memory systems correspond to procedural and declarative memory systems, respectively. The *procedural memory* system is involved in perceptual learning and the learning of new habits and skills. Temperament can thus be defined in terms of individual differences in associative learning in response to, for example, reward or danger, reflecting the temperamental dimensions reward dependence (see above) and harm avoidance (see below). While genetic influences on the development of temperamental characteristics are increasingly identified, additional influences most probably occur during infancy. Animal studies have clearly shown that stress early in life, by separation of the infant from its mother, produces a reaction in the infant that is stored primarily by the procedural memory system. This is the only well-differentiated memory system that the infant has early in its life, but this action of the procedural memory system leads to a cycle of changes that ultimately damages the hippocampus and thereby results in a persistent change in declarative memories (Kandel 1999).

The *declarative memory* system may well be involved in the predisposition to suicidal behaviour because of its role in autobiographical memory and in the development of self-concepts via insight learning. The (medial) temporal lobe and the hippocampus are involved in one component of the declarative memory system, namely episodic or autobiographical memory. In addition to these structures, the prefrontal cortex is also involved in the storage of declarative memory through its role in working memory (a short-term component of autobiographical memory). In particular, the dorsolateral area of the prefrontal cortex mediates the generation of multiple response alternatives, which are needed in order to prevent the development of a perception that there is 'no escape' from psychosocial adversity. Declarative memory systems may thus serve to modify the unconscious automatic responses to stimuli as determined by temperamental characteristics, by using information that is stored in the autobiographical memory system. It is now clear that glutamate and gamma-aminobutyric acid (GABA) are involved in the development of declarative memory (Nutt 2000), which is a crucial aspect of psychotherapeutic strategies aimed at gaining mastery over temperament-driven behaviour (Gabbard 2000).

The psychobiology of 'no rescue'

As described above, fluency tasks have demonstrated that the tendency to perceive no rescue following exposure to psychosocial adversity reflects a deficient capacity for generating positive future events. In addition, fluency in generating positive events was found to correlate with levels of hopelessness, that is the less fluent patients were in generating positive events, the higher were their levels of hopelessness. A recent comparative functional neuroimaging study by our group used a fluency paradigm and showed blunted activation in the dorsolateral prefrontal cortex in patients who had recently attempted suicide (Audenaert *et al.* 2002). Using PET, Oquendo *et al.* (2003) demonstrated that higher verbal fluency correlates positively with regional cortical glucose metabolism in the prefrontal cortex. Using SPECT, we were able to demonstrate a (negative) correlation between (mainly dorsolateral) prefrontal binding to 5-HT$_{2a}$ receptors in the brains of attempted suicide patients, on the one hand, and their levels of hopelessness and harm avoidance (i.e. behavioural inhibition, characterized by uncertainty and worrying about the future) on the other (Van Heeringen *et al.* 2003). Meyer *et al.* (2003) subsequently demonstrated that there is serotonergic modulation of dysfunctional attitudes about the future in self-harm patients.

It thus appears that the third psychobiological component of the predisposition to suicidal behaviour is associated with a decreased serotonergic functioning in the prefrontal cortex, which may become manifest as increased levels of hopelessness and behavioural inhibition following exposure to adverse circumstances. Based on these findings, it can be hypothesized that increased behavioural inhibition (i.e. anxiety-based avoidance) is the primary mechanism involved, which may lead to suicidal behaviour only in the presence of a (dopamine-driven?) force that is strong enough to break through this inhibition and which may manifest itself as hostility, anger, or aggression. This may explain the association between serotonergic dysfunction and impulsivity or dysregulation of aggression, as found in combined psychological autopsy–post-mortem brain tissue studies of individuals who died by suicide (Mann *et al.* 1999). Serotonin acts in an antagonistic way to dopamine, so that a depletion of the serotonergic system may, indeed, disinhibit aggressive behaviour.

Implications for treatment and prevention

There is thus increasing evidence that the predisposition to suicidal behaviour comprises three components that can be described in cognitive psychological, neuropsychological, neuroanatomical, and neurobiological terms. The converging nature of findings in these divergent research domains allows for the description of a hypothetical psychobiological model of the predisposition to suicidal behaviour.

The first component (attention-related perceptual biases related to the sensitivity to particular life events) appears to be mediated by the frontotemporal cortex (in conjunction with the hippocampus) and modulated by the 5-HT_{1a} and noradrenergic neurotransmission systems. Sensitivity to life events is associated with hyper-reactivity of the neurobiological stress system, resulting in increased production of cortisol.

The neurobiological aspects of the second component of the predisposition (reduced problem-solving capacity related to deficient autobiographical memory) are less clear, but research outside the suicidological domain suggests involvement of the frontal cortex and the glutamate and GABA-ergic systems.

The third component (perceived 'no rescue' following exposure to particular life events due to a reduced fluency in generating positive future events) appears to be related to dysfunctioning of the 5-HT_{2a} system in the (dorsolateral) prefrontal cortex in conjunction with the amygdala, resulting in increased behavioural inhibition and hopelessness.

The dissection of the predisposition to suicidal behaviour into these components is, at least in part, supported by studies of the neurobiological modulation of involved neuropsychological dysfunctions. For instance, drugs that influence 5-HT_{1a} function (such as buspirone) selectively affect performance on neuropsychological tests of memory and learning without affecting executive functions (mediated by the dorsolateral prefrontal cortex), while the reverse appears to be the case for drugs that influence the 5-HT_{2a} system (Deakin 1996). Animal studies have shown that a balance between (hippocampal) 5-HT_{1a} and (cortical) 5-HT_{2a} functioning is essential for an adequate response to social stress (McKittrick et al. 1995).

Although the proposed psychobiological model of the predisposition to suicidal behaviour is thus to be regarded as largely hypothetical, it can be used to guide clinicians in their difficult task of predicting and treating suicidal behaviour. With regard to the prediction of suicidal behaviour, it follows from the model that the assessment of suicide risk among depressed patients should include the assessment of interpersonal sensitivity, problem-solving capacities, and hopelessness, respectively. Further research is clearly needed to determine whether neuropsychological measurement of attention, working memory, and fluency can be used to assess suicide risk among depressed individuals. The few available studies on the subject indicate that personality assessment using, for example, the Temperament and Character Inventory (Cloninger et al. 1993), particularly with regard to the reward dependence and harm avoidance temperament dimensions, can be useful in view of their involvement in the first and third components of the predisposition model.

The psychobiological model of the predisposition to suicidal behaviour suggests that in order for treatment to be effective, its three components have to be addressed. Williams and Pollock (2001) have formulated cognitive psychological strategies for the treatment of each of the components. In short, these strategies include, first, teaching patients to understand their attentional processes by helping them to identify when their hypersensitivity to stimuli signalling 'loser' status may be occurring. Secondly, the therapist should help patients to identify the reasons why, and the moments when, they may be having difficulties in generating alternative solutions to problems. This means that patients are encouraged to practise detailed recollection of past events. Such a rehearsal practice is also part of dialectical behaviour therapy, and serves to decrease generalization of autobiographical memories. In view of the beneficial effect of mindfulness-based cognitive therapy on overgeneral autobiographical memory, its application in the treatment of the predisposition to suicidal behaviour should also be considered. The cognitive psychological approach to the treatment of the third component of the predisposition aims to encourage patients to practise generating positive (rescue) events (focusing on the next few days, rather than being drawn into discussing the next few years).

Psychobiological theory (Cloninger *et al.* 1993) states that in order to achieve permanent changes in trait-dependent predisposition characteristics, psychotherapeutic approaches may benefit from adjunctive psychopharmacological treatment. While recent studies have provided evidence for a beneficial effect in the treatment of depression, it is currently unclear whether such a combined approach indeed increases the efficacy of treatment in terms of preventing (repetition of) suicidal behaviour. It is also unclear whether psychotherapy and drug treatment should be simultaneously provided, or whether drug therapy should precede psychotherapy. The latter approach might be useful in view of the fact that functional neuroimaging studies of depressed and suicidal individuals commonly show markedly decreased activity in the areas of the brain that are involved in learning. Such observations suggest that drug treatment should precede psychotherapeutic approaches in order to be effective.

The neurotransmission systems involved in the modulation of the components of the predisposition to suicidal behaviour, as described above, may provide guidelines with regard to the choice of appropriate pharmacological facilitation of the cognitive psychological treatment of these components. The involvement of the serotonergic system suggests that drugs targeting this system, such as SSRI antidepressants, lithium, and atypical antipsychotic drugs, may be particularly effective. Results of the few studies that have been carried out provide support for choosing serotonergic drugs (Malone and Moran 2001).

Drug treatment may thus be useful through its facilitating effect on psychotherapy, but recent findings indicate that such treatment may even be necessary. More particularly, it has been shown recently that cortisol has a detrimental effect on working memory (involved in the second component of the predisposition; Lupien *et al.* 1999) and on the recall of pleasant words, and not negative or neutral words (involved in the third component; Tops *et al.* 2004). It is therefore hypothesized that cortisol enhances behavioural inhibition (Tops *et al.* 2004), and thus, in view of the demonstrated association between behavioural inhibition and hopelessness (Van Heeringen *et al.* 2003), levels of hopelessness. These findings suggest that our relative inability to prevent (repetition of) suicidal behaviour may be due to detrimental effects of increased cortisol production (related to the first component of the predisposition) on the neuropsychological functions involved in the second and, particularly, the third component. In order for cognitive psychological treatment of the second and third components to be successful, it may thus well be necessary to counteract the increased production of cortisol.

In conclusion, psychobiological theory states that stable behavioural change requires that conceptual insights modify habits by disciplined practice, perhaps facilitated by pharmacotherapy (Cloninger *et al.* 1993). This chapter has described, first, how cognitive psychotherapeutic practice can target the characteristics associated with the predisposition to suicidal behaviour. Secondly, currently available information on the neurobiological underpinnings of this predisposition was reviewed. In addition, it has been shown that there is increasing evidence of an association between biological and cognitive psychological characteristics of the predisposition, thus allowing for the description of a psychobiological model. In view of the magnitude of the problem of (repeated) self-harm, the current lack of knowledge about efficacious treatment, and the potential effect of pharmacotherapy on the outcome, there is an urgent need for research into the effects of combined treatment approaches. It is suggested that adding pharmacotherapy to cognitive psychotherapy may not only have a facilitating effect, but that it may even be necessary in order to prevent suicidal behaviour.

References

Arato, M., Banki, C.M., Bissette, G., Nemeroff CB (1989). Elevated CSF CRF in suicide victims. *Biological Psychiatry*, 25, 355–9.

Åsberg, M., Träskman, L., and Thoren, P. (1976). 5-HIAA in the cerebrospinal fluid. A biochemical suicide predictor? *Archives of General Psychiatry*, 33, 1193–7.

Audenaert, K., Van Laere, K., Dumont, F., Slegers, G., Mertens, J., Van Heeringen, C., *et al.* (2001). Decreased frontal serotonin 5-HT2a receptor binding index in deliberate self harm patients. *European Journal of Nuclear Medicine*, 28, 175–82.

Audenaert, K., Goethals, I., Van Laere, K., Lahorte, P., Brans, B., Versijpt, J., *et al.* (2002). SPECT neuropsychological activation procedure with the Verbal Fluency Test in attempted suicide patients. *Nuclear Medicine Communications*, 23, 907–16.

Beautrais, A.L., Joyce, P.R., Mulder, R.T., Fergusson, D.M., Deavoll, B.J., and Nightingale, S.K. (1996). Prevalence and comorbidity of mental disorders in persons making serious suicide attempts: a case-control study. *American Journal of Psychiatry*, 153, 1009–14.

Beck, A.T., Brown, G.K., Steer, R.A., Dahlsgaard, K.K., and Grisham, J.R. (1999). Suicide ideation at its worst point: A predictor of eventual suicide in psychiatric outpatients. *Suicide and Life-Threatening Behavior*, 29, 1–9.

Becker, E.S., Strohbach, D., and Rinck, M. (1999). A specific attentional bias in suicide attempters. *Journal of Nervous and Mental Disease*, 18, 730–5.

Brunner, J., Keck, M.E., Landgraf, R., Uhr, M., Nahmendorf, C., and Bronisch, T. (2002). Vasopressin in CSF and plasma in depressed suicide attempters: preliminary results. *European Neuropsychopharmacology*, 12, 489–94.

Carter, C.S. (1998). Neuroendocrine perspectives on social attachment and love. *Psychoneuroendocrinology*, 23, 779–818.

Cavanagh, J.T.O., Carson, K.J., Sharpe, M., and Lawrie, S.M. (2003). Psychological autopsy studies of suicide: systematic review. *Psychological Medicine*, 33, 395–404.

Cloninger, C.R. (1994). Temperament and personality. *Current Opinions in Neurobiology*, 4, 266–73.

Cloninger, C.R., Svrakic, D.M., and Przybeck, T.R. (1993). A psychobiological model of temperament and character. *Archives of General Psychiatry*, 30, 975–90.

Coryell, W. and Schlesser, M. (2001). The dexamethasone suppression test and suicide prediction. *American Journal of Psychiatry*, 158, 748–53.

Deakin, J.F.W. (1996). 5-HT, antidepressant drugs and the psychosocial origins of depression. *Journal of Psychopharmacology*, 10, 31–8.

Engström, G., Nymann, G.E., and Träskman-Bendz, L. (1996). The Marke-Nymann Temperament Scale in suicide attempters. *Acta Psychiatrica Scandinavica*, 94, 320–5.

Evans, J., Williams, J.M.G., O'Loughlin, S., and Howells, K. (1992). Autobiographical memory and problem-solving strategies of parasuicide patients. *Psychological Medicine*, 22, 399–405.

Gabbard, G.O. (2000). A neurobiologically informed perspective on psychotherapy. *British Journal of Psychiatry*, 177, 117–22.

Harris, E.C. and Barraclough, B. (1997). Suicide as an outcome for mental disorders. A meta-analysis. *British Journal of Psychiatry*, 170, 205–28.

Hawton, K., Arensman, E., Townsend, E., Bremmer, S., Feldman, E., Goldney, R., *et al.* (1998). Deliberate self harm: a systematic review of the efficacy of psychosocial and pharmacological treatment in preventing repetition. *British Medical Journal*, 137, 441–7.

Hawton, K., Houston, K., Haw, C., Townsend, E., and Harriss, L. (2003). Comorbidity of axis-I and axis-II disorders in patients with attempted suicide. *American Journal of Psychiatry*, 160, 1494–500.

Heinrichs, M., Baumgartner, T., Kirschbaum, C., and Ehlert, U. (2003). Social support and oxytocin interact to suppress cortisol and subjective responses to psychosocial stress. *Biological Psychiatry*, 54, 1389–98.

Inder, W.J., Donald, R.A., Prickett, T.C.R., Frampton, C.M., Sullivan, P.F., and Mulder, R.T. (1997). Arginine vasopressine is associated with hypercortisolemia and suicide attempts in depression. *Biological Psychiatry*, 42, 744–7.

Kandel, E.R. (1999). Biology and the future of psychoanalysis revisited: a new intellectual framework for psychiatry revisited. *American Journal of Psychiatry*, 156, 589–96.

Keilp, J.G., Sackeim, H.A., Brodsky, B.S., Oquendo, M.A., Malone, K.M., and Mann, J.J. (2001). Neuropsychological dysfunction in depressed suicide attempters. *American Journal of Psychiatry*, 158, 735–41.

King, D.A., Conwell, Y., Cox, C., Henderson, R.E., Denning, D.G., and Caine, E. (2000). A neuropsychological comparison of depressed suicide attempters and non-attempters. *The Journal of Neuropsychiatry and Clinical Neurosciences*, 12, 64–70.

Kodama, T., Honda, Y., and Watanabe, M. (2002). Release of neurotransmitters in the monkey frontal cortex is related to the level of attention. *Journal of Psychiatry and Clinical Neurosciences*, 56, 341–2.

Linehan, M.M., Rizvi, S.L., Welch, S.S., and Page, B. (2000). Psychiatric disorders of suicidal behaviour: personality disorders. In *The international handbook of suicide and attempted suicide*, (ed. K. Hawton and C. van Heeringen), pp. 147–79. Wiley, Chichester.

Lupien, S.J., Gillin, C.J., and Hauger, R.L. (1999). Working memory is more sensitive than declarative memory to the acute effects of corticosteroids: a dose–response study in humans. *Behavioral Neuroscience*, 113, 420–30.

Malone, K.M. and Moran, M. (2001). Psychopharmacological approaches to the suicidal process. In *Understanding suicidal behaviour: the suicidal process approach to research, treatment and prevention,* (ed. C. van Heeringen), pp. 255–73. Wiley, Chichester.

Mann, J.J. (2002). A current perspective of suicide and attempted suicide. *Annals of Internal Medicine,* 136, 302–11.

Mann, J.J. (2003). Neurobiology of suicidal behaviour. *Nature Neuroscience Reviews,* 4, 819–28.

Mann, J.J., Waternaux, C., Haas, G.L., and Mallone, K.M. (1999). Toward a clinical model of suicidal behavior in psychiatric patients. *American Journal of Psychiatry,* 156, 181–9.

McKittrick, C.R., Blanchard, R.J., and Blanchard, B.S. (1995). Serotonin receptor binding in a colony model of chronic social stress. *Biological Psychiatry,* 37, 383–96.

McLeod, A.K., Rose, G.S., and Williams, J.M.G. (1993). Components of hopelessness about the future in parasuicide. *Cognitive Therapy and Research,* 17, 441–55.

Meyer, J.H., Kapur, S., Houle, S., Da Silva, J., Owczarck, B., Brown, G.M., *et al.* (1999). Prefrontal cortex 5-HT$_2$ receptors in depression: an [F-18] setoperone PET imaging study. *American Journal of Psychiatry,* 156, 1029–34.

Meyer, J.H., McMain, S., Kennedy, S.H., Korman, L., Brown, G.M., DaSilva, J.N., *et al.* (2003). Dysfunctional attitudes and 5-HT$_2$ receptors during depression and self-harm. *American Journal of Psychiatry,* 160, 90–9.

Nutt, D.J. (2000). The psychobiology of posttraumatic stress disorder. *Journal of Clinical Psychiatry,* 61 (suppl. 5), 24–9.

Oquendo, M., Placidi, G.P.A., Malone, K.M., Campbell, C., Keilp, J., Brodsky, B., *et al.* (2003). Positron emission tomography of regional brain metabolic responses to a serotonergic challenge and lethality of suicide attempts in major depression. *Archives of General Psychiatry,* 60, 14–22.

Sidley, G.L., Whitaker, K., Calam, R.M., and Wells, A. (1997). The relationship between problem-solving and autobiographical memory in parasuicide patients. *Behavioural and Cognitive Psychotherapy,* 25, 195–202.

Sugiori, M., Kawashima, R., Nakagawa, M., Okada, K., Sato, T., Goto, R., *et al.* (2000). Correlation between human personality and neural activity in cerebral cortex. *NeuroImage,* 11, 541–6.

Tops, M., van der Pompe, G., Wijers, A.A., den Boer, J.A., Meijman, T.F., and Korf, J. (2004). Free recall of pleasant words from recency positions is especially sensitive to acute administration of cortisol. *Psychoneuroendocrinology,* 29, 327–38.

Van Heeringen, C. (2001). *Understanding suicidal behaviour: the suicidal process approach to research, treatment and prevention.* Wiley, Chichester.

Van Heeringen, C. (2003). The neurobiology of suicide and suicidality. *Canadian Journal of Psychiatry,* 48, 13–21.

Van Heeringen, C. and Marušič, A. (2003). Understanding the suicidal brain. *British Journal of Psychiatry,* 183, 282–4.

Van Heeringen, C., Audenaert, K., Van de Wiele, L., and Verstraete, A. (2000). Cortisol in violent suicidal behaviour: association with personality and monoaminergic activity. *Journal of Affective Disorders,* 60, 181–9.

Van Heeringen, C., Audenaert, K., Van Laere, K., Dumont, F., Slegers, G., Mertens, J., *et al.* (2003). Prefrontal 5-HT$_{2a}$ receptor binding index, hopelessness and personality characteristics in attempted suicide. *Journal of Affective Disorders,* 74, 149–58.

Williams, J.M.G. and Pollock, L. (2001). Psychological aspects of the suicidal process. In *Understanding suicidal behaviour: the suicidal process approach to research, treatment and prevention*, (ed. C. van Heeringen), pp. 76–94. Wiley, Chichester.

Yatham, L.N., Liddle, P.F., Shiah, I.S., Scarrow, G., Lam, R.W., Adam, M.J., *et al.* (2000). Brain serotonin(2) receptors in major depression: a positron emission tomography study. *Archives of General Psychiatry*, 57, 850–8.

7

Interplay of genes and environment as contributory factors in suicidal behaviour

Andrej Marušič and Peter McGuffin

Introduction

In this chapter a rather new field will be discussed, the genetics of suicidal behaviour, from the definition of the phenotypes to molecular genetic investigations. On the way we will consider the interplay of genes and environment, concluding with likely future and ethical implications. There is an increasing number of publications about genetics of suicide ideation and behaviour, and an increasing number of reviews on genetic aspects of suicidality as well as a recent meta-analysis (Lalovic and Turecki 2002). Despite this, many suicidologists do not hide their reservations about the genetics of suicidal behaviour. This, we suggest, arises out of misconceptions, such as the idea that discovering a genetic contribution means that proneness to suicide cannot be altered, whereas in fact genes operate in a probabilistic rather than deterministic way in complex traits that increase vulnerability to suicide or self-harm.

From a definition of phenotype to the molecular genetic investigation

Phenotype

Before any genetic analysis takes place, a phenotype has to be defined. And here is a potential strength of the genetics of suicidal behaviour. Completed suicide is most probably the most precisely defined phenotype in behavioural genetics. Although some false negatives will occur (especially in countries with underestimated suicide rates), false-positive cases will be rare. More difficulty arises in the category of attempted suicides, and even more so when suicide ideation is studied as a phenotype. It has therefore been suggested that genetic studies are more likely to end up with positive results if focused on the completed end of the suicidality spectrum (Linkowski *et al.* 1985).

Quantitative genetics

Family studies show that the risk of suicide is increased when there is a suicide in the family (Pfeffer *et al.* 1994), particularly when a violent method is used (Linkowski *et al.* 1985). A very recent familial study was conducted in a region with a high suicide rate. The suicidality of young men was closely associated with suicidality among their first-degree relatives. Again, the more explicit the suicidal behaviour, the stronger the effect became (Marušič *et al.* 2004). One of the limitations of family studies is that they do not differentiate between genetic and other factors, as family members share both genetic and environmental factors.

Classical research methods, which differentiate between that which is genetic and that which is acquired within the family, are the 'natural experiments' of twin and adoption studies. If the concordance of a given behaviour (that is simultaneous appearance of certain behaviour in both twins) in identical twins is significantly greater than between fraternal twins, we can conclude that there exists a certain genetic predisposition towards such behaviour. In the case of identical twins the concordance of suicide is much greater than is the case with fraternal twins (Roy *et al.* 1991). Genetic model fitting on one of the largest studies of twins showed that 43% of the variability of suicidal behaviour can be explained by genetics, while the remaining 57% reflects environmental factors (McGuffin *et al.* 2001).

Data relating to adopted children are rare, but what there is shows a similar picture. Wender *et al.* (1986) showed increased rates of suicide in the biological rather than adopting relatives of depressed adoptees, whereas Schulsinger *et al.* (1979) found that more biological relatives of adopted-away suicides die by suicide compared with biological relatives of control adoptees. Therefore family twin and adoption data are consistent in suggesting a genetic predisposition towards behaviour leading to suicide. Having established this fact, two questions remain to be answered.

The first question is how can genetic factors increase the probability of suicidal behaviour in an individual. Suicide does not, of course, show a simple Mendelian pattern of transmission; there is not a 'suicide gene'. As in the case of other complex behaviour patterns, it is likely that the predisposition towards suicide consists of numerous genetic and environmental factors, which manifest themselves as suicidal behaviour only when a certain threshold of liability is crossed. According to this model, relatives of people who have committed suicide will be more liable to suicide and will thus cross the threshold that triggers the expression of suicidal behaviour to a correspondingly greater extent (Falconer 1965). The genome and the environment are interrelated in various ways and it is hard to speak deterministically about the influence of one or the other, particularly as it appears that some complex behavioural patterns are connected with many genetic factors (polygenetically), which interact with numerous environmental effects (multifactorially). In other words, we can talk about a polygenetic multifactorial aetiological model of suicidal behaviour.

The other question is about the specificity of the genetic suicide risk factors. It is difficult on present evidence to decide about the extent to which such genetic factors are specific to suicide or whether they more generally confer a liability to different mental disorders. For example, it remains unclear whether the genes predisposing to suicide are identical with those predisposing to affective disorder but, since only about half of those committing suicide have a diagnosis of depression, it seems probable that the overlap is incomplete.

Molecular genetics

How do we locate and identify genes that are involved in suicidal behaviour? Thus far, one of the major benefits to biomedical science of the advance in molecular genetics has been in enhancing the feasibility of so-called positional cloning. This process begins with genome scans, studies of a disorder segregating in families and examining the co-segregation with genetic markers that are roughly evenly spread throughout the genome. Using a few hundred of such markers allows the detection of linkage for any single gene trait, given the right number of families of suitable structure, containing multiply affected members. Linkage studies of disease allow the position of loci to be discovered and it is then possible to move from identifying the position of genes to actually cloning and identifying the genes themselves. The main problem when we come to studies of suicide is that linkage studies of the completed act are unlikely to be feasible because we need to have access to the DNA of multiple families with multiple affected members.

An alternative approach is to carry out association studies that, in their classic form, simply depend upon comparing a sample of cases with a sample of unaffected controls. Association studies also have an advantage over linkage studies of being much better at detecting genes that may only have small effects. The disadvantage at present is that comprehensive genome scans using association are not feasible because they require many thousands of markers to be genotyped (Sham and McGuffin 2002). Therefore the most practicable approach currently is to focus on so-called candidate genes; that is, genes involved in metabolic pathways in the brain that could plausibly have something to do with suicidal behaviour.

Altered serotonergic function

As it is thought that the variability of serotonergic neurotransmitters plays a pivotal role in individual differences in mood, impulsiveness, and aggression, it is no surprise that molecular genetic studies of suicide and suicidal behaviour focus on serotonergic genes. Genetically determined variation in neurotransmitter systems most probably interacts with environmental influences during different development stages of suicidal behaviour, from depressive states to suicidal thoughts and plans, to actual attempts and fatal suicidal acts. It has been suggested that variation in the $5-HT_{1a}$ receptor is associated with general depressive thoughts, and the related $5-HT_2$ with despair, frequently followed by suicidal thoughts (Deakin 1996). Some genetic factors in suicide may be related to aggressiveness and impulsivity (New *et al.* 1998), which have their effects independently of, or additively to, a mental disorder.

Overall, polymorphisms in some relevant genes could contribute to alterations in protein function that are part of the neurochemical underpinnings of psychopathologies that are related to suicide risk, such as affective disorders, alcohol-related mental disorders, psychoses, personality disorders or aggressive-impulsive traits, or perhaps even suicidal behaviour itself. Altered serotonergic function is indeed implicated in the aetiology and pathogenesis of several major psychiatric conditions, and in particular, there is evidence for an association of lower serotonergic function and suicidal behaviour. Thus genes related to the serotonergic system are candidate genes worthy of study as part of the genetic diathesis for suicidal behaviour. Accordingly, more than 100 international peer-reviewed publications on molecular genetic investigations of suicidal behaviour have been already published and almost all of them investigated various parts of the serotonergic tree. These candidate genes can be classified into three subgroups:

- gene involved in *synthesis of serotonin*—tryptophan hydroxylase (TPH) is the rate-limiting enzyme in serotonin synthesis;
- genes involved in *serotonergic neurotransmission*—serotonin transporter (5-HTT), which regulates reuptake of serotonin into presynaptic neurons, and different serotonin receptors that also regulate neurotransmission; and
- genes involved in *serotonin catabolism*—monoaminoxidase (MAO).

Synthesis of serotonin

In one of the pioneering publications in this field, Nielsen *et al.* (1994)— continued in Nielsen *et al.* (1998)—showed an association between a variant in an intron, or non-coding region, of the tryptophan hydroxylase gene (TPH) and suicidality, severity of suicide attempts, and alcoholism. An association with a polymorphism in an intron poses some difficulty for interpretation.

Although variations in introns were thought originally not to be functionally significant, it is now known that they can influence the pattern of gene splicing. Alternatively, a variant in an intron may be pointing to a variation elsewhere in the gene that does alter enzyme activity. Rotondo *et al.* (1999) have examined the possible role of TPH in more detail by screening its promoter region. They found four variants that could modulate the activity of the gene, and one of these was significantly associated with suicidality in a sample of offenders of different Caucasian nations. Most recently, Arango *et al.* (2003) reported another significant association for the TPH gene. The less common A allele variant of the A779C polymorphism was associated with suicide attempts. Abbar *et al.* (2001) studied the entire TPH gene in a case-control study, including 231 individuals who had attempted suicide and 281 controls. Significant associations were found between variants in introns 7, 8 and 9 and in the 3' non-coding region and suicide attempts (the association was strongest for subjects who had attempted suicide by violent means and who had a history of major depression). On the other hand, no significant association was observed between suicide attempts and polymorphisms in the promoter, intron 1 and intron 3. Bass *et al.* (2002) investigated the TPH gene and reported another allelic association with poor pre-morbid social and work adjustment and with violent suicide, this time specifically for a subgroup of subjects with bipolar affective disorder. Although a great majority of positive results presented here, and those of previous studies (e.g. Mann *et al.* 1996; Gelernter *et al.* 1998), suggest that a genetic variant at the 3' end of the TPH gene may be a susceptibility factor for a phenotype combining serious suicidal behaviour and impulsive aggression (e.g. suicide by violent means only, severity of suicide attempt, and offending), several studies have reported negative findings (e.g. Bennet *et al.* 2000; Du *et al.* 2000*a*), albeit with suicide ideation rather than serious suicidal behaviour.

Serotonin neurotransmission—the serotonin transporter (5-HTT)

A 44 bp insertion/deletion in the 5' flanking promoter region of the serotonin transporter (5-HTT) gene affects 5-HTT expression and probably 5-HT reup-take. Baca-Garcia *et al.* (2002) tested the association between suicide attempts and a polymorphism in the promoter area of the 5-HTT with the two allelic variants, the long (l) variant and the short (s) variant. Individuals with low expression of the serotonin transporter (s/s or s/l) were significantly over-represented in female attempters. Lethality appeared to have a significant influence on the effects of the genotype in suicide, since females with low expression of the 5-HTT were over-represented among non-lethal female attempters. Some support for an association with variation in a serotonin transporter gene also comes from work by Bondy *et al.* (2000), Bellivier *et al.* (2000), and Courtet *et al.* (2001), who have found a relationship specifically with violent suicide or very severe suicide attempts. On the other hand, when this promoter region was studied in other samples around the world, no significant genotypic or allelic association with suicidal behaviour was found (e.g. Rujescu *et al.* 2001; Zalsman *et al.* 2001; Yen *et al.* 2003).

Serotonin neurotransmission—serotonin receptors (5-HT_{1A}, 5-HT_{2A}, 5-HT_{1B})

More than 40 molecular genetic suicidology studies have focused on three serotonin receptor genes, half of them focusing on the 5-HT_{2A} receptor gene. There are two common 5-HT_{2A} receptor gene polymorphisms in humans. Du *et al.* (2000*b*) have reported an association between a T102C polymorphism in the first exon, or expressed region, of the serotonin receptor 5-HT_{2A} and suicidal ideation in patients with depression. Some support for an association with variation in the 5-HT_{2A} also comes from work by Arias *et al.* (2001), who have found a relationship with suicide behaviour in the Spanish population. No association was found when Ono *et al.* (2001) examined whether the A1438G polymorphism of the 5-HT_{2A} receptor gene was associated with suicide itself, using Japanese completed suicides. 5-HT_{2A} receptor expression is reported to be increased in suicide (Arango *et al.* 2003). Functional polymorphisms involving the promoter region that affect gene expression may explain this finding.

Nishiguchi *et al.* (2002) examined the association between the structural polymorphisms, Pro16Leu and Gly272Asp, of the 5-HT_{1A} receptor gene and completed suicide, and found no significant difference in genotype distribution or allele frequencies between suicide victims and controls. Their findings suggested that it is unlikely that the 5-HT_{1A} receptor gene is implicated in the susceptibility to suicide.

Another serotonin receptor, namely 5-HT_{1B}, is also of interest. Thus far, evidence exists that the uncommon T371G (Phe124Cys) and the common promoter region A161T polymorphisms may exhibit functional effects, and possibly that the common synonymous G861C does as well. From the 18 reported population-based case-control studies of 5-HT_{1B} in a range of disorders, two important associations stand out: with antisocial alcoholism in the Finnish population and a history of suicide attempts in European–American personality disorder patients (Sanders *et al.* 2002). Huang *et al.* (1999) and Arango *et al.* (2003) also studied polymorphisms for the 5-HT_{1B} receptor. However, no association between either polymorphism and depression, suicide, aggression, or alcoholism was observed.

Serotonin catabolism

Malafosse *et al.* (1997) suggested that the MAO-A gene may be involved in susceptibility to suicide behaviour and to traits such as impulsivity and aggression. Du *et al.* (2002) reported an association between the *EcoRV* polymorphism of the MAO-A gene with alleles associated with enzyme activity in male but not female post-mortem brain samples from 44 depressed suicide victims and 92 control subjects of the same ethnic background. Their results provide evidence that genetic factors may modulate risk for depression, suicide, or both, by influencing monoaminergic activity in a sexually dimorphic manner.

Some reservations, meta-analysis, RNA analysis, and future directions

Studies such as those discussed above can so far be regarded as only suggestive, and need to be followed up by further work. One of the problems that has pervaded association studies in psychiatry, and indeed studies of many other common forms of disease, has been that attempted replications have been on so small a scale as to have little power to confirm original positive findings (Owen *et al.* 1997). Most associations so far with suicidal behaviour have had small effect sizes, as would be predicted for a trait resulting from a combined affect of multiple genes. Therefore, serious regard needs to be paid to effect sizes, and power calculations appropriate to these need to be performed before future studies of genetic association and suicidality are undertaken. A consequence of not paying attention to power would be, as already has been the case in some areas, the worst of both worlds. That is, authors end up with uninteresting negative results, but are unable to say whether these reflect a true absence of an association (an association ruled out) or simply a low chance of detecting an effect that actually exists (i.e. a spurious negativity because of a type II error).

In an attempt to overcome these shortcomings and problems of genetic studies of suicide, the first meta-analysis of association studies of the TPH gene and suicide behaviour was reported recently. Lalovic and Turecki (2002) reported negative results for intron 7, based on 17 publications with an overall number of 1290 cases and 2295 controls. On the other hand, an analysis by Rujescu *et al.* (2003), including only those studies that were performed on samples of similar ethnic origins and geographic closeness, provides strong evidence for an association of suicide-related behaviour with an A218 nucleotide polymorphism in the TPH gene in Caucasians.

So far little attention has been paid to the possible interplay of genes with environmental factors such as life events and social support. As such, a simultaneously performed candidate gene and psychological autopsy study might be a way forward. As a nice example of such simultaneously performed research, Caspi *et al.* (2003) tested why stressful experiences lead to depression in some people but not in others, by using a prospective-longitudinal study of a representative birth cohort. The functional polymorphism mentioned earlier in the promoter region of the serotonin transporter (5-HTT) gene was found to moderate the influence of stressful life events on depression. Individuals with one or two copies of the short allele of the 5-HTT promoter polymorphism exhibited more depressive symptoms, diagnosable depression, and suicidality in relation to stressful life events than individuals homozygous for the long allele. This epidemiological study provides evidence of a gene-by-environment interaction, in which an individual's response to environmental insults is moderated by his or her genetic make-up.

From proximal to ultimate causation for suicide

Human suicide directly contradicts the generally held views that evolution selects for behaviour that promotes the existence of the organism and its genes. Human suicide, unlike most other behaviour, acts against the survival of the behaving organism. De Catanzaro (1980) offered some explanations for this, including the limited circumstances in which suicide may occur because of beneficial effects it has on other, surviving individuals who share the suicidal individual's genes. A distinction between proximal and ultimate causation for suicide behaviour can be made. While determining the proximal causation can only address the question of how suicide happens in a biopsychosocial sense, formulation of the ultimate causation of suicide could also incorporate the question of why it exists (Abed 2000).

Many functional mental disorders strongly associated with suicidal behaviour most probably represent accentuation or dysregulation of normal human traits (such as impulsivity, aggression, and emotional lability) or misplaced psychological or behavioural coping strategies (Marks and Nesse 1994). Similarly, we could try to generate some hypotheses about ultimate causation of suicide behaviour. For example, a type of suicidal behaviour specific to so-called atypical depression could represent initial accentuation and later dysregulation of aggressive and impulsive behaviour. Males who were more aggressive and brave were better warriors and, as such, more often rewarded for their actions. Furthermore, the more disinhibited and violent they were, the easier it was for them to spread their genes during and after conquest of new territories. Overall, these traits had been selected and, as such, accentuated in some parts of the world. In a more contemporary society, the behavioural manifestations of the same traits have become regarded as pathological. One way of coping, for subjects who inherited these traits, is continuous suppression. However, it is particularly likely that these traits will escape from control (potentially with a more acceptable self-aggressive outcome) when an individual is under the influence of alcohol or some other disinhibiting substance.

Some basis for the above hypothesis could be found in the recent investigation by Voracek *et al.* (2003), who studied the marked variation regarding the suicide rate in 34 European countries—where the suicide rate for men varies by a factor of 28—and described it well by regressing the national suicide rate on the capital cities' latitudes and on an interaction term of squared latitude multiplied by longitude. The interaction term explained more than 40% of male and almost 30% of female suicide rates. Latitude explained a further significant increment of more than 10% in the variance of both male and female suicide rates. This regression model quantifies the Finno-Ugrian suicide hypothesis of Kondrichin (1995) and Marušič and Farmer (2001).

Kondrichin (1995) suggested that high suicide rates in Finno-Ugrians could be due to the fixation in the gene pool of certain behavioural traits predisposing to suicide during the early stages of ethnogenesis. It is also noteworthy that both Finns and Hungarians share the same proportion of European (90%) to Uralic (10%) genes (Cavalli-Sforza *et al.*, 1994). Marušič and Farmer (2001) noted that nations with a high suicide rate (European countries with rates above 20/100 000/year) occur along a J-shaped curve from Finland to Austria. This J-curve pattern also supports the thesis that genetic predisposition could have influenced the suicide rates in these neighbouring countries. It is also possible that the people in these neighbouring countries may also share similar proportions of Uralic genes to Finns and Hungarians. This area maps on to the second principal component identified for European gene distribution, representing the ancestral adaptation to cold climates and the Uralic language dispersion (Cavalli-Sforza and Cavalli-Sforza 1995; Sykes 2001). It is of note that in terms of orientation, shape, and steepness of these gradients, the spatial pattern of European suicide rates is very different from that found in ecological analyses of geographic areas of comparable size in other continents; for example, the United States, Canada, or Australia (Lester 1985; Lester and Shephard 1998).

From present science to future practice, with some ethical implications

Until we know more about the genetic factors significant in the development of suicidal behaviour, most of the work related to suicide prevention will be directed at improving environmental conditions, particularly with respect to those individuals where the tendency towards suicidal behaviour is most pronounced. However, even these activities do not touch upon just one aspect of the tendency towards suicidal behaviour (that is the environmental factors) and neglect the other (genetic factors). By influencing the environment we are always, at the same time, tackling the process of the interaction of the genome and the envirome, which may consequently reduce the development of some at-risk personality characteristics, and the trigger of risky behaviour. The focus of our research is thus directed not only at discovering genetic factors in the development of suicidal behaviour, but also at the search for protective background factors (family, school, working environment, relations between the sexes, religion, etc.).

Nevertheless, if the genetics of suicide continues developing as quickly as it has in the past decade, its future is indeed promising. It is very likely that evidence in future will show some genetic risk factors for suicide behaviour of small effect, which will be specific for certain groups or certain populations. This will, in turn, lead to upgrading traditional preventive measures into more focused and effective tasks. Knowledge of genetic risk factors will allow screening and allocating help to those particularly at risk, which means an increase in cost-effectiveness; and knowledge about molecular genetic risk factors is almost essential for the development of pharmacological ways of preventing suicide behaviour.

On the other hand, one should not forget that identifying people at risk has societal implications and, therefore, raises a number of ethical issues regarding public policy (Meltzer 2000). First of all, it will soon become very important to protect the confidentiality of data on individuals (both suicidal cases and their controls), from whom material for molecular genetic research on suicide will have been taken. Secondly, as with any other investigation in behavioural genetics, we must make sure that potential subjects can provide informed consent. They have to be informed that their participation is voluntary and that they may withdraw at any time. The risks and the benefits of the study must be clearly stated, and alternatives to the study should be made available to the participants. Thirdly, in collaboration with the pharmaceutical industry, anyone involved in the genetic investigation of suicide behaviour will have to be aware of their precise roles as researchers, as opposed to those of clinicians. Finally, the question of to whom (suicidal subjects, their relatives, relatives of suicide victims?), when (sufficient validity?) and how (with or without education and genetic counselling) to present information once genetic testing becomes more commonplace will have to be addressed.

The genetics of suicidal behaviour has developed significantly over the past couple of years. Sooner or later results of similar impact to those recently published in genetic investigations of schizophrenia (Elkin *et al.* 2004) will be available. A much more narrowly defined phenotype (e.g. completed suicides versus living people of the same age) will prove to be helpful in this respect. It is unwise to wait for the first strongly replicated results to appear without being prepared 'ethically' for their implications.

References

Abbar, M., Courtet, P., Bellivier, F., Leboyer, H., Boulenger, J.P., Castelhau, D., *et al.* (2001). Suicide attempts and the tryptophan hydroxylase gene. *Molecular Psychiatry*, 6, 268–73.

Abed, R.T. (2000). Psychiatry and darwinism—Time to reconsider? *British Journal of Psychiatry*, 177, 1–3.

Arango, V., Huang, Y.Y., Underwood, M.D., and Mann, J.J. (2003). Genetics of the serotonergic system in suicidal behavior. *Journal of Psychiatric Research*, 37, 375–86.

Arias, B., Gasto, C., Catalan, R., Gutierrez, B., Pintor, L., and Fananas, L. (2001). The 5-HT(2A) receptor gene 102T/C polymorphism is associated with suicidal behavior in depressed patients. *American Journal of Medical Genetics*, 105, 801–4.

Baca-Garcia, E., Vaquero, C., Diaz-Sastre, C., Saiz-Ruiz, J., Fernandez-Piqueras, J., and de Leon, J. (2002). A gender-specific association between the serotonin transporter gene and suicide attempts. *Neuropsychopharmacology*, 26, 692–5.

Bass, N., McQuillin, A., Lawrence, J., Darragh, N., Kalsi, G., Curtis, D., *et al.* (2002). Investigation of the gene encoding tryptophan hydroxylase (TPH) and suicide behaviour in bipolar affective disorder shows allelic association with poor pre-morbid social and work adjustment and with violent suicide. *American Journal of Medical Genetics*, 114, 6.

Bellivier, F., Szoke, A., Henry, C., Lacoste, J., Bottos, C., Nosten-Bertrand, M., *et al.* (2000). Possible association between serotonin transporter gene polymorphism and violent suicidal behavior in mood disorders. *Biological Psychiatry*, 48, 319–22.

Bennett, P.J., McMahon, W.M., Watabe, J., Achilles, J., Bacon, M., Coon, H., *et al.* (2000). Tryptophan hydroxylase polymorphisms in suicide victims. *Psychiatric Genetics*, 10, 13–17.

Bondy, B., Erfurth, A., de Jonge, S., Kruger, M., and Meyer, H. (2000). Possible association of the short allele of the serotonin transporter promoter gene polymorphism (5-HTTLPR) with violent suicide. *Molecular Psychiatry*, 5, 193–5.

Caspi, A., Sugden, K., Moffitt, T.E., Taylor, A., Craig, I.W., Harrington, H., *et al.* (2003). Influence of life stress on depression: Moderation by a polymorphism in the 5-HTT gene. *Science*, 301 (5631), 386–9.

Cavalli-Sforza, L.L., Menozzi, P., and Piazza, A. (1994). *The history and geography of human genes*. Princeton University Press, Princeton.

Cavalli-Sforza, L.L. and Cavalli-Sforza, F. (1995). *The great human diasporas: the history of diversity and evolution*. Perseus Books, Cambridge, Massachusetts.

Courtet, P., Baud, P., Abbar, M., Boulenger, J.P., Castelnau, D., Mouthon, D., *et al.* (2001). Association between violent suicidal behavior and the low activity allele of the serotonin transporter gene. *Molecular Psychiatry*, 6, 338–41.

Deakin, J.F.W. (1996). 5-HT, antidepressant drugs and the psychosocial origins of depression. *Journal of Psychopharmacology*, 10, 31–8.

de Catanzaro, D. (1980). Human suicide: A biological perspective. *Behavioral and Brain Sciences*, 3, 265–90.

Du, L.S., Faludi, G., Palkovits, M., Bakish, D., and Hrdina, P.D. (2000a). Tryptophan hydroxylase gene 218A/C polymorphism is not associated with depressed suicide. *International Journal of Neuropsychopharmacology*, 3, 215–20.

Du, L., Bakish, D., Lapierre, Y.D., Ravindran, A.V., and Hrdina, P.D. (2000b). Association of polymorphism of serotonin 2A receptor gene with suicidal ideation in major depressive disorder. *American Journal of Medical Genetics*, 96, 56–60.

Du, L.S., Faludi, G., Palkovits, M., Sotonyi, P., Bakish, D., and Hrdina, P.D. (2002). High activity-related allele of MAO-A gene associated with depressed suicide in males. *Neuroreport*, 13, 1195–8.

Elkin, A., Kalidindi, S., and McGuffin, P. (2004). Have schizophrenia genes been found? *Current Opinion in Psychiatry*, 17, 107–13.

Falconer, D.S. (1965). The inheritance of liability to certain diseases, estimated from the incidence among relatives. *Annals of Human Genetics*, 29, 51–76.

Gelernter, J., Kranzler, H., and Lacobelle, J. (1998). Population studies of polymorphisms at loci of neuropsychiatric interest (tryptophan hydroxylase (TPH), dopamine transporter protein (SLC6A3), D3 dopamine receptor (DRD3), apolipoprotein E (APOE), mu opioid receptor (OPRM1), and ciliary neurotrophic factor (CNTF)). *Genomics*, 52, 289–97.

Huang, Y.Y., Grailhe, R., Arango, V., Hen, R., and Mann, J.J. (1999). Relationship of psychopathology to the human serotonin 1B genotype and receptor binding kinetics in postmortem brain tissue. *Neuropsychopharmacology*, 21 (2), 238–46.

Kondrichin, S.V. (1995). Suicide among Finno-Ugrians [letter]. *Lancet*, 346, 1632–3.

Lalovic, A. and Turecki, G. (2002). Meta-analysis of the association between tryptophan hydroxylase and suicidal behavior. *American Journal of Medical Genetics*, 114 , 533–40.

Lester, D. (1985). Variation of suicide and homicide rates by latitude and longitude in the United States, Canada, and Australia [letter]. *American Journal of Psychiatry*, 142, 523–4.

Lester, D. and Shephard, R. (1998). Variation of suicide and homicide rates by longitude and latitude. *Perceptual and Motor Skills*, 87, 186.

Linkowski, P., de Maertelaer, V., and Mendlewicz, J. (1985). Suicidal behavior in major depressive illness. *Acta Psychiatrica Scandinavica*, 72, 233–8.

Malafosse, A., Leboyer, M., Preisig, M., Maller, I., Ferrero, F., and Guimon, J. (1997). Association studies between manic depressive illness and suicidal behaviour and 'serotonergic' genes. *European Psychiatry*, 12(S2), 119s.

Mann, J.J., Malone, K.M., Nielsen, D.L., Goldman, D., Erdos, J., and Gelernter, J. (1996). Molecular genetics of suicidal behavior. *European Neuropsychopharmacology*, 6(S3), 22.

Marks, I. and Nesse, R. (1994). Fear and fitness: An evolutionary analysis of anxiety disorders. *Ethology and Sociobiology*, 15, 247–61.

Marušič, A. and Farmer, A. (2001). Genetic risk factors as possible cause of the variation in European suicide rates. *British Journal of Psychiatry*, 179, 194–6.

Marušič, A., Roskar, S., and Hughes, R.H. (2004). Familial study of suicide behaviour among adolescents in Slovenia. *Crisis*, 25, 74–7.

McGuffin, P., Marušič, A., and Farmer, A. (2001). What can psychiatric genetics offer suicidology? *Crisis*, 22, 61–5.

Meltzer, H.Y. (2000). Genetics and etiology of schizophrenia and bipolar disorder. *Biological Psychiatry*, 47, 171–3.

New, A.S., Gelernter, J., Yovell, Y., Trestman, R.L., Nielsen, D.A., Silverman, J., et al. (1998). Tryptophan hydroxylase genotype is associated with impulsive–aggression measures: A preliminary study. *American Journal of Medical Genetics*, 81, 13–17.

Nielsen, D.A., Goldman, D., Virkkunen, M., Tokola, R., Rawlings, R., and Linnoila, M. (1994). Suicidality and 5-hydroxyindoleacetic acid concentration associated with a tryptophan hydroxylase polymorphism. *Archives of General Psychiatry*, 51, 34–8.

Nielsen, D.A., Virkkunen, M., Lappalainen, J., Eggert, M., Brown, G.L., Long, J.C., et al. (1998). A tryptophan hydroxylase gene marker for suicidality and alcoholism. *Archives of General Psychiatry*, 55 (7), 593–602.

Nishiguchi, N., Shirakawa, O., Ono, H., Nishimura, A., Nushida, H., Ueno, Y., et al. (2002). Lack of an association between 5-HT1A receptor gene structural polymorphisms and suicide victims. *American Journal of Medical Genetics*, 114, 423–5.

Ono, H., Shirakawa, O., Nishiguchi, N., Nishimura, A., Nushida, H., Ueno, Y., and Maeda, K. (2001). Serotonin 2A receptor gene polymorphism is not associated with completed suicide. *Journal of Psychiatric Research*, 35, 173–6.

Owen, M.J., Holmans, P., and McGuffin, P. (1997). Association studies in psychiatric genetics. *Molecular Psychiatry*, 2, 270–3.

Pfeffer, C.R., Normandin, L., and Kakuma, T. (1994). Suicidal children grow up: Suicidal behavior and psychiatric disorders among relatives. *Journal of American Academy of Child and Adolescent Psychiatry*, 33, 1087–97.

Rotondo, A., Schuebel, K., Bergen, A., Aragon, R., Virkkunen, M., Linnoila, M., et al. (1999). Identification of four variants in the tryptophan hydroxylase promoter and association to behavior. *Molecular Psychiatry*, 4, 360–8.

Roy, A., Segal, N.L., Centerwall, B.S., and Robinette, C.D. (1991). Suicide in twins. *Archives of General Psychiatry*, 48, 28–32.

Rujescu, D., Giegling, I., Sato, T., and Moeller, H.J. (2001). A polymorphism in the promoter of the serotonin transporter gene is not associated with suicidal behavior. *Psychiatric Genetics*, 11, 169–72.

Rujescu, D., Giegling, I., Sato, T., Hartmann, A.M., and Moller, H.J. (2003). Genetic variations in tryptophan hydroxylase in suicidal behavior. Analysis and meta-analysis. *Biological Psychiatry*, 54, 465–73.

Sanders, A.R., Duan, J., and Gejman, P.V. (2002). DNA variation and psychopharmacology of the human serotonin receptor 1B(HTR1B) gene. *Pharmacogenomics*, 3, 745–62.

Schulsinger, F., Kety, S.S., Rosenthal, D., and Wender, P.H. (1979). A family study of suicide. In *Origin, prevention and treatment of affective disorders*, (ed. M. Schou and E. Stromgren). Academic Press, London.

Sykes, B. (2001). *The seven daughters of Eve*. Norton, New York.

Voracek, M., Fisher, M.L., and Marušič, A. (2003). The Finno-Ugrian Hypothesis: variation in European suicide rates by lattitude and longitude. *Perceptual and Motor Skills*, 97, 401–6.

Wender, P.H., Kety, S.S., Rosenthal, D., Schulsinger, F., Ortmann, J., and Lunde, I. (1986). Psychiatric disorders in the biological and adoptive families of adopted individuals with affective disorders. *Archives of General Psychiatry*, 43, 923–9.

Yen, F.C., Hong, C.J., Hou, S.J., Wang, J.K., and Tsai, S.J. (2003). Association study of serotonin transporter gene VNTR polymorphism and mood disorders, onset age and suicide attempts in a Chinese sample. *Neuropsychobiology*, 48, 5–9.

Zalsman, G., Frisch, A., Bromberg, M., Gelernter, J., Michaelovsky, E., Campino, A., *et al.* (2001). Family-based association study of serotonin transporter promoter in suicidal adolescents: no association with suicidality but possible role in violence traits. *American Journal of Medical Genetics*, 105, 239–45.

8

Traumatic stress and suicidal behaviour: an important target for treatment and prevention

Lars Mehlum

Introduction

Traumatic stress syndromes are often overlooked in those clinical settings where they are not the presenting complaint or where the trauma belongs to the patients' past life (Brady *et al.* 2000). This also seems to be a tendency when it comes to patients presenting with suicidal behaviours (Zimmerman and Mattia 1999). There is not a lack of recognition of stressful life events in general as risk factors for suicidal behaviour, but most of the research attention in this field has focused on life events such as loss and separation, death, divorce, conflicts, and family problems. Less attention has, however, been paid to the connection that often exist between exposure to *traumatic* stress and subsequent suicidal behaviour. Clinical experience and growing research evidence suggest that a longstanding vulnerability for suicidal behaviour may be a sequel of traumatic exposure. There is a need to take the possibility of such exposure into consideration in clinical settings when assessing suicide risk and planning interventions and treatments, since traumatic stress syndromes and related problems may greatly influence the outcome. Furthermore, research into traumatic stress may enhance our understanding of the interplay between individual vulnerability factors and environmental stress in the development of suicidality. Psychotraumatology addresses the profound influence of traumatic exposure on the individual's perception of self and others, and the ability to form and maintain stable nourishing interpersonal relationships. This is of particularly great relevance to our current challenges of fully understanding and preventing the highly prevalent deliberate self-harm in the young (Santa Mina and Gallop 1998; Hawton *et al.* 2002). This chapter will focus on traumatic stress and suicidal behaviours, including examining what evidence there is for an association between these phenomena, and discussing possible mediating mechanisms between traumatic exposure and subsequent suicidal behaviour.

What is traumatic stress?

There is ample research evidence that both acute and chronic stressors have the potential to increase the risk of suicidal behaviour and that multiple stressful events have a cumulative effect (Heikkinen *et al.* 1994). However, some events seem to have a particular psychological toxicity—they have a capacity to create fear and an intense sense of threat. Such events are potentially traumatic. Whereas previously we required traumatic events—when used as a diagnostic criterion—to be 'outside the range of usual human experience' (American Psychiatric Association 1980), we currently do not perceive them as categorically different from less severe stressful events. In determining the traumatic effect on the individual, we now consider collectively the type and nature of the event, the intensity of fear and helplessness experienced, the personal coping resources and, finally, the support available to the individual in order to overcome the event.

How common is traumatic stress?

A number of studies, including the US National Comorbidity Survey (Kessler *et al.* 1995), show that surprisingly high proportions of the general population (50–70%) report having been exposed to trauma that meets the DSM-IV (American Psychiatric Association 1994) stressor criterion for post-traumatic stress disorder (PTSD). These are events that are so severe that they are likely to cause distress in almost anyone, although only between 15% and 25% of those exposed will actually develop PTSD (Breslau *et al.* 1991; Kessler *et al.* 1995). The most common events are sudden, unexpected death of a close friend or relative, accidents, exposure to various forms of assaultive violence, other injury, rape, sexual or physical abuse or shocking experience, or being witness to someone being killed or seriously injured (Breslau *et al.* 1998).

It is important to understand that the prevalence figures above are derived from epidemiological studies in Western societies during peacetime. In other regions of the world, during earlier periods in our history, and under specific conditions, the prevalence can be very different. The International Red Cross Federation has estimated that in the 25-year period from 1967 to 1991 disasters killed 7 million people and affected another 3 billion (International Federation of the Red Cross 1993). The vast majority of affected people live in developing countries. So far we have not mentioned the consequences of warfare. Since the Second World War there have been more than 140 wars in which an estimated 40 million people have been killed.

Even in peaceful developed countries, however, trauma invoked by disasters or terrorism may affect huge numbers of people. This was demonstrated through the attacks on New York on 11 September 2001. It is estimated that more than 100 000 people directly witnessed the disaster (Schuster *et al.* 2001). Furthermore, the attack was followed by the strongly perceived danger of subsequent acts of terrorism and hostilities, and even the prospect of war. Studies have shown that the population of New York has had a substantially higher prevalence of PTSD than other US metropolitan areas in the 1–2 years after the attack (Schlenger *et al.* 2002; Yehuda, 2002) and that children, in particular, have been affected. A substantial proportion of children in New York had severe (18%) or moderate (66%) post-traumatic stress reactions (Fairbrother *et al.* 2003). It is important to realize that it is not only those who are wounded in accidents, disasters, wars, or acts of terrorism who run the risk of developing traumatic stress reactions, but also survivors, rescued and evacuated individuals, leaders, rescue workers, and health-care personnel, not to mention families, friends, and colleagues.

Types of traumatic stress

Post-traumatic stress responses, with their secondary ill-effects, may be caused by brief or single overwhelming events, such as accidents, disasters, violent assault, etc. When the trauma has been fairly circumscribed and of limited duration—what we usually label as type I traumatic stress—manifest and enduring symptoms of PTSD are usually only seen in those who have been exposed to particularly intense traumatization or who have been more vulnerable. However, additional secondary problems, such as affective disorder, substance abuse, and social and relational problems, are frequently seen, and these conditions all increase the risk of suicide, which has, indeed, been observed in a number of studies of traumatized groups (Davidson *et al.* 1991; Adams and Lehnert 1997). Examples of type II traumatic stress exposure—the long-lasting or chronic traumatization—are prolonged childhood abuse, long-term violent relationships, combat stress, concentration camp experiences, and torture (Herman 1992). Under such conditions the person must adapt in some way to a situation where further traumatic exposure is very likely and where there is little support or protection, or possibility for recovery (Adams and Lehnert 1997). Type II traumatic stress seems to have the tendency to create more complex clinical stress responses, such as personality disturbances, dissociation, and behavioural changes (Herman 1992; Allen 2001), and to be associated with self-destructive behaviour ranging from self-mutilation to completed suicide (Molnar *et al.* 2001; Ystgaard *et al.* 2004).

Post-traumatic stress disorder

To be given a diagnosis of PTSD according to DSM-IV (American Psychiatric Association 1994) a person must have been exposed to an extremely stressful event involving intense fear, helplessness, or horror. The diagnosis also requires that the person shows symptoms within three different categories, namely: (1) re-experiencing of the stressful event; (2) avoidance of stimuli that remind them of the event; and (3) symptoms of hyperarousal. Re-experiencing of the event includes distressing and intrusive recollections of the event, such as images, dreams, or flashbacks. Avoidance symptoms include avoiding persons, places, or things that set off feelings about the incident. Symptoms of hyperarousal refer to reactions such as sleep disturbances, concentration problems, irritability or aggressiveness, hypervigilance, and increased startle reactions. Symptoms must lead to impairment in important areas of function, the duration must be at least 1 month, and the symptoms usually start within 3 months after the trauma. Other traumatic stress-related syndromes include acute stress disorder (duration of symptoms less than 1 month) (American Psychiatric Association 1994) and complex PTSD (Roth *et al.* 1997).

As mentioned previously, not all individuals who are exposed to traumatic stress develop PTSD or other stress-related syndromes. A range of additional factors are involved in the pathogenesis of these disorders, and, although it is beyond the scope of this chapter to give a complete description of these factors, I will discuss some of them in the following. First, however, we will take a closer look at what evidence there is for a connection between exposure to traumatic stress and later suicidal behaviour in various segments of the population.

Suicidal behaviour in different groups exposed to traumatic stress

Our knowledge of the possible association between traumatic stress and suicidal behaviour stems not only from specific studies of this issue but also from parts of the suicidological research literature containing indirect relevant information on this topic. The emphasis of specific studies has predominantly been on the relationship between suicidal behaviour and exposure to childhood adversities and to war-zone trauma, whereas studies of disaster survivors or victims of violence, such as assault, rape, and torture, are relatively scarce. One of the few population-based investigations analysing both the prevalence of traumatic events in general and the prevalence of suicidal behaviour, including the association between these phenomena, is the study carried out by Goldney and co-workers (Goldney *et al.* 2000). They found that traumatic events had a substantial association with suicidal ideation, with a population-attributable risk of 38%. The population-attributable risk is a measure expressing the proportion of a disease that can be associated with exposure to a risk factor (Caughlin *et al.* 1994).

Traumatic loss and separation

Turning to specific types of trauma, one classic variant is traumatic loss by death or other separation. A large fraction of the suicide research literature provides evidence that both suicide attempters and completers have experienced such trauma significantly more often than the general population, either early in life (Wasserman and Cullberg 1989; Bron *et al.* 1991) or at a later stage (Qin and Mortensen 2003). However, such an increased risk of suicidal behaviour may not necessarily be due to a direct traumatic effect. There is evidence that the consequences for a child of a parental loss is primarily a function of how the remaining parent copes with the situation and whether or not the child's daily environment is changed for the worse as a consequence of the loss (Adams *et al.* 1982). The remaining parent's ability to help the child to cope with the bereavement is of crucial importance. Direct traumatic effects are, however, commonly seen in cases where people are made witness to the sudden, unexpected, or violent death of others, and in particular of people with which they have a close relationship. That this exposure is associated with later suicidal behaviour has been particularly well documented in studies of people bereaved by suicide (Ness and Pfeffer 1990; Prigerson *et al.* 1999).

Childhood physical and sexual abuse

Perhaps the clearest indication of an association between traumatic exposure and an increased risk of suicidal behaviour is derived from research into childhood adversities. There is strong evidence that childhood physical and sexual abuse increase the risk of both adolescent and adult self-harm and suicidal behaviours; this has been demonstrated in a range of studies over the past decade, both in community samples (Davidson *et al.* 1996; Silverman *et al.* 1996; Bensley *et al.* 1999; Molnar *et al.* 2001) and various clinical settings, including primary care (Gould *et al.* 1994), general hospital care (Ystgaard *et al.* 2004) and psychiatric care (Briere and Zaidi 1989; Brown and Anderson 1991; Kaplan *et al.* 1995; Briere *et al.* 1997; Lipschitz *et al.* 1999). However, one of the questions that remains unresolved is whether childhood sexual abuse (CSA) leads to an increased risk of *completed suicide* (White and Widom 2003). The odds ratio for *attempted suicide* in adults with a past history of abuse has been found to be up to 25 (Santa Mina and Gallop 1998). The prevalence of childhood sexual abuse is high. In the US National Comorbidity Survey (Molnar *et al.* 2001) of a large and representative sample from the general population, it was reported to be 2.5% among men and 13.5% in women. Thus it is not surprising that the population attributable risk for child sexual abuse has been estimated to be 9–20% of suicide attempts (Brown *et al.* 1999; Molnar *et al.* 2001). The risk of attempted suicide on the basis of adverse childhood experiences seems to be elevated throughout the life span (Dube *et al.* 2001), although a number of other risk factors, such as mental disorders, substance abuse, and additional stressful life events, not surprisingly, plays an equally important role. The risk of repeated suicidal behaviour has been particularly well documented in individuals having been exposed to child-hood *sexual* abuse (Brown and Anderson 1999, Ystgaard *et al.* 2004). Many clinicians tend to regard repeated or chronic suicidal behaviour in a young female patient as a relatively strong indicator of history of CSA. A large proportion of these chronically self-destructive young patients have been shown to have cluster B personality disorders and/or PTSD. The combination of these characteristics has been proposed as a separate syndrome—complex PTSD. There is growing evidence that chronically self-destructive or self-mutilating individuals with a history of CSA also tend to have characteristics such as problems with aggression and impulsivity, and other behaviours consistent with borderline personality disorder (Stanley *et al.* 2001).

Violence, rape, and torture

Regrettably, there is no end to the variation in the types of violence encountered among humans, even during peacetime in developed societies; in private homes, in the streets, in schools, and other institutions such as jails. The problem increases considerably if we include other regions of the world or take a look back into our own, not too remote, past. Despite the magnitude of the problem of violence, there is a great lack of systematic knowledge about the consequences of violence for the individual, in terms of the risk of suicidal behaviour. Some studies have demonstrated an association between rape and subsequent suicidal ideation (Dahl 1989) and suicidal behaviour (Ullman and Brecklin 2002). Women who have been the victims of CSA and then suffer adult sexual assault seem to have a particularly high lifetime risk of suicide attempts, controlling for demographic factors and other psychosocial characteristics (Cloitre *et al.* 1997; Ullman and Brecklin 2002).

Ferrada-Noli *et al.* (1998*a*) found a clear co-variation between traumatic exposure, PTSD, and suicidal behaviour in their interview study of refugees having experienced imprisonment, torture, mock executions, and/or sexual violence. In the group of torture victims having displayed manifest suicidal behaviour, these researchers were actually able to demonstrate an association between the torture method the victim had been exposed to and the subject's preference for suicide attempt method (Ferrada-Noli *et al.* 1998*b*); for example, water torture was associated with attempted suicide by drowning, and torture with the use of sharp instruments was associated with suicide methods such as stabbing or cutting.

War-zone trauma

Durkheim's classical observation that, during times of war, suicide rates will decline in the general population—particularly in the male population— (Durkheim 1897) seems still to be valid and has been confirmed in studies from recent wars (Grubisic-Ilic *et al.* 2002). This is explained as an effect of increased social integration and social cohesion within society taking place during periods of external threat. It is interesting to note that these mechanisms seem also to be operative under conditions such as the 11 September 2001 attacks on New York. In a study by Salib (2003) on suicide rates in England and Wales, the month of September 2001 was characterized by a significantly lower rate than in September of any of the preceding 22 years. When discussing the possible effects of war on suicide rates in those affected it is important therefore to remember that protective mechanisms, such as increased social cohesion, might be operative. However, for those who have actually been exposed directly to war-zone trauma, effects at a group level seem to be predominantly detrimental.

The best epidemiological evidence for this has been established through studies in the United States after the Vietnam War. The very large US Vietnam veterans population (of more than 5 million individuals) has been shown to have a significantly increased standardized mortality ratio (SMR) for suicide, particularly those who had a diagnosis of PTSD (Bullman and Kang 1994) or had been wounded (Bullman and Kang 1996). In other studies, Vietnam veterans have also been shown to have increased levels of suicidal ideation and history of suicide attempts, and again these phenomena seem to be highly correlated with a diagnosis of PTSD. With additional diagnoses, particularly depression, there is an even stronger association (Hendin and Haas 1991; Kramer *et al.* 1994). The problems of modern warfare, the complex roles and tasks of military personnel, and the problems veterans have in readjusting to a peaceful society, have been highlighted in recent studies on peace-keeping. Exposure to combat and other war-zone stress has indeed been found to be a very strong predictor of the development of PTSD in veterans from such military operations, both in a short- (Litz *et al.* 1997) and long-term perspective (Mehlum and Weisæth

2002). In a recent study by Thoresen *et al.* (2003), investigating the mortality up to 17 years after completion of service, with a trace rate of 97% of the cohort, a significantly elevated suicide mortality (SMR = 1.4) was found. In this cohort the SMR seemed to increase with the number of years after service.

We have focused on some of the areas in which research into the possible association between traumatic stress and suicide has reached an acceptable level, both in terms of quantity and quality. Many other specific types of trauma or exposed groups could have been mentioned, but in the majority of these cases the research evidence is still too weak. Whereas there is obviously a continued need for research into these areas, we can conclude at this point that there is sound proof from clinical and epidemiological studies of an association between exposure to traumatic stress and an increased risk of a range of suicidal behaviours. However, so far we have not discussed the nature of this association.

Traumatic stress and suicidal behaviour: possible pathways and mediating mechanisms

When discussing possible mediating mechanisms, we are faced with the problem that there might be multiple simultaneous trauma. To disentangle the effects of one trauma from another is often impossible. In this section we will limit ourselves to discussing some possible pathways to suicide, or mediating mechanisms between traumatic stress in general and suicide, remembering that it is possible that several parallel or combined mechanisms may exist.

Dose–response relationship

For several types of traumatic exposure there seems to exist a dose–response relationship concerning the capacity of a stressor to increase the risk of suicidal behaviour. The 'dose' might be considered in terms of the severity of the trauma, the duration, the number of incidents, the degree of threat to life, and even such factors as whether or not the trauma was a result of a wilful act or an accident. Studies have demonstrated a dose–response relationship for CSA (Santa Mina and Gallop 1998, Molnar *et al.* 2001). Regarding war-related traumatic exposure, there is clear evidence of a dose–response relationship for the risk of developing PTSD (Fontana and Rosenheck 1994), but a direct correlation with suicide risk has not been documented firmly.

Via development of mental disorder

Some studies have suggested that PTSD functions as a mediating variable between traumatic exposure and depression and suicidal behaviour (Mazza and Reynolds 1999). As we have indicated above, in many groups having been exposed to traumatic stress there seems to be a substantial overlap between the presence of suicidal behaviour and PTSD; one of these groups is victims of CSA, who run an increased risk of developing PTSD (Widom 1999). In the DSM-IV field trial for PTSD, when subjects with PTSD were checked for a wide range of factors that might be related to the disorder, two-thirds of subjects who had been exposed to abuse before the age of 14 were found to have a history of suicidal behaviour. Fewer of those who had been exposed to abuse later in life reported such behaviours. In subjects with PTSD who had been exposed to a disaster, substantially fewer had a reported history of suicidal behaviour (van der Kolk *et al.* 1991). Wunderlich and co-workers (Wunderlich *et al.* 1998) investigated psychiatric co-morbidity and suicidal behaviour in a random sample of 3021 adolescents and young adults aged 14–24 years, and indicated that there was a particularly high risk of suicide attempts in subjects diagnosed with PTSD. Oquendo *et al.* (2003) found the same, but added that there was a significantly increased rate of suicide attempts among patients with co-morbid PTSD and major depressive episode. There is generally a very high co-morbidity between PTSD and depressive disorder (van der Kolk *et al.* 1991) and there is probably a cumulative effect of these disorders on risk of suicide.

The question whether or not suicide risk is completely mediated through the development of mental disorder has been debated. Studies addressing this question within the context of traumatized individuals have mainly been performed in the field of CSA. In the comprehensive longitudinal study by Ferguson and co-workers (2000), where 1265 children in New Zealand were followed over the course of 21 years, the researchers found that none of the childhood trauma predicted suicidal behaviour independent of mental illness and stressful life events in adolescence. In contrast, data of Molnar and co-workers from the US National Comorbidity Study (Molnar *et al.* 2001) indicated that a significant proportion (20–30%) of suicide attempts were not related to psychopathology. When discussing the role of mental disorder in the wake of traumatic exposure, we should avoid oversimplifying matters. A diagnosis such as PTSD must, of course, be broken down and analysed in detail, in order to understand better what specific aspects of the syndrome could play a role in a complex suicidal process. One example of such an approach is the clinical study of Amir *et al.* (1999) of patients with and without PTSD, which indicated that the increased suicide risk of PTSD patients was significantly correlated with unfavourable scores on coping dimensions.

Dissociative mechanisms

Dissociative symptoms are frequently seen in individuals who have been exposed to traumatic stress, although the relationship between trauma and dissociation is far from linear. One common definition of dissociation is that it is a disruption in the usually integrated functions of consciousness, memory, identity, and perception of the environment (American Psychiatric Association 1994). It includes phenomena such as amnesia, depersonalization, derealization, personality disturbances (such as multiple personality), and, in extreme cases, psychotic reactions. One way of understanding dissociative symptoms is to view them as methods of detachment from the trauma; this serves at least in a short time perspective as a psychological, and often also physical, survival strategy and defensive mechanism against unbearable and otherwise inescapable physical and mental pain. However, with repeated or prolonged traumatic exposure this often develops into an habitual response, representing a highly inadequate coping strategy. Studies have demonstrated that individuals with repeated self-harm or chronic self-mutilation tend to have an increased number of dissociative symptoms (van der Kolk *et al.* 1991). According to Orbach (1994), this tendency to choose escape instead of encounter may enhance a sense of hopelessness and helplessness and the development of self-destructive behaviour. Thus, in the long run, dissociation constitutes part of the vulnerability state. This may predispose to self-destructive behaviour in subjects who are exposed to repeated trauma while trapped in an invalidating, non-supportive environment.

Overgeneral autobiographical memory

How this dysfunctional coping strategy leads to suicidal behaviour has been described from a different perspective by Mark Williams and co-workers. They have demonstrated that suicidal patients have problems with recalling specific autobiographic memories (Williams *et al.* 1996). Suicidal individuals tend to respond in a more general, or less specific, way than control subjects when asked to recall an event from their past that made them happy. Williams hypothesizes that such patients may suffer a bombardment of intrusive memories from past trauma and that their overgeneral memory may then be viewed as a strategy to regulate emotion: 'They stop short of recalling specific memories lest it brings up a traumatic event' (Williams *et al.* 1996). Whereas this defensive tendency of retrieving memories in a less specific way may give an instantaneous protection and relief, it has been claimed that in the long run it may also reduce the person's efficient use of their memory database in daily problem-solving challenges (Raes *et al.* 2003). Deficiency in problem solving is typical for many suicidal individuals. This way of viewing dissociative symptoms probably seems very plausible to many clinicians as it fits well with experiences from clinical practice, but it remains to be confirmed in clinical studies. An interesting observation was made by Startup and co-workers

(2001) in a study of patients with borderline personality disorder, where those who showed greatest overgeneral recall reported fewest parasuicidal acts. The researchers hypothesized that overgeneral autobiographical recall may serve as a defensive mechanism for borderline individuals, helping them to avoid otherwise intruding and distressing memories, and thus possibly reducing the tendency towards self-destructive behaviour.

Research into traumatic stress is currently being carried out along several different lines involving the brain's memory systems. Hopefully, some of this research will lead to therapeutic measures that can help reduce the frequency with which traumatized individuals succumb to suicide. This example is the suicide note of a 17-year-old boy:

> Why I have chosen to take my own life? From I was four years old till I became 9, I was sexually abused. I just can't stand it any more. It is something that I will never be able to put behind me. The memories and inner pictures are so vivid. And it is as if my self-confidence has been crushed against a rock.

Other cognitive mechanisms and maladaptive coping

To complete our consideration of cognitive mechanisms possibly linking trauma and suicidal behaviour, we should also mention some very well-known disturbances often described in groups of suicidal individuals encountered in clinical settings. Such cognitive disturbances include (among others) low self-esteem, helplessness, hopelessness, rigid or dichotomous thinking, selective perceptions, and false attributions of causality to oneself. We commonly describe these psychological disturbances as parts of depressive states. However, in some studies they have been analysed within a trauma perspective. Cognitive disturbances are most frequently seen in the wake of type II trauma, particularly CSA (Kendall-Tackett 2002). Abused children are regrettably often trapped in a chronic state of helplessness, powerlessness, and intense fear, making them victims, not survivors. Such an inescapable dead-end life situation probably has a very powerful influence over basic patterns of thinking, coping, and regulation of emotions, through which self-destructive behaviour may evolve as one maladaptive solution. Hopelessness and an external locus of control (Allen and Tarnowski 1989; Brown *et al.* 1998) have indeed been found as frequent features of abused children who display suicidal behaviour. This also holds for low self-esteem and a negative attributional style (Fergusson *et al.* 2000). Although less evidence exists from studies of other groups exposed to type II trauma, it is natural to assume that similar mechanisms may also exist in these contexts.

When discussing pathways to suicidal behaviour, we very often put our emphasis on the perspective of *causality*. We should, however, also consider suicidal processes from a perspective of *intentionality*. Maladaptive as it may be, self-destructive behaviour can be viewed as a self-regulatory mechanism with respect to mood and behaviour. Many chronically self-destructive individuals report that their main reasons for self-harm are to ease tension and to get relief from intense feelings of pain, emptiness, or numbing that have built up, or even to obtain a feeling of euphoria. Others report that self-harm helps them acquire a sense of control over themselves or get a firmer grip over reality when faced with dissociative symptoms. Other, not uncommon, motives for suicidal behaviour include obtaining or maintaining influence over the behaviour of others, or expressing anger or revengeful feelings towards others. In a study by Mehlum and co-workers (2003), motives and intentions such as those mentioned here were significantly more frequently reported by suicide attempters who were diagnosed as having PTSD than by other suicide attempters.

This presentation of possible pathways from trauma to suicide, and the mediating mechanisms involved, could have been extended substantially. We might, for example, have discussed the possibilities of trauma leading to increased suicide risk through the potentially harmful effects on social attachment capacity and the ability to form intimate and stable relationships with others. Trauma victims frequently report that they lack the normal feeling of invulnerability that the majority of people have ('It can't happen to me' or 'It can't happen here') and instead they are stuck with a feeling of foreboding. Finally, there are some existential aspects that might have been mentioned, such as the perception of profound loss of meaning and cohesion, or the lost sense of having value and identity, that are seen in numerous traumatized individuals. Even existentially-linked guilt feelings may be associated with suicidal behaviour in the wake of trauma, as demonstrated in studies of Hendin and Haas (1991) and Fontana and Rosenheck (1994) in combat veterans from the Vietnam War, where things the veterans had done as soldiers haunted them in the years afterwards and increased the risk of suicidal behaviour.

Rather than examining all these issues further, the rest of this chapter is devoted to discussion of some implications of these findings for suicide prevention and clinical practice.

Some implications for suicide prevention and clinical practice

That suicidal behaviour in a wide range of groups and settings, both in the general population and in clinical populations, may have origins in various forms of traumatic stress seems well documented. However, mediating mechanism and pathways are still not well understood and there is a great need for increased research into these complex conditions. This research should attempt to integrate knowledge from both the psychotraumatological and suicidological fields, and with a biopsychosocial approach. However, in clinical, everyday reality, many patients risk not having the traumatic origins of their problems addressed when they present with suicidal symptoms. Or, conversely, symptoms of suicide risk are overlooked when traumatic stress is the presenting problem. A reason for this poorly integrated practice may be that both suicide and many forms of traumatic stress (CSA, intrafamilial violence, etc.) are still fairly taboo themes, hence clinicians and patients, as well as relatives, may wish to avoid them if possible, because of their tendency to create unpleasant feelings, such as anxiety, guilt feelings, or helplessness. Another obvious reason for the lack of an integrative approach is that many clinicians lack adequate knowledge about the link between traumatic stress and suicidal behaviour. Perhaps the most important thing we could do to improve practice is to increase the knowledge in gatekeepers and clinicians who have the responsibility for evaluating suicidal patients and planning their treatments in both the short and longer term.

Another way to ensure that traumatic stress is not overlooked in the clinical evaluation process is to create better instruments for systematic assessment that identify the different types of trauma and the role they may play in the development of self-destructive behaviour. Some such instruments do exist, but they appear not to be in very widespread use. They are also poorly integrated with assessment instruments for general psychiatric symptomatology. Assessment of traumatic origins of symptoms is also important for planning treatment for patients in suicidal crises.

Only a fraction of those at risk for suicide at any given time will undergo an expert evaluation of their suicidality and related problems. Furthermore, if it is true that not all suicidal behaviour in the wake of traumatic stress is mediated through psychopathology, we need to develop screening or detection procedures that can be applied in non-clinical populations in a variety of settings. One such obvious arena is the school system, where increased attention must be paid to the needs of children who have been exposed to sexual and/or other abuse, and those who may be experiencing ongoing abuse. Since the link between CSA and suicidal behaviour is particularly well documented, early detection and intervention for *all* traumatized children and adolescents is of utmost importance. School is, however, the only arena on which we can hope to reach some of the most at-risk groups of children—those who have parents with severe mental disorders, substance abuse, or other problems impairing their capacity to protect their children against abuse.

How treatment programmes for victims of CSA and the many other groups of individuals who have been exposed to traumatic stress should be designed falls outside the scope of this text. However, the general need to incorporate suicide risk assessments in the clinical evaluation and treatment planning for these groups must be underlined. Fortunately, over the past decade we have seen substantial improvements in preventive intervention models and treatments for trauma-exposed groups (for a recent update, see Orner and Schnyder 2003) and in some programmes suicide risk has indeed been addressed more systematically (Andreassen *et al.* 2002; Ekblad and Wasserman 2002).

Conclusion

With some significant exceptions, the field of traumatic stress research has, so far, only included the study of suicidal behaviour related to trauma to a very limited degree. One reason may be that suicidality in this context may be linked to some of the most problematic aspects of psychological trauma; namely helplessness, lack of control, sense of worthlessness, and loss of meaning. For clinicians to encounter such feelings in patients is potentially very painful and frightening, and hence they often avoid addressing them and the associated suicide themes. Similarly, since traumatic exposure is often overlooked in clinical settings where it is not the presenting complaint, it often goes undetected in groups of suicidal patients. In the years to come we need to increase clinicians' knowledge and develop more treatment models that integrate knowledge from trauma-focused therapies with important knowledge from suicidology.

References

Adams, D.M. and Lehnert, K.L. (1997). Prolonged trauma and subsequent suicidal behaviour: child abuse and combat trauma reviewed. *Journal of Traumatic Stress*, 10, 619–34.

Adams, K.S., Buckoms, A., and Streiner, D. (1982). Parental loss and family stability in attempted suicide. *Archives of General Psychiatry*, 39, 1081–5.

Allen, D.M. and Tarnowski, K.J. (1989). Depressive characteristics of physically abused children. *Journal of Abnormal Child Psychology*, 17, 1–11.

Allen, J.G. (2001). *Traumatic relationships and serious mental disorders*. John Wiley & Son, Chichester.

American Psychiatric Association (1980). *Diagnostic and statistical manual of mental disorders: DSM-III*. American Psychiatric Press, Washington, DC.

American Psychiatric Association (1994). *Diagnostic and statistical manual of mental disorders: DSM-IV*. American Psychiatric Press, Washington, DC.

Amir, M., Kaplan, Z., Efroni, R., and Kotler, M. (1999). Suicide risk and coping styles in posttraumatic stress disorder patients. *Psychotherapy and Psychosomatics*, 68, 76–81.

Andreassen, A.L., Thoresen, S., and Mehlum, L. (2002). Veterans from peacekeeping: evaluation of a follow-up programme. *Prehospital and Disaster Medicine*, 17, 7.

Bensley, L.S., Van Eenwyk, J., Spieker, S.J., and Schoder, J. (1999). Self-reported abuse history and adolescent problem behaviors. I. Antisocial and suicidal behaviors. *Journal of Adolescent Health*, 24, 63–172.

Brady, K.T., Killeen, T.K., Brewerton, T., and Lucerini, S. (2000). Comorbidity of psychiatric disorders and posttraumatic stress disorder. *Journal of Clinical Psychiatry*, 61 (suppl. 7), 22–32.

Breslau, N., Davis, G.C., Andreski, P., and Peterson, E.L. (1991). Traumatic events and posttraumatic stress disorder in an urban population of young adults. *Archives of General Psychiatry*, 48, 216–22.

Breslau, N., Kessler, R.C., Chilcoat, H.D., Schultz, L.R., Davis, G.C., and Andreski, P. (1998). Trauma and posttraumatic stress disorder in the community: The 1996 Detroit Area Survey of Trauma. *Archives of General Psychiatry*, 55, 626–32.

Briere, J. and Zaidi, L.Y. (1989). Sexual abuse history and sequelae in female psychiatric emergency room patients. *American Journal of Psychiatry*, 146, 1602–6.

Briere, J., Woo, R., McRae, B., Foltz, J., and Sitzman, R. (1997). Lifetime victimization history, demographics, and clinical status in female psychiatric emergency room patients. *Journal of Nervous and Mental Disease*, 185, 95–101.

Bron, B., Strack, M., and Rudolph G. (1991). Childhood experiences of loss and suicide attempts: Significance in depressive states of major depressed and dysthymic or adjustment disordered patients. *Journal of Affective Disorders*, 23, 165–72.

Brown, G.R. and Anderson, B. (1991). Psychiatric morbidity in adult inpatients with childhood histories of sexual and physical abuse. *American Journal of Psychiatry*, 148, 55–61.

Brown, J., Cohen, P., Johnson, J.G., and Salzinger, S. (1998). A longitudinal analysis of risk factors for child maltreatment: Findings of a 17-year prospective study of officially recorded and self-reported child abuse and neglect. *Child Abuse and Neglect*, 22, 1065–78.

Brown, J., Cohen, P., Johnson, J.G., and Smailes, E.M. (1999). Childhood abuse and neglect: specificity of effects on adolescent and young adult depression and suicidality. *Journal of the American Academy of Child and Adolescent Psychiatry*, 38, 1490–6.

Bullman, T.A. and Kang, H.K. (1994). Posttraumatic stress disorder and the risk of traumatic deaths among Vietnam veterans. *Journal of Nervous and Mental Disease*, 182, 604–10.

Bullman, T.A. and Kang, H.K. (1996). The risk of suicide among wounded Vietnam veterans. *American Journal of Public Health*, 86, 662–7.

Caughlin, S., Benichou, J., and Weed, D.L. (1994) Attributable risk estimation in case-control studies. *Epidemiological Review*, 16, 51–63.

Cloitre, M., Scarvalone, P., and Difede, J.A. (1997). Posttraumatic stress disorder, self-and interpersonal dysfunction among sexually retraumatized women. *Journal of Traumatic Stress*, 10, 437–52.

Dahl, S. (1989). Acute response to rape—a PTSD variant. *Acta Psychiatrica Scandinavica*, Suppl., 355, 56–62.

Davidson, J.R.T., Hughes, D., Blazer, D.G., and George, L.K. (1991). Post-traumatic stress-disorder in the community – an epidemiological study. *Psychological Medicine*, 21, 713–21.

Davidson, J.R.T., Huges, D.C., George, L.K., and Blazer, D.G. (1996). The association of sexual assault and attempted suicide within the community. *Archives of General Psychiatry*, 53, 550–5.

Dube, S.R., Anda, R.F., Felitti, V.J., Chapman, D.P., Williamson, D.F., and Giles, W.H. (2001). Childhood abuse, household dysfunction, and the risk of attempted suicide throughout the life span: findings from the Adverse Childhood Experiences Study. *Journal of the American Medical Association*, 286, 3089–96.

Durkheim, É. (1897). *Suicide – a study in sociology* (republished in 1952 by Routledge and Kegan Paul, London).

Ekblad, S. and Wasserman, D. (2002). *Tidig upptäckt och preventiv behandling av asylsökande i riskzonen för självmord*. National Institute of Psychosocial Medicine, Stockholm.

Fairbrother, G., Stuber, J., Galea, S., Fleischman, A.R., and Pfefferbaum, B. (2003). Posttraumatic stress reactions in New York City children after the September 11, 2001, terrorist attacks. *Ambulatory Pediatrics*, 3, 304–11.

Fergusson, D.M., Woodward, L.J., and Horwood, L.J. (2000). Risk factors and life processes associated with the onset of suicidal behaviour during adolescence and early adulthood. *Psychological Medicine*, 30, 23–39.

Ferrada-Noli, M., Asberg, M., Ormstad, K., Lundin, T., and Sundbom, E. (1998*a*). Suicidal behavior after severe trauma. Part 1: PTSD diagnoses, psychiatric comorbidity, and assessments of suicidal behavior. *Journal of Traumatic Stress*, 11, 103–12.

Ferrada-Noli, M., Asberg, M., and Ormstad, K. (1998*b*). Suicidal behavior after severe trauma. Part 2: The association between methods of torture and of suicidal ideation in posttraumatic stress disorder. *Journal of Traumatic Stress*, 11, 113–24.

Fontana, A. and Rosenheck, R. (1994). Traumatic war stressors and psychiatric symptoms among World War II, Korean, and Vietnam War veterans. *Psychology of Aging*, 9, 27–33.

Goldney, R.D., Wilson, D., Dal Grande, E., Fisher, L.J., and McFarlane, A.C. (2000). Suicidal ideation in a random community sample: attributable risk due to depression and psychosocial and traumatic events. *Australia and New Zealand Journal of Psychiatry*, 34, 98–106.

Gould, D.A., Stevens, N.G., Ward, N.G., Carlin, A.S., Sowell, H.E., and Gustafson, B. (1994). Self-reported childhood abuse in an adult population in a primary care setting. Prevalence, correlates, and associated suicide attempts. *Archives of Family Medicine*, 3, 252–6.

Grubisic-Ilic, M., Kozaric-Kovacic, D., Grubisic, F., and Kovacic, Z. (2002). Epidemiological study of suicide in the Republic of Croatia—comparison of war and post-war periods and areas directly and indirectly affected by war. *European Psychiatry*, 17, 259–64.

Hawton, K., Rodham, K., Evans, E., and Weatherall, R. (2002). Deliberate self harm in adolescents: self report survey in schools in England. *British Medical Journal*, 23, 1207–11.

Heikkinen, M., Aro, H., and Lonnqvist, J. (1994). Recent life events, social support and suicide. *Acta Psychiatr Scand Suppl.*, 377, 65–72.

Hendin, H. and Haas, A.P. (1991). Suicide and guilt as manifestations of PTSD in Vietnam combat veterans. *American Journal of Psychiatry*, 148, 586–91.

Herman, J.L. (1992). *Trauma and recovery*. Basic Books, New York.

International Federation of Red Cross and Red Crescent Societies. (1993). *World Disasters Report 1993*. Genera, IFRCRC.

Kaplan, M.L., Asnis, G.M., Lipschitz, D.S., and Chorney, P. (1995). Suicidal behavior and abuse in psychiatric outpatients. *Comprehensive Psychiatry*, 36, 229–35.

Kendall-Tackett, L. (2002). The health effects of childhood abuse: four pathways by which abuse can influence health. *Child Abuse and Neglect*, 26, 715–29.

Kessler, R.C., Sonnega, A., Bromet, E., Hughes, M., and Nelson, C.B. (1995). Posttraumatic stress disorder in the National Comorbidity survey. *Archives of General Psychiatry*, 52, 1048–60.

Kramer, T.L., Lindy, J.D., Green, B.L., Grace, M.C., and Leonard, A.C. (1994). The comorbidity of post-traumatic stress disorder and suicidality in Vietnam veterans. *Suicide and Life Threatening Behavior*, 24, 58–67.

Lipschitz, D.S., Winegar, R.K., Nicolaou, A.L., Hartnick, E., Wolfson, M., and Southwick, S.M. (1999). Perceived abuse and neglect as risk factors for suicidal behaviour in adolescent inpatients. *Journal of Nervous and Mental Disease*, 187, 32–9.

Litz, B.T., Orsillo, S.M., Friedman, M., Ehlich, P., and Batres, A. (1997). Posttraumatic stress disorder associated with peacekeeping duty in Somalia for U.S. military personnel. *American Journal of Psychiatry*, 154, 178–84.

Mazza, J.J. and Reynolds, W.M. (1999). Exposure to violence in young inner-city adolescents: relationships with suicidal ideation, depression, and PTSD symptomatology. *Journal of Abnormal Child Psychology*, 27, 203–13.

Mehlum, L. and Weisæth, L. (2002). Predictors of post-traumatic reactions in Norwegian UN peace-keepers seven years after service. *Journal of Traumatic Stress*, 15, 17–26.

Mehlum, L., Ystgaard, M., and Hestetun, I. (2003). Traumatic stress symptomatology – its influence on the clinical outcome in suicide attempters – a follow-up study. Paper presented at XXIIth congress of the International Association for Suicide Prevention, Stockholm, 10–14 September 2003.

Molnar, B.E., Buka, S.L., and Kessler, R.C. (2001) Child sexual abuse and subsequent psychopathology: results from the National Comorbidity Survey. *American Journal of Public Health*, 91, 753–60.

Ness, D.E. and Pfeffer, C.R. (1990). Sequelae of bereavement resulting from suicide. *American Journal of Psychiatry*, 147, 279–85.

Oquendo, M.A., Friend, J.M., Halberstam, B., Brodsky, B.S., Burke, A.K., Grunebaum, M.F., *et al.* (2003). Association of comorbid posttraumatic stress disorder and major depression with greater risk for suicidal behavior. *American Journal of Psychiatry*, 160, 580–2.

Orbach, I. (1994). Dissociation, physical pain, and suicide: a hypothesis. *Suicide and Life Threatening Behavior*, 24, 68–79.

Orner, R. and Schnyder, U. (ed.). (2003). *Reconstructing early intervention after trauma – Innovations in the care of survivors*. Oxford University Press, Oxford.

Prigerson, H.G., Bridge, J., Maciejewski, P.K., Beery, L.C., Rosenheck , R.A., Jacobs, S.C., *et al.* (1999). Influence of traumatic grief on suicidal ideation among young adults. *American Journal of Psychiatry*, 156, 1994–5.

Qin, P. and Mortensen, P.B. (2003). The impact of parental status on the risk of completed suicide. *Archives of General Psychiatry*, 60, 797–802.

Raes, F., Hermans, D., de Decker, A., Eelen, P., and Williams, J.M.G. (2003). Autobiographical memory specificity and affect regulation: an experimental approach. *Emotion*, 3, 201–6.

Roth, S., Newman, E., Pelcovitz, D., van der Kolk, B.A., and Mandel, F.S. (1997). Complex PTSD in victims exposed to sexual and physical abuse: results from the DSM-IV Field Trial for Posttraumatic Stress Disorder. *Journal of Traumatic Stress*, 10, 539–55.

Salib, E. (2003). Effect of 11 September 2001 on suicide and homicide in England and Wales. *British Journal of Psychiatry*, 183, 207–12.

Santa Mina, E.E. and Gallop, R.M. (1998). Childhood physical and sexual abuse and adult self-harm and suicidal behaviour: A literature review. *Canadian Journal of Psychiatry*, 43, 793–800.

Schlenger, W.E., Caddell, J.M., Ebert, L., Jordan, B.K., Rourke, K.M., Wilson, D., *et al.* (2002). Psychological reactions to terrorist attacks: findings from the National Study of Americans' Reactions to September 11. *Journal of the American Medical Association*, 288, 581–8.

Schuster, M.A., Bradley, D., Stein, B.D., Jaycox, L., Collins, R.L., Marshall, G.N., *et al.* (2001). A national survey of stress reactions after the September 11, 2001, terrorist attack. *New England Journal of Medicine*, 345, 1507–12.

Silverman, A.B., Reinherz, H.Z., and Giaconia, R.M. (1996). The long-term sequelae of child and adolescent abuse: A longitudinal community study. *Child Abuse and Neglect*, 20, 709–23.

Stanley, B., Gameroff, M.J., Michalsen, V., and Mann, J.J. (2001). Are suicide attempters who self-mutilate a unique population? *American Journal of Psychiatry*, 158, 427–32.

Startup, M., Heard, H., Swales, M., Jones, B., Williams, J.M.G., and Jones, R.S. (2001). Autobiographical memory and parasuicide in borderline personality disorder. *British Journal of Clinical Psychology*, 40, 113–20.

Thoresen, S., Mehlum, L., and Moller, B. (2003). Suicide in peacekeepers. A cohort study of mortality from suicide in 22,275 Norwegian veterans from international peacekeeping operations. *Social Psychiatry and Psychiatric Epidemiology*, 38, 605–10.

Ullman, S.E. and Brecklin, L.R. (2002). Sexual assault history and suicidal behavior in a national sample of women. *Suicide and Life Threatening Behavior*, 32, 117–30.

Van der Kolk, B.A., Perry, J.C., and Herman, J.L. (1991). Childhood origins of self-destructive behavior. *American Journal of Psychiatry*, 148, 1665–71.

Wasserman, D. and Cullberg, J. (1989). Early separation and suicidal behaviour in the parental homes of 40 consecutive suicide attempters. *Acta Psychiatrica Scandinavica*, 79, 296–302.

White, H.R. and Widom, C.S. (2003). Does childhood victimization increase the risk of early death? A 25-year prospective study. *Child Abuse and Neglect*, 27, 841–53.

Widom, C.S. (1999). Posttraumatic stress disorder in abused and neglected children grown up. *American Journal of Psychiatry*, 156 (8), 1223–9.

Williams, J.M., Ellis, N.C., Tyers, C., Healy, H., Rose, G., and MacLeod, A.K. (1996). The specificity of autobiographical memory and imageability of the future. *Memory and Cognition*, 24, 116–25.

Wunderlich, U., Bronisch, T., and Wittchen, H.U. (1998). Comorbidity patterns in adolescents and young adults with suicide attempts. *European Archives of Psychiatry and Clinical Neuroscience*, 248, 87–95.

Yehuda, R. (2002). Post-traumatic stress disorder. *New England Journal of Medicine*, 348, 108–14.

Ystgaard, M., Hestetun, I., Loeb, M., Schjelderup, G., and Mehlum, L. (2004). Does there exist a specific relationship between childhood sexual abuse and repeated suicidal behaviour. *Child Abuse and Neglect*, 28, 863–75.

Zimmerman, M. and Mattia, J.I. (1999). Is posttraumatic stress disorder underdiagnosed in routine clinical settings? *Journal of Nervous and Mental Disease*, 187 (7), 420–8.

9

Making mental health services safer

Louis Appleby, Nicola Swinson, and Navneet Kapur

Introduction

Suicide is among the top three causes of death among 15–34-year-olds world-wide (World Health Organization 2001). The World Health Organization has identified suicide prevention as a key priority. The reversal of rising trends in suicide and attempted suicide in Europe is a target as part of the 'Health for All' strategy. In the UK *Our Healthier Nation* targets a 20% reduction in the general population rate from 1997 to 2010 (Department of Health 1999*a*) and the *National Suicide Prevention Strategy for England* was published in 2002 (Department of Health 2002*a*). In the USA the Surgeon General released a 'Call to Action to Prevent Suicide' and a 'National Strategy for Suicide Prevention' in 1999, with the explicit goal of achieving a significant reduction in suicidal behaviour (Vastag 2001).

The National Confidential Inquiry into Suicide and Homicide by People with Mental Illness (Appleby *et al.* 2001) showed that 24% of suicides had been in recent contact with mental health services, approximately 1200 cases annually.

In order to move towards achieving the above targets, a broadly based suicide prevention strategy is required (Appleby 2001; De Leo 2002). However, statutory services do have an important role to play.

The aim of this chapter is to assess how we might make mental health services safer. Specifically, what role might mental health services have in reducing the rate of suicide? We address this question by general reference to previously published work and by specific reference to our own national survey of suicides by the mentally ill.

The role of mental illness in suicide

The lack of compelling evidence, in the form of controlled intervention studies, regarding the efficacy of suicide prevention measures in the mentally ill has led critics to doubt the efficacy of interventions (Geddes 1999). The following framework may be helpful when considering how mental health services might contribute to prevention:

- Who is at risk?
- When are they at risk?
- How do patients commit suicide?
- What is the link to mental health service activity?

Who is at risk?

Risk factors for suicide have low sensitivity and specificity, and therefore have limited clinical utility (Kapur 2000). Given the rarity of suicide, even in this high-risk group, accurate prediction of the majority of suicides without an unacceptably high false-positive rate is not possible (Powell *et al.* 2000). Consequently, services may have to accept that many patients may need to be targeted to prevent a few suicides. However, the components of suicide prevention, such as increased clinical supervision, encouragement of compliance, and improved patient management, will result in improved clinical care for severely ill patients.

Diagnoses

Severe mental illness has been shown, consistently to increase the risk of suicide (Foster *et al.* 1999; Mann 2002). A recent meta-analysis (Harris and Barraclough 1997) estimated that mental illness conferred a risk 11 times that of the general population, the highest risks occurring in anorexia nervosa, substance dependence, and depression. A case-control study of 149 suicides in Greater Manchester found risks higher than in many previous studies, and the extent of increased risk varied according to diagnosis and gender (Table 9.1) (Baxter and Appleby 1999). Risk was found to be increased more than tenfold in schizophrenia, affective disorders, and personality disorders in both genders, and in males with substance

Table 9.1 Common mental disorders and the risk of suicide compared to that of the general population (from Baxter and Appleby 1999)

Diagnosis	RR (95%CI), males	RR (95%CI), females
Schizophrenia	14.2 (9.19-α)	14.6 (8.80-α)
Affective disorders	12.2 (8.5-α)	16.3 (12.2-α)
Neuroses	2.1 (0.25-α)	7.9 (2.9-α)
Personality disorders	12.8 (6.6-α)	20.9 (9.6-α)
Substance dependence	14.29 (4.64-α)	0
Organic brain disease	3.3 (0.8-α)	0

RR, rate ratios.

dependence. Neurotic disorders carried an increased risk in females, but not males, and no increased risk was associated with organic brain disorders. Of particular note was the increased risk in personality disorders, particularly in females, where it was the highest for any diagnosis. Co-morbid secondary diagnoses have been shown to increase risk (Henriksson *et al.* 1993). A case-control psychological autopsy study in Northern Ireland reported odds ratios of 52.4 for Axis I (psychiatric) disorders but odds ratios of 346 if co-morbid with an Axis II (personality) disorder (Foster *et al.* 1999).

Independent risk factors

These diagnoses confer an increased risk generally, but a broader range of variables needs to be considered in order to identify and target effectively those at greatest risk. Clinical factors shown to increase risk independently in all diagnostic groups are: a history of deliberate self-harm (Appleby *et al.* 1999; Foster *et al.* 1999; King *et al.* 2001*a,b*), suicidal ideas during aftercare (Appleby *et al.* 1999), a family history of suicide or recent bereavement (Powell *et al.* 2000). Socio-demographic risk factors identified are: living alone (King *et al.* 2001*a*,) and current unemployment (Foster *et al.* 1999). However, some evidence suggests that conventional population risk factors for suicide do not adequately identify the potential for suicide in people with severe mental illness (King and Barraclough 1990; Beautrais *et al.*1998).

Variation in risk factors

Risk is dynamic; it can easily change, particularly as a result of an alteration in circumstances. Suicidal plans or deliberate self-harm during admission are known to increase risk (Powell *et al.* 2000). Other features shown to predict increased risk include low mood, hopelessness (King *et al.* 2001*b*), severe anhedonia, and severe anxiety or panic (Fawcett *et al.* 1987). Admission subsequent to worsening substance abuse (even in the absence of clinical evidence of relapse) has been shown to independently increase the risk of suicide (Fawcett *et al.* 1987).

Adverse life events

Traumatic or adverse life events, especially of an interpersonal nature, have also been shown to independently increase risk (Foster *et al.* 1999; Goldney *et al.* 2000; King *et al.* 2001*a*). A recent prospective longditudinal cohort study has further clarified the impact of traumatic events (Caspi *et al.* 2003). This study showed that individuals with either one or two copies of the short allele of the 5-HT T promoter polymorphism of the serotonin transporter gene, which promotes serotonin reuptake in cell membranes, exhibited more depressive symptoms, diagnosable depression, and suicidality after life events than individuals homozygous for the long allele. Although clearly posing ethical challenges, this evidence of gene-by-environment interaction may ultimately lead to identification of individuals most at risk of suicide.

When are they at risk?

Course of illness

Increased suicide risk is lifelong in people with mental illness, being present across age ranges and duration of illness. However, risk is not uniform and is highest in patients below the age of 30 years. In severe mental illness, risk is highest early on in the illness, being greatest during the 3 years after first contact. Indeed, the risk in the first year of illness is increased by 20 times for females and 30 times for males, compared with general population rates (Baxter and Appleby 1999). However, this may not apply to alcohol dependence and chronic conditions, where suicide risk is associated with long-term illness (Runeson *et al.* 1996).

In-patients

Individuals are at elevated risk during periods of in-patient care, with suicide rates of 137 per 100 000 in-patients being reported (Powell *et al.* 2000), or over 10 times the general population rate. Further in-patient data indicated that 47% of suicides occurred during the first admission, and 43% within the first week of admission (Busch *et al.* 2003).

After discharge

High rates of suicide following discharge from psychiatric care are well documented (Appleby *et al.* 1999; Ho 2003). A recent case-control study showed that over one-third of discharged patient suicides occurred within 1 month of discharge (King *et al.* 2001a). Increased risks of over 100 times the general population risk have been found in the month after discharge (Goldacre *et al.* 1993; Lewis *et al.* 1997). Risk has been shown to remain elevated at around 30–60 times the population rate for 1 year after discharge (Goldacre *et al.* 1993).

There are several possible explanations for the high risk following discharge from psychiatric care. Individuals may be re-exposed to stressors that may have precipitated the admission, may have increased access to means of suicide, and clinically may not have completely recovered. Insight may return, leading to a realization of the impact of mental illness. Although it is likely that the above have a cumulative effect, the predominant factor may be the rapid withdrawal of supervision. This may have implications for service delivery with regard to closer integration between in-patient and community mental health services, early access in crisis, and early follow-up of patients with severe mental illness.

How do patients commit suicide?

The methods of suicide predominantly used by psychiatric patients have clear implications for preventive strategies. In a large-scale, long-term follow-up study of suicide in psychiatric patients in Salford, the proportion of drug overdose was higher in women than in men (61.8% against 37.8%). Poisoning by gas (generally car exhaust) was mainly used by men (12.2% against 1.1%). Hanging was used in 12.9% of all suicides, with a preponderance of males, and jumping was the method in 14.6% of all suicides (Baxter and Appleby 1999). This contrasts with in-patient suicides, where hanging is the most common method used, followed by jumping from a height or in front of a moving vehicle (Busch *et al.* 2003).

What is the link to mental health service activity?

Intensity of care

An association has been shown between suicide rates and number of admissions (Baxter and Appleby 1999). A case-control study of aftercare in suicides showed that suicides were over three times more likely to have had their level of care reduced at their final outpatient appointment. This included decreasing frequency of outpatient clinic attendances and decreasing doses of medication. In over half of this sample the suicide occurred within 3 months of their care being reduced (Appleby *et al.* 1999).

Reasons for the association between reduction of care and subsequent suicide may include the fact that, for individuals who clinically deteriorated after the reduction in care, services were unable to detect or respond quickly to relapse. It is also possible that the level of care at the final appointment was necessary to prevent relapse and protect the patient from persistent suicide risk; hence, when the protective influence of intensity of care decreased, risk increased.

Breakdown of care is also independently associated with an increase in suicide risk in psychiatric in-patients (King *et al.* 2001*b*). Risk was shown to increase by a factor of 16 when significant professionals were on leave or leaving. If predisposed to suicide, this break in continuity of carer may be a final precipitating factor. A change in consultant since their previous admission was another independent risk factor, with continuous contact between discharge and follow-up exerting a protective influence.

This would seem to support the need for adequate continuity of care, early intervention where possible, and close supervision of patients, including encouragement with compliance, particularly at times of high risk.

Pharmacological interventions

There is a need for improved detection and adequate treatment of depression. Suicide has been linked to a lack of recognition, and therefore treatment, of depression (Rihmer *et al.* 1990; Isometsä *et al.* 1994). Swedish data showed a significant association between a 3.5-fold increase in antidepressant prescribing and reduction in suicide rates (Isacsson 2000). Hall *et al.* (2003) reported a clear relationship (which the authors suggested was causal) between increased antidepressant prescribing and decreased suicide mortality in Australia, with groups with the highest antidepressant exposure exhibiting the largest reductions in suicide rates.

Although it is not necessarily antidepressants *per se* that lead to the reduction in suicide, increased antidepressant prescribing may be a proxy measure for improved clinical management of depression, with closer supervision, regular risk assessment, support, and liaison with the family. Moreover, GPs are unlikely to use pharmacological therapy without psychosocial assessment and support. Their increase in prescribing of antidepressants would therefore appear to reflect increased recognition, diagnosis, and treatment of depression (Hall *et al.* 2003).

Broadly speaking, effectiveness within classes of medication are similar. However, interesting findings are emerging regarding patients on clozapine treatment. Reid *et al.* (1998) showed decreased suicide rates in schizophrenic patients receiving clozapine, but there was no randomization to treatment groups. This preliminary finding has been further investigated by the Inter-SePT trial; a 2-year, multicentre, randomized, controlled trial of clozapine compared with olanzapine (Meltzer *et al.* 2003). Patients on clozapine had significantly less suicidal behaviour, suicide attempts, and required fewer interventions or admissions to prevent suicide or concomitant antidepressants or anxiolytics. This is consistent with an increasing body of evidence from the US and the UK (Munro *et al.* 1999).

In the absence of satisfactory trials, some evidence exists that compliance with lithium therapy decreases suicide risk once prophylaxis is established (Tondo *et al.* 1998). There is a reduction in suicide rate in the long term for individuals attending lithium clinics. It is unclear whether this is influenced by other factors, such as compliance or clinic attendance *per se*, but it would appear that the combination of medication and attendance at specialized clinics is effective with regard to reduction of suicide risk.

A national survey of suicides by the mentally ill

The relatively low incidence of suicide means that, if it is used as an outcome measure in randomized trials, thousands of patients would be required in each treatment arm. There is, therefore, little evidence from intervention studies with respect to effective strategies in suicide prevention. An alternative strategy might be a comprehensive survey of suicides to establish patient characteristics and antecedents of suicide, including aspects of clinical care, thus allowing effective targeting of resources.

The National Confidential Inquiry into Suicide and Homicide by People with Mental Illness provides this in a comprehensive, national sample of all suicides and homicides by those with previous contact with psychiatric services in the UK (Appleby *et al.* 2001). This commenced in 1992, in association with the Royal College of Psychiatrists, and was re-established at the University of Manchester in 1996. The National Confidential Inquiry into Suicide and Homicide by People with Mental Illness now holds a comprehensive, national database. It is funded by the National Institute for Clinical Excellence, the Scottish Office (now the Scottish Executive), the Welsh Office, and the HSS Executive in Northern Ireland.

The main aims of the suicide inquiry are to collect detailed clinical data on people who die by suicide and have been in recent contact (within 12 months) with mental health services. Specific recommendations are then made for clinical practice and policy that may help to reduce the risk of suicide by people under the care of mental health services.

The Inquiry is particularly interested in the circumstances of suicide in specific 'priority groups'. Priority groups were selected on the basis of being at high risk or having greater treatment needs, or being likely to experience difficulty in maintaining contact with services. Examples of priority groups include patients who were in-patients at the time of the incident, were discharged from in-patient care less than 3 months earlier, or were subject to the Care Programme Approach at a level of supervision requiring regular multidisciplinary review. Other priority groups are patients who were not compliant with treatment, had missed their final appointment with services, were from an ethnic minority, or were homeless.

Methodology

Subjects and method

Data collection on suicides has three stages (Hunt *et al.* 2003): the collection of a comprehensive national sample, irrespective of mental health history; the identification of people within the sample who have been in contact with mental health services in the 12 months before death; and the collection of clinical data about these people.

Information on all deaths in England and Wales receiving a verdict of suicide or an open verdict at coroner's inquest is obtained from the Office for National Statistics (ONS) in England and Wales, and the General Register Offices (GRO) in Scotland and Northern Ireland. The cases presented here consist of suicides registered from 1 April 1996 until 31 March 2000. In the Inquiry open verdicts are included unless it is clear that suicide was not considered at inquest—for example, in deaths from an unexplained medical cause. Open verdicts are often reached in cases of suicide and are conventionally included in research on suicide (O'Donnell and Farmer 1995; Neeleman and Wessley 1997; Linsley *et al.* 2001) and in official suicide statistics.

Identifying details on each suicide are submitted to the main hospital and community trusts providing mental health services to the deceased's district of residence. When trust records show that contact has occurred in the 12 months before suicide, the person becomes an 'inquiry case'. All local mental health services in England and Wales regularly return data to the inquiry. Procedures are in place for direct reporting from units that have multi-district catchment areas, including regional forensic psychiatry units, or that have no catchment area, including national units and private hospitals.

For each inquiry case, the consultant is sent a questionnaire and asked to complete it after discussion with other members of the mental health team. The questionnaire consists of sections covering identification of priority groups, social/demographic characteristics, clinical history, details of suicide, aspects of care, details of final contact with services, and respondents' views on prevention. The social and clinical items reflect many of the most frequently reported risk factors for suicide. The majority of items are factual; a number (e.g. compliance) are based on the judgements of clinicians.

Findings

The National Confidential Inquiry has been notified of 36 683 suicides and probable suicides in England and Wales since April 1996, which corresponds to an average annual general population suicide rate of 10.0 per 100 000. Three-quarters were male, giving a male to female ratio of 3:1. This ratio was highest in 25–34-year-olds and lowest in the over 75 year group and is consistent with higher reported suicide rates among males, compared with females, worldwide (Cantor 2000). Three methods of suicide accounted for 71% of suicides—hanging (the most common overall), self-poisoning, and carbon monoxide poisoning. Frequencies varied between the sexes, hanging being most common in men and self-poisoning most common in women.

The Inquiry currently holds information on 8446 suicides known to have been in contact with mental health services in the preceding 12 months. The figures presented below refer to the 4859 cases collected during the first 4 years of data collection, starting in 1996 (a 95% response rate for the total of 5099 suicides in contact with services). This represents 24% of the total number of suicides in the general population during this time period, i.e. around 1250 suicides annually in England and Wales.

Socio-demographic and clinical characteristics

What are the socio-demographic and clinical characteristics of patients with mental disorder who complete suicide? Table 9.2 presents some data from the National Confidential Inquiry. Like suicides in the general population, males were over-represented. However, there was a smaller male to female ratio, 1.9:1. The age profile varied between sexes, with a peak incidence for males in the 25–34-year age group and a later, flatter peak for females (peak incidence in the 35–44-year age group).

The distribution of primary diagnoses is shown in Fig. 9.1. Over half of patients also had a secondary psychiatric diagnosis. Sixteen per cent of patients had been admitted to a psychiatric bed on more than five occasions. Two-thirds had a history of deliberate self-harm. Violence and substance misuse also featured prominently.

There were differences in clinical characteristics across age groups (Table 9.3). Suicides in young patients were more often characterized by schizophrenia, personality disorder, and alcohol or drug misuse. These diagnoses decreased proportionally with increasing age, whereas the proportion of affective disorders increased with age. Rates of co-morbidity were highest in younger age groups.

Table 9.2 Sociodemographic characteristics, clinical characteristics and aspects of care for 4859 suicides in contact with mental health services in England and Wales

Number	(*n* = 4859)	% (95% confidence interval)
Socio-demographic characteristics		
Median age (range)		41 (13–95)
Male	3198	66 (64–67)
Ethnic minority	282	6 (5–7)
Not currently married	3405	71 (70–73)
Unemployed/long-term sick	2765	58 (58–60)
Living alone	2006	43 (41–44)
Clinical characteristics		
Any secondary diagnosis	2460	52 (51–54)
Over 5 previous admissions	712	16 (15–17)
History of previous self-harm	3077	64 (63–66)
History of violence	920	19 (18–21)
History of alcohol misuse	1899	40 (38–41)
History of drug misuse	1348	28 (27–30)
Aspects of clinical care		
Last contact with services within 7 days	2308	48 (47–50)
Symptoms at last contact	2990	64 (63–65)
Out of contact with services	1153	29 (27–30)
Non-compliant with treatment	929	22 (21–24)

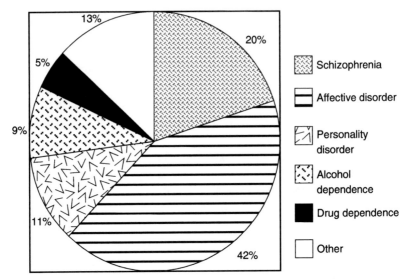

Fig. 9.1 Distribution of primary diagnoses among suicides by people with recent contact with mental health services, 1996–2000.

Suicides appeared to cluster in the first year after onset of illness: 21% occurred at this time and this was more common in those under 25 years and those over 65 years. The latter group tended to suffer from affective disorder and lower rates of previous deliberate self-harm, violence, and substance misuse.

A quarter of cases had never been admitted to psychiatric in-patient care and 16% had more than five previous admissions. This 'multiple admissions' group was larger in the 35–64-year range and was characterized by more severe mental illness and indicators of risk.

Table 9.3 Comparison of younger (35 years and under) and older (65 years and over) suicides in cases in the Confidential Inquiry, in terms of methods of suicide and psychiatric and other characteristics

	Younger	Older
Method	Hanging and overdose Jumping–height/moving vehicle	Hanging and overdose Drowning
Characteristics	Psychosis, personality disorder Substance abuse, co-morbidity Recent loss of contact with services Unemployed	Depression Physical illness Recent bereavement Isolation Suicide pacts (2%)

Methods of suicide

The most common methods of suicide in males and females in the Inquiry sample are shown in Fig.9.2.

Aspects of clinical care

Table 9.2 also shows aspects of clinical care for mentally ill suicides. Nineteen per cent had been in contact with services in the 24 hours prior to death and almost half within 7 days. Two-thirds had active symptoms at their last contact. Almost one-third of the sample were out of contact with services and one-fifth were non-compliant with treatment.

Immediate risk of suicide was reported by the clinicians to be low or absent in 85% of patients at the last contact. High immediate risk was identified in only 2%. This could be taken to suggest that once high risk is identified, preventive actions usually take place. However, long-term risk was judged to be moderate or high in 43% cases. In the majority of cases, the care plan was unchanged at the final contact and only 2% were detained under the Mental Health Act.

When asked regarding their views on prevention, respondents believed that suicide could have been prevented in over 20% cases. Features associated with these cases were a diagnosis of affective disorder, in-patient status, detectable symptoms at final contact, and being seen as moderate or high risk. Factors seen as decreasing the likelihood of suicide were: better compliance with treatment, closer patient supervision, closer contact with the family, and better staff training.

Antecedents to suicide

Common antecedents to suicide are shown in Table 9.4. The nature of adverse life events differed between age groups: relationship, family, childcare, and accommodation problems predominating in the young, whereas more older

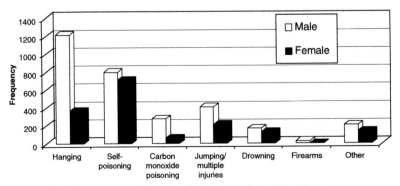

Fig. 9.2 Methods of suicide in the mentally ill, by gender, 1996–2000.

suicides experienced bereavement or anniversaries of bereavements, physical and family problems, and health problems in someone else.

Population subgroups

Ethnic minorities The data suggest that suicides in ethnic minorities were more often preceded by non-compliance or missed contact with services. Compared with the Inquiry sample as a whole, there was a much higher proportion of patients with schizophrenia and previous violence in the group of ethnic minorities, particularly in those of Caribbean origin, whereas Asians were less likely to be living alone.

Homeless Almost half of the homeless suicides were in-patients at the time of the suicide. This may be because they were less likely to be in contact with services in the community and were therefore more severely ill when admitted. A quarter had recently been discharged from in-patient care. The most common primary diagnosis was schizophrenia, followed by affective disorder and alcohol dependence. There were high rates of co-morbidity, substance misuse, and violence.

In-patients and those recently discharged

Those who die by suicide while in-patients, or shortly after discharge from hospital, are a particularly important group as, being in close proximity to care, they are potentially amenable to intervention.

Table 9.4 Common antecedents to suicide in patients with recent contact with mental health services (n = 4859)

Antecedent (last 3 months)	Number of suicides in contact with mental health services (%)
Adverse life events	2138 (44)
Suicidal ideation	1409 (29)
Disengagement	1312 (27)
Deliberate self-harm	1215 (25)
Non-compliance with treatment	923 (19)
Increased alcohol misuse	875 (18)
Bereavement	243 (5)
Clear evidence of relapse	1312 (27)
'Proxy indicators' of risk, e.g. increase substance misuse, self-harm, non-compliance	2381 (49)

In-patients A surprisingly high proportion of the Inquiry sample (16%) were in-patients at the time of death. This represents over 180 patients annually. They were a group with higher morbidity than the sample as a whole, the majority having severe mental illness (either schizophrenia or affective disorder) with significant levels of co-morbidity, deliberate self-harm, and social isolation. A quarter of in-patient suicides occurred during the first week of admission. The majority of ward suicides occurred by hanging. Most cases were voluntary patients on general adult psychiatry open wards under routine observation.

However, significant numbers were on higher levels of observation, absent without leave, or on agreed leave when the suicide occurred. A substantial minority of suicides occurred during intermittent observation (e.g. every 15 min). This method of ensuring safety is widely used across the UK, but has not been subject to rigorous testing and its value must be in doubt. A quarter of wards reported problems observing patients because of ward design. Most patients were seen as being at no or low immediate risk at the final contact prior to suicide.

Recently discharged patients Almost a quarter of the Inquiry cases had died by suicide within 3 months of discharge from psychiatric in-patient care, around 275 patients annually in England and Wales. Post-discharge suicides were most frequent (32%) in the 2 weeks after leaving hospital, the highest number occurring on the day after discharge. Most patients (92% of the post-discharge group) had a follow-up appointment arranged. However, in 40% of cases suicide took place before this appointment.

This group of patients was characterized by frequent indicators of risk, such as high levels of co-morbidity, substance misuse, self-harm, and violence. They tended to have a more disrupted pattern of care, with the most recent admission likely to be of short duration and ending in patient-initiated discharge. They were more likely to be non-compliant with treatment, symptomatic at last contact, but disengaged at the time of suicide.

Non-compliance

Non-compliance with medication was reported immediately prior to suicide, in around one-fifth of the sample in the month before death. Nearly one-third of these patients had a diagnosis of schizophrenia, and they were more likely to come from an ethnic minority, be socially isolated, and have higher rates of psychiatric morbidity (particularly substance misuse, co-morbid diagnoses, and previous admissions). Face-to-face attempts to encourage compliance with treatment were made in under two-thirds of cases.

Loss of contact with services was also common, occurring in one-third of community suicides, including in 17% with schizophrenia. Assertive attempts at re-engagement were made in just over half the cases.

It is clearly unrealistic to expect an assertive response by services to every patient who refuses treatment or fails to attend an appointment. However, the findings show that in a number of cases, despite severe mental illness and previous evidence of risk, services relied on letters rather than direct contact to re-establish care, or did not attempt to re-establish compliance by face-to-face interview.

Comparisons between countries

The findings highlighted above are derived from data from England and Wales. However, data are now available for Scotland and Northern Ireland. When findings from one country are confirmed in another, they can be viewed as more robust. When they differ, they highlight areas for more detailed comparative studies. Comparisons can be seen in Table 9.5.

Recommendations

The National Confidential Inquiry is essentially a descriptive study, with the methodological limitations inherent in this kind of research (Hunt *et al.* 2003). First, this study is a survey of clinical circumstances preceding suicide. Although aetiological conclusions cannot be drawn without a comparison sample, uncontrolled national studies can be informative for service planning

Table 9.5 Comparisons between countries for suicides in contact with mental health services

	England and Wales (*n*=4859)	Scotland (*n*=613)	Northern Ireland (*n*=134)
General population suicide rate	10.0	17.3	9.9
Number of suicides in contact with mental health services:			
Male [*n* (%)]	3198(66)	404(69)	91(68)
Method:			
Drowning [n (%)]	298(6)	60(10)	22(16)
Firearms [*n* (%)]	33(0.6)	10(1.7)	3(2.2)
Primary diagnosis:			
Schizophrenia [n (%)]	960(20)	99(17)	18(14)
Affective disorder [*n* (%)]	2036(42)	194(33)	54(41)
Alcohol dependence [*n* (%)]	439(9)	100(17)	30(23)
In-patient [*n* (%)]	754(16)	70(12)	13(10)
Post discharge [*n* (%)]	1100(23)	134(23)	36(27)
Non-compliance [n (%)]	929(22)	82(17)	24(21)

(Lönnqvist 1988). Secondly, the information from clinicians was based on case records and clinical judgements rather than standardized methods. However, a large number of suicide studies have relied on similar methods. Thirdly, the clinicians who provided the information were not blinded to the outcome and this may have resulted in a bias in their responses. However, the majority of the questionnaire consisted of factual items, which should help to reduce the bias from this source.

Data from the current study were used to inform national recommendations. The main aims of these were to make mental health services safer generally, and to facilitate suicide prevention in the mentally ill.

The most important clinical recommendations are included in 'Twelve points to a Safer Service' (Appleby *et al.* 2001). Recommendations applicable to suicide prevention are outlined in Table 9.6. Local mental health services will be supported by the National Institute for Mental Health in England to implement these (Department of Health 2002*a*).

In the absence of major intervention studies with conclusive evidence, the Inquiry's findings and subsequent recommendations indicate components of good clinical practice.

Risk management training

The fact that the majority of suicides were seen to be at low or no immediate risk at last contact prior to the suicide is of concern and suggests that, in some suicides, there are opportunities for prevention, possibly by accurate risk assessment.

Table 9.6 Specific strategies to reduce suicide in the mentally ill (Appleby *et al.* 2001)

- ◆ Regular staff risk management training
- ◆ Patients with severe mental illness and self-harm to receive the most intensive level of care
- ◆ Individualized care plans
- ◆ Prompt access to services for patients in crises
- ◆ Assertive outreach teams
- ◆ Availability of atypical antipsychotics
- ◆ Strategies for dual diagnosis
- ◆ In-patient wards to remove all likely ligature points
- ◆ Prompt follow-up following discharge from in-patient care
- ◆ Careful prescribing of medication
- ◆ Multidisciplinary post-incident review

In addressing this, the National Service Framework states that training in risk assessment is a priority and should be updated every 3 years. Recently launched in-patient guidance by the Department of Health supports staff training in risk assessment and management (Department of Health 2002*b*).

Improved recognition of risk and depression by health professionals has been shown to decrease suicides rates (Rutz *et al.* 1992). Evaluation of a suicide risk assessment programme (Appleby *et al.* 2000) demonstrated promising results.

Assertive outreach teams

The disrupted pattern of care and high levels of disengagement that characterize many of the Inquiry sample, especially the post-discharge group, needs to be addressed. Assertive outreach services to prevent loss of contact with high-risk patients are of potential utility. With a view to this, government plans to modernize mental health services include 170 assertive outreach teams and a further 50 teams to deliver care and treatment to the small number of people who are difficult to engage.

Several studies worldwide have supported the benefits of assertive outreach services and of maintenance of contact with patients, both generally (Stein and Test 1980; Motto and Bostrom 2001; Eagles *et al.* 2003) and within specific subgroups, such as the homeless (Dixon *et al.* 1997) and elderly (De Leo *et al.* 2002).

Availability of atypical antipsychotic medication

The use of atypical antipsychotic medication is supported by recent National Institute for Clinical Excellence guidelines (National Institute for Clinical Excellence 2002).

Evidence shows a reduction in relapse rates with certain atypical antipsychotics such as risperidone (Csernansky *et al.* 2002). Studies have also shown that atypical antipsychotics have an antidepressant action in schizophrenic patients with depression, and may contribute to a reduction in suicidality (Collaborative Working Group on Clinical Trial Evaluations 1998). As noted earlier, it has been shown that clozapine may contribute to a reduction in suicidal behaviour (Meltzer *et al.* 2003).

This clearly requires further evaluation, but the beneficial actions with regard to side-effect profile, and therefore improved compliance alone, suggest that atypical antipsychotics should be widely available.

Strategies for dual diagnosis

It is well established that co-morbidity confers an increased risk of suicide (Barraclough *et al.* 1974). It is also well documented that traditional services cater poorly for this group, often with little in the way of integrated work between general adult psychiatry services and specialist substance misuse services. Studies have demonstrated the potential benefits of an integrated approach, in improvements in patient engagement, hospital use, psychotic symptoms, and quality of life (Drake *et al.* 1997). There is a lack of conclusive evidence on the impact on suicide rates but, given that suicide clusters around episodes of illness, the above benefits may result in a reduction in suicide risk.

Removal of ligature points on in-patient wards

There is a large body of evidence showing that reducing access and availability to means does not invariably result in widespread substitution of method, and can effect a reduction in suicide rates (Oliver and Hetzel 1973; Kreitman 1976; Gunnell and Frankel 1994; Lester 1990; Amos *et al.* 2001).

Safety and access to means of suicide on in-patient wards is clearly highly concerning, given the high rates of suicide by hanging in in-patients. Following the publication of the Chief Medical Officer's report *An organisation with a memory* (Department of Health 2000), all services were required to remove all non-collapsible curtain rails by March 2002. Recently there has been a decrease in in-patient suicide rates, proportionally greater than the decrease in the general population suicide rates. The reduction in rates is not accounted for solely by declining in-patient numbers, and it may be that reduced access to ligature points has contributed to this fall.

Prompt follow-up following discharge

Suicide is significantly associated with a reduction in care at last contact (Appleby *et al.* 1999) and with disrupted continuity of care (King *et al.* 2001*b*). There is a high rate of suicide immediately after discharge. Taking these findings together, it may be that early follow-up with maintenance of care would help to reduce risk in this group.

Careful prescribing of medication

A prospective cross-sectional study of deliberate self-harm showed that, of deliberate self-harm patients prescribed antidepressants in the preceding year, one-third overdosed on their most recently prescribed antidepressant (Donovan *et al.* 2000). Further evidence indicates that overprescription by GPs is often the source of medication taken in overdose (Oyefeso *et al.* 1999). Thus, restriction of medication prescribed to those with a recent history of deliberate self-harm might help to reduce the mortality associated with self-poisoning.

The impact of recommendations

One of the main criticisms levelled at the Inquiry recommendations is the lack of conclusive evidence from intervention studies demonstrating their efficacy. Providing more intensive care and supervision to many patients who would not go on to commit suicide may be seen as a waste of resources (Geddes 1999). However, the clinical recommendations outlined are aspects of high-quality care and, therefore, although the primary aim is reduction in risk, a secondary benefit is inevitably improved care and management for those who need it.

The impact of Inquiry recommendations can be monitored in various ways. The National Confidential Inquiry database allows temporal monitoring of suicide rates, generally and in specific subgroups. Preliminary results indicate a fall in in-patient suicide rates that is not merely a result of a decrease in in-patient numbers.

The Inquiry is currently investigating the relationship between service configuration and suicide rates. This ongoing study aims to evaluate the extent of compliance of trusts with Inquiry recommendations and looks at both changes within individual trusts as well as aggregate changes.

Inquiry recommendations also helped to inform the *National Service Framework for Mental Health* (Department of Health 1999*b*) and the *National Suicide Prevention Strategy for England* (Department of Health 2002*a*).

Conclusions

Mental health services can be made safer. The National Confidential Inquiry findings suggest that suicide prevention requires services to be strengthened as a whole. Components of this include increasing the intensity of service activity at times of risk (for instance, early follow-up after discharge), assertive outreach for patients who are non-compliant or disengaged, improved access to services in crisis, and better use of the Care Programme Approach. High-risk patients for priority intervention, such as dual diagnosis patients and young males, need to be identified and targeted. Specific measures ensuring effective and acceptable treatment, with appropriate medication in limited supply to minimize risk, are required, along with reducing the access to means of suicide, particularly hanging on in-patient wards. Finally, supervision of patients clearly warrants attention, potentially facilitated by regular, rigorous staff training in risk management.

These measures, while having suicide prevention as a primary aim, are components of high-quality care and, therefore, as a secondary benefit, should result in the provision of a better-quality service for all patients who need it most.

References

Amos, T., Appleby, L., and Kiernan, K. (2001). Changes in rate of suicide by car exhaust asphyxiation in England and Wales. *Psychological Medicine*, 31, 935–9.

Appleby, L. (2001). Preventing suicide must remain a priority. *British Medical Journal*, 323, 808–9.

Appleby, L., Dennehy, J., Thomas, C., Faragher, B., and Lewis, G. (1999). Aftercare and clinical characteristics of people with mental illness who commit suicide: a case-control study. *Lancet*, 353, 1397–400.

Appleby, L., Morriss, R., Gask, L., Roland, M., Perry, B., Lewis, A., *et al.* (2000). An educational intervention for front-line health professionals in the assessment and management of suicidal patients (The STORM Project). *Psychological Medicine*, 30 (4), 805–9.

Appleby, L., Shaw, J., Sherrat, J., Amos, T., Robinson, J., and McDonnell, R. (2001). safety first: five-year report of the National Confidential Inquiry into Suicide and Homicide by People with Mental Illness. Department of Health, London.

Barraclough, B., Bunch, J., Nelson, B., and Sainsbury, P. (1974). A hundred cases of suicide: Clinical aspects. *British Journal of Psychiatry*, 125, 355–73.

Baxter, D. and Appleby, L. (1999). Case register study of suicide risk in mental disorders. *British Journal of Psychiatry*, 175, 322–6.

Beautrais, A.L., Joyce, P.R., and Mulder, R.T. (1998). Unemployment and serious suicide attempts. *Psychological Medicine*, 28, 209–18.

Busch, K.A., Fawcett, J., and Jacobs, D. (2003). Clinical correlates of in-patient suicide. *Journal of Clinical Psychiatry*, 64, 14–19.

Cantor, C.H. (2000). Suicide in the Western World. In *The international handbook of suicide and attempted suicide*, (ed. K. Hawton and K. van Heeringen) pp. 9–28. John Wiley and Sons, Chichester.

Caspi, A., Sugden, K., Moffitt, T.E., Taylor, A., Craig, I.W., Harrington, H., *et al.* (2003). Influence of life stress on depression: moderation by a polymorphism in the 5-HTT gene. *Science*, 301, 386–9.

Collaborative Working Group on Clinical Trial Evaluations (1998). Atypical antipsychotics for treatment of depression in schizophrenia and affective disorders. *Journal of Clinical Psychiatry*, 59 (suppl. 12), 41–5.

Csernansky, J.G., Mahmoud, R., Brenner, R. and the Risperidone–USA-79 Study (2002). A companion of risperidone and haloperidol for the prevention of relapse in patients with schizophrenia. *New England Journal of Medicine*, 346, 16–22.

De Leo, D. (2002). Why are we not getting any closer to preventing suicide? *British Journal of Psychiatry*, 181, 372–4.

De Leo, D., Dello Buono, M., and Dwyer, J. (2002). Suicide among the elderly: long term impact of a telephone support and assessment intervention in northern Italy. *British Journal of Psychiatry*, 181, 226–9.

Department of Health (1999a). *Saving Lives: Our Healthier Nation*. The Stationery Office, London.

Department of Health (1999b). *National Service Framework for Mental Health*. Department of Health, London.

Department of Health (2000). *An organisation with a memory*. Report of an expert group on learning from adverse events in the NHS chaired by the Chief Medical Officer. Department of Health, London.

Department of Health (2002a). *National Suicide Prevention Strategy for England*. Department of Health, London.

Department of Health (2002*b*). *Mental Health Policy Implementation Guide: Adult Acute In-patient Care Provision.* Department of Health, London.

Dixon, L., Weiden, P., Torres, M., and Lehman, A. (1997). Assertive community treatment and medication compliance in the homeless mentally ill. *American Journal of Psychiatry,* 154, 1302–4.

Donovan, S., Clayton, A., Beeharry, M., Jones, S., Kirk, C., Waters, K., *et al.* (2000). Deliberate self harm and antidepressant drugs. Investigation of a possible link. *British Journal of Psychiatry,* 177, 551–6.

Drake, R.E., Yovetich, N.A., Bebout, R.R., Harris, M., and McHugo, G.J. (1997). Integrated treatment for dually diagnosed homeless adults. *Journal of Nervous and Mental Disease,* 185, 298–305.

Eagles, J.M., Carson, D.P., Begg, A., and Naji, S.A. (2003). Suicide prevention: a study of patients' views. *British Journal of Psychiatry,* 182, 261–5.

Fawcett, J., Scheftner, W.A., Clark, D.C., Hedeker, D., Gibbons, R., and Coryell, W. (1987). Clinical predictors of suicide in patients with affective disorder: a controlled prospective study. *American Journal of Psychiatry,* 144, 35–40.

Foster, T., Gillespie, K., McClelland, R., and Patterson, C. (1999). Risk factors for suicide independent of DSM-III-R axis 1 disorder. Case control psychological autopsy study in Northern Ireland. *British Journal of Psychiatry,* 175, 175–9.

Geddes, J. (1999). Suicide and homicide by people with mental illness. We still don't know how to prevent most of these deaths. *British Medical Journal,* 318, 1225–6.

Goldacre, M., Seagrott, V., and Hawton, K. (1993). Suicide after discharge from psychiatric inpatient care. *Lancet,* 342, 283–6.

Goldney, R.D., Wilson, D., Dal Grande, E., Fisher, L.J., and McFarlane, A.C. (2000). Suicidal ideation in a random community sample; attributable risk due to depression and psychosocial and traumatic events. *Australian and New Zealand Journal of Psychiatry,* 34, 98–106.

Gunnell, D. and Frankel, S. (1994). Prevention of suicide: aspirations and evidence. *British Medical Journal,* 308, 1227–33.

Hall, W.D., Mant, A., Mitchell, P.B., Rendle, V.A., Hickie, I.B., and McManus, P. (2003). Association between antidepressant prescribing and suicide in Australia, 1991–2000: trend analysis. *British Medical Journal,* 326, 1008.

Harris, E.C., and Barraclough, B. (1997). Suicide as an outcome for mental disorders: a meta-analysis. *British Journal of Psychiatry,* 170, 205–28.

Hawton, K. (2002). Sex and suicide. Gender differences in suicidal behaviour. *British Journal of Psychiatry,* 177, 484–5.

Henriksson, M.M., Aro, H.M., Marttunen, M.J., Heikkinen, M.E., Isometsa, E.T., Kuoppasalmi, K.I., *et al.* (1993). Mental disorders and comorbidity in suicide. *American Journal of Psychiatry,* 150, 935–40.

Ho, T.P. (2003). The suicide risk of discharged psychiatric patients. *Journal of Clinical Psychiatry,* 64, 702–7.

Hunt, I., Robinson, J., Bickley, H., Meehan, J., Parsons, R., McCann, K., *et al.* (2003). Suicide in ethnic minorities within 12 months of contact with mental health services. National clinical survey. *British Journal of Psychiatry,* 183, 155–60.

Isacsson, G. (2000). Suicide prevention – a medical breakthrough? *Acta Psychiatrica Scandinavia,* 103, 238–9.

Isometsä, E.T., Aro, H.M., Henriksson, M.M., Heikkinen, M.E., and Lönnqvist, J.K. (1994). Suicide in major depression in different treatment settings. *Journal of Clinical Psychiatry,* 55, 523–7.

Kapur, N. (2000). Evaluating risks. *Advances in Psychiatric Treatment,* 6, 399–406.

King, E. and Barraclough, B. (1990). Violent death and mental illness: a study of a single catchment area over 8 years. *British Journal of Psychiatry,* 156, 714–20.

King, E.A., Baldwin, D.S., Sinclair, J.M.A., Baker, N.G., Campbell, M.J., and Thompson, C. (2001*a*). The Wessex Recent In-Patient Suicide Study, case-control study of 234 recently discharged psychiatric patient suicides. *British Journal of Psychiatry,* 178, 531–6.

King, E.A., Baldwin, D.S., Sinclair, J.M.A., and Campbell, M.J. (2001*b*). The Wessex Recent In-Patient Suicide Study, case-control study of 59 in-patient suicides. *British Journal of Psychiatry,* 178, 537–42.

Kreitman, N. (1976). The coal gas story: United Kingdom suicide rates, 1960–1971. *British Journal of Preventative and Social Medicine,* 30, 86–93.

Lester, D. (1990). The availability of firearms and the use of firearms for suicide. *Acta Psychiatrica Scandinavia,* 81, 146–7.

Lewis, G., Hawton, K., and Jones, P. (1997). Strategies for preventing suicide. *British Journal of Psychiatry,* 171, 351–4.

Linsley, K.R., Schapira, K., and Kelly, T.P. (2001). Open verdict v. suicide – importance to research. *British Journal of Psychiatry,* 178, 465–8.

Lönnqvist, J. (1988). National suicide prevention project in Finland: a research phase of the project. *Psychiatrica Fennica,* 19, 125–32.

Mann, J.J. (2002). A current perspective of suicide and attempted suicide. *Annals of Internal Medicine,* 136, 302–11.

Meltzer, H.Y., Alphs, L., Green, A.I., Altamura, A.C., Anand, R., Bertoldi, A., *et al.* International Suicide Prevention Trial Study Group (2003). Clozapine treatment for suicidality in schizophrenia. International Suicide Prevention Trial (InterSePT). *Archives of General Psychiatry,* 60, 82–91.

Motto, J.A. and Bostrom, A.G. (2001). A randomized controlled trial of postcrisis suicide prevention. *Psychiatric Services,* 52, 828–33.

Munro, J., O'Sullivan, D., Andrews, C., Arana, A., Mortimer, A., and Kerwin, R. (1999). Active monitoring of 12 760 clozapine recipients in the UK and Ireland. Beyond pharmacovigilance. *British Journal of Psychiatry,* 175, 576–80.

National Institute for Clinical Excellence (2002). *Guidance on the use of newer (atypicals) antipsychotic drugs for the treatment of schizophrenia.* Technology Appraisal Guidance no.43. NICE, London.

Neeleman, J. and Wessley, S. (1997). Changes in classification of suicide in England and Wales: time trends and associations with coroners' professional background. *Psychological Medicine,* 27, 467–72.

O'Donnell, I. and Farmer, R. (1995). The limitations of official suicide statistics. *British Journal of Psychiatry,* 166, 458–61.

Oliver, R.G. and Hetzelm, B.S. (1973). An analysis of recent trends in suicide rates in Australia. *International Journal of Epidemiology,* 2, 91–101.

Oyefeso, A., Ghodse, H., Clancy, C., and Corkery, J.M. (1999). Suicide among drug addicts in the UK. *British Journal of Psychiatry,* 175, 277–82.

Powell, J., Geddes, J., Deeks, J., Goldacre, M., and Hawton, K. (2000). Suicide in psychiatric hospital in-patients. Risk factors and their predictive power. *British Journal of Psychiatry,* 176, 266–72.

Reid, W.H., Mason, M., and Hogan, T. (1998). Suicide prevention effects associated with clozapine therapy in schizophrenia and schizoaffective disorder. *Psychiatric Services,* **49,** 1029–33.

Rihmer, Z., Barsi, J., and Katona, C.L.E. (1990). Suicide rates in Hungary correlate negatively with reported rates of depression. *Journal of Affective Disorders,* **20,** 87–91.

Runeson, B., Beskow, J., and Waern, M. (1996). The suicidal process among young people. *Acta Psychiatrica Scandinavia,* **93,** 35–42.

Rutz, W., von Knorring, L., and Walinder, J. (1992). Long term effects of an educational program for general practitioners given by the Swedish Committee for the Prevention and Treatment of Depression. *Acta Psychiatrica Scandinavia,* **85,** 83–8.

Stein, L.I. and Test, M.A. (1980). Alternative to mental hospital treatment. I. Conceptual model, treatment program, and clinical evaluation. *Archives of General Psychiatry,* **37** (4), 392–7.

Tondo, L., Baldessarini, R.J., Hennen, J., Floris, G., Silvetti, F., and Tohen, M. (1998). Lithium treatment and risk of suicidal behaviour in bipolar disorder patients. *Journal of Clinical Psychiatry,* **59,** 405–14.

Vastag, B. (2001). Suicide prevention plan calls for physicians' help. *Journal of the American Medical Association,* **285,** 2701–3.

World Health Organisation (2001). *The World Health Report 2001: Mental health: new understanding, new hope.* World Health Organisation, Geneva.

10

Risk factors for suicidal behaviour: translating knowledge into practice

Robert. D. Goldney

Risk factors for suicidal behaviour have been recognized for over 200 years and practitioners have used their contemporaneous knowledge in their endeavours to prevent it. However, the manner in which knowledge has been implemented in practice has been the subject of considerable debate. In order to gain insight into the present state of the science and art of suicide prevention, it is useful to have an historical perspective (Goldney and Schioldann 2002).

The historical perspective

In 1892 Tuke reviewed risk factors and his focus on mental illness, male gender, divorce, and interpersonal distress, alcohol, incarceration, and rural employment has stood the test of time. Other risk factors that have proved enduring, and which were reported by earlier writers, were those of gambling by Moore in 1790, and the potential influence of the media by Burrows in 1828. Burrows also described what has become known as the medical model of suicide prevention, when he stated that 'the medical treatment of the propensity to suicide, whether prophylactic or therapeutic, differs not from that which is applicable in cases of ordinary insanity'. However, social issues were not ignored, and in 1838, Peuchet referred to suicide as a 'deficient organization of our society'. Subsequently in 1897 Durkheim elaborated on the sociological views of earlier researchers.

Other influential authors of the nineteenth century included Lisle, whose report in 1856 on over 52 000 suicides is probably still the largest data set to be published. He provided a list of no fewer than 48 causes, including debt, 'disappointed love', and the 'desire to avoid legal pursuit', as well as the evocative descriptions of 'debauchery', 'nostalgia', and 'disgust with marriage'.

In contrast to such social and personal issues, it was even apparent to Moore in 1790 that occasionally suicide 'by attacking successive generations of the same family proves itself to be hereditary', a particularly prescient observation which was to be confirmed almost 200 years later by adoption (Schulsinger *et al.* 1979) and twin studies (Statham *et al.* 1998).

Other factors found to be associated with suicidal behaviour in the twentieth century included previous suicidal behaviour, early parental loss, other adverse early life experiences, substance abuse, the degree of suicidal intent and planning, hopelessness, unemployment, and what has been described as 'terminal malignant alienation' (Morgan and Priest 1991).

With the acquisition of such knowledge about suicidal behaviour, along with an increasing awareness of the magnitude of the challenge of suicide prevention worldwide, it was not unexpected when, in 1993, the World Health Organization promulgated what it described as 'Six basic steps for suicide prevention'. These were: the treatment of psychiatric patients; control of possession of guns; detoxification of domestic gas; detoxification of car emissions; control of toxic substance availability; and toning down reports in the press (World Health Organization 1993).

Evidence-based medicine

While the World Health Organization recommendations appeared to be logical and non-controversial, being based on clinical wisdom of the time, within a year Wilkinson (1994) had stated that 'the reality is that there is no convincing evidence that education, improved social conditions and support, or better training play a substantive part in preventing suicide', and, in a similar pessimistic vein, Gunnel and Frankel (1994), in a paper entitled 'The prevention of suicide: aspirations and evidence', concluded that 'no single intervention has been shown in a well conducted randomised controlled trial to reduce suicide'.

That such comments were technically correct was subsequently substantiated by systematic reviews of the treatment literature. Thus Hawton *et al.* (1998), in a review of the efficacy of psychosocial and pharmacological treatments for the prevention of repetition of suicidal behaviour, concluded that 'currently there is insufficient evidence on which to make firm recommendations about the most effective forms of treatment for patients who have recently deliberately harmed themselves'. Similarly, in a review of the role of lithium maintenance treatment of mood disorders in preventing suicide, Burgess *et al.* (2001) concluded that 'there is no definitive evidence from this review as to whether or not lithium has an anti-suicidal effect'.

These reviews and comments were prompted by the desirable focus on evidence-based medicine in the latter part of the twentieth century. However, such a focus needs to be considered in the perspective that suicide, for all its drama and the clarity with which retrospective analyses provide, has a low base rate, with the attendant clinical and research limitations that this imposes, particularly in terms of demonstrating the effectiveness of treatments (Goldney 2000; Cuijpers 2003).

The challenge of detecting those who may die by suicide, which is a necessary requirement if one is to mount a research methodology to prevent such behaviour, has been well recognized for 50 years. Rosen (1954) was probably the first to draw attention to the limitations of the prediction of infrequent events in suicidal subjects, with a cogent description of the interaction between the low incidence of suicide itself and the large number of false positives that are predicted on the basis of those subjects possessing the conventional risk factors associated with suicide. At the individual level this was later emphasized by Pokorny (1983), who stated that 'We do not possess any item of information or any combination of items that permits us to identify to a useful degree the particular persons who will commit suicide'.

Because of the lack of specificity of the risk factors for suicide, the numbers required for conclusive aggregate data analysis are particularly daunting. For example, Gunnel and Frankel (1994) calculated that to demonstrate a 15% reduction in suicide in those discharged from psychiatric hospitals, where there is a 0.9% chance of suicide in the subsequent year, over 140 000 patients would be required in the sample. Similarly, to demonstrate a 15% reduction in suicide for those who have attempted suicide, where there is a 2.8% chance of suicide in the subsequent 8 years, would require a sample size of almost 45 000 subjects. This was also illustrated well by Lewis *et al.* (1997), who provided a mathematical model for deriving the numbers needed to treat to demonstrate the effectiveness of suicide prevention measures in high-risk populations, and noted that for an intervention that would reduce the suicide rate in doctors and farmers by 25%, 25 000 and 33 000 subjects, respectively, would be required. Not unexpectedly, they expressed reservations about the feasibility and affordability of studies to demonstrate such effectiveness.

It is acknowledged that the numbers required to demonstrate the effectiveness of the prevention of repetition of suicidal behaviour are appreciably less than for suicide *per se*. However, they are still daunting, and Hawton *et al.* (1998), in their previously noted review on the prevention of repetition of suicidal behaviour, reported that even when data from 20 randomized controlled trials were combined in a meta-analysis, numbers were too small to detect differences in outcome. Indeed, they advised that for future research in preventing repetition of suicidal behaviour, 'If the predicted rate were 10% in the experimental group vs 15% in the control, with α set at 0.05 and β set at 0.2, a total of 687 subjects would be required in each treatment group, while if the rates were 20% and 30%, 293 subjects would be required in each group'.

It could be argued that multi-centre, collaborative trials could be utilized to fulfil the need for sufficient numbers to demonstrate the effectiveness of intervention programmes in preventing repeated attempted suicide. However, the logistical demands, let alone the financial requirements, are daunting. For example, in a World Health Organization/European Union study (Bille-Brahe *et al.* 1996) of 4163 persons who had attempted suicide, for a variety of reasons only 2432 subjects were asked to participate in a follow-up study, and of those only 1145 were re-assessed after 1 year. This provided what the researchers termed as a 'gross completion rate' of 28% of the original sample, or a 'net completion rate' of 47% of those who agreed to participate. When one considers these figures with the need for randomization of treatment and control subjects in future studies, the challenge in designing outcome research in this area is quite evident, even with highly motivated researchers in dedicated centres, such as in this study.

The importance of this for future research has been further emphasized by Hawton (1998), who has gone so far as to state that unless sufficient numbers are utilized, it 'is a waste of scientific time and funding, and could be deemed unethical in terms of patient participation'.

Those charged with responsibility for suicide prevention could be forgiven for being pessimistic following the above reviews. However, the results of such reviews not only fail to support long-held clinical beliefs, but they also ignore research methodologies other than the randomized controlled trial, the so-called gold standard. Investors are aware of the fluctuations of the price of gold, and there are fluctuations in the value of randomized controlled trials, particularly when such trials are logistically impractical. When that is the case, obstacles to elucidating a valid result need to be circumvented by other research methodologies.

Therefore a more pragmatic approach needs to be adopted in considering other research that could give clinicians confidence in their practice to reduce suicidal behaviour.

Pragmatic evidence-based medicine

It is logical to consider that by alleviating risk factors there should be an impact on suicidal behaviour. It should be noted at this point that the words 'suicidal behaviour' have been used, not just 'suicide' or 'attempted suicide'. It is acknowledged that there are some differences between these groups, but there are also major similarities, and their overlapping nature has been accepted (Lester *et al.* 1979; Beautrais 2001), to the extent that Ottoson (1979) stated 'that they are expressions of a common suicidal process'. Also included in suicidal behaviour is suicidal ideation, although sometimes its importance is minimized (Goldney *et al.* 2001). However, it is, at the very least, a necessary, though not sufficient, requirement for suicide, and its association with suicide attempts (Sokero *et al.* 2003) and suicide (Joiner *et al.* 2003) indicates that it is appropriate to also consider studies that have used suicidal ideation as an outcome measure.

In the past few decades a number of studies using different methodologies have more clearly delineated and quantified important risk factors. Psychological autopsy studies have demonstrated consistently across countries with different cultures that 80–90% of suicides had mental disorders, particularly depression and substance abuse (Cheng 1995); twin studies have confirmed the importance of inherited as well as environmental factors (Statham *et al.* 1998); case-control studies of serious suicide attempts have demonstrated the importance of mood disorders and substance abuse (Beautrais *et al.* 1996); large retrospective cohort studies have demonstrated 'a strong, graded relationship to attempted suicide' of adverse childhood experiences, including emotional, physical, and sexual abuse, household substance abuse, mental illness, and incarceration, and parental domestic violence, separation, or divorce (Dube *et al.* 2001); longitudinal cohort analyses have shown that 'vulnerability/resiliency to suicidal responses among those depressed (and those not depressed) is influenced by an accumulation of factors including: family history of suicide, childhood sexual abuse, personality factors, peer affiliations and school success' (Fergusson *et al.* 2003); and large population-based nested case-control studies based on Danish register data have found the strongest risks for suicide to be mental illness necessitating hospitalization, unemployment, and low income (Mortensen *et al.* 2000; Qin *et al.* 2003).

It is evident that many of these risk factors, particularly those in childhood and adolescence, are not specific for suicidal behaviours, as they are related to adult mental disorders in general (Fergusson *et al.* 2003). Furthermore, one does not have to invoke the risk of future suicide as a reason for addressing them. Such issues, for example childhood sexual abuse, parental domestic violence and unemployment, are important in their own right, and they demand the attention not only of health professionals, but also of the community as a whole.

Clinicians cannot influence what has happened in the past, although they may wish to lobby for social change that might influence future generations. However, in regard to the contemporaneous practice of suicide prevention, it is important to ensure that a correct perspective be maintained on the relative importance of various risk factors. In this regard the Danish register studies of Mortensen *et al.* (2000) and Qin *et al.* (2003) are particularly valuable, as they have used the population attributable risk (PAR) statistic. This is a singularly appropriate statistic for research assessing the differing impact of various contributing factors to suicidal behaviour, as it has the potential to place risk factors in perspective at the population level. The PAR provides a measure of the proportion of a condition that can be associated with exposure to a risk factor, or the proportion of the condition that would be eliminated if the risk factor was not present. It can be illustrated by considering the association between smoking and lung cancer. It is accepted that smoking causes lung cancer, but not in everyone who smokes. The PAR of smoking for lung cancer is about 80%, which means that if all smoking were eliminated, approximately 80% of all lung cancer cases would also be eliminated (Lilienfeld and Lilienfeld 1980). In an analogous manner, the various PARs for suicidal behaviour can be calculated.

Qin *et al.* (2003) examined data for 21 169 suicides and 423 128 comparison subjects, and the PAR for having ever had a psychiatric admission was 40.3%, whereas those PARs for other statistically significant contributors, including unemployment, having a sickness-related absence from work, being in the lowest income quartile, and being on a disability or age pension were 2.8%, 6.4%, 8.8%, 3.2%, and 10.2%, respectively. While these other issues can not be ignored, clearly the focus of attention needs to be on those persons who have required psychiatric hospitalization. Indeed, using the same database, Agerbo *et al.* (2002) emphasized that for suicide in 496 young people between 10 and 21 years of age, the strongest risk factor was mental illness, and that the effect of the parents' socio-economic factors decreased after adjusting for family history of mental illness and suicide.

The PAR statistic has been used in other studies with broadly similar results. For example, Beautrais *et al.* (1996) stated that 'population attributable risk estimates suggest that elimination of mood disorders would result in very substantial reductions, up to 80%, in risk of a serious suicide attempt.' Beautrais (1999) also re-analysed data from the American work on suicide of Shaffer *et al.*, Gould *et al.*, and Brent *et al.*, and calculated a PAR of mood disorders for suicide to be 46% for the first two studies and 37% for the third.

Other PAR studies, utilizing different measures of depression and suicidal ideation (Goldney *et al.* 2000, 2003; Pirkis *et al.* 2000), have found PARs of 47%, 57%, and 39%, respectively, of depression for suicidal ideation, and 40% of depression for attempted suicide (Pirkis *et al.* 2000). Indeed, perhaps counter-intuitively, in a study examining the contribution of clinical depression, traumatic and psychosocial events to suicidal ideation, Goldney *et al.*

(2000) found that when multivariate analyses of results were undertaken, which allowed for the interaction of different variables, only clinical depression was significantly associated with suicidal ideation, with a PAR of 47%. Thus no individual traumatic (e.g. war, life-threatening accident, torture, serious physical attack) or psychosocial (unplanned loss of job, marriage breakdown, burglary, death of someone close) event remained statistically significant. Furthermore, although the lifetime summation of traumatic events attained statistical significance (PAR = 38%), even the summation of psychosocial events did not achieve a statistically significant association with suicidal ideation. This does not mean that those events are not important in themselves; it simply means that they need to be placed in perspective when considering factors contributing to suicidal ideation.

Other research methodologies have also pointed to the importance of the recognition and adequate treatment of mental diseases in suicide prevention. Isacsson *et al.* (1999) and Marzuk *et al.* (1995) have emphasized the lack of congruence between the use of psychotropic medication at the time of suicide and the patterns of diagnoses made at psychological autopsy; Hulten and Wasserman (1998) have commented on the lack of continuity of care; Waern *et al.* (1999) have reported on the absence of enquiry about suicidal thoughts in elderly suicides; and in two large surveys of suicides in England (National Confidential Inquiry 2001) and Australia (Burgess *et al.* 2000), no fewer than 21% and 20% in the respective studies were considered to have been preventable, but for poor assessment and treatment, poor staff–patient communication and relationships, inadequate supervision, and lack of continuity of care.

Such findings add weight to the view of Whitlock (1977), who stated that 'putting it bluntly, we can do a lot to prevent suicide if we make use of the medical facts associated with the behaviour', a comment virtually identical to that of Burrows, made in 1828. However, it is all too clear that this has not always occurred, and that a sense of pessimism has prevailed, in part engendered by the absence of randomized controlled trials to have proven the efficacy of our interventions. Nevertheless, there are intervention studies which give considerable confidence that suicidal behaviours can be prevented. The remainder of this chapter presents selected reports, which are by no means exhaustive, but which illustrate the diverse paths to suicide prevention.

Standard treatments

That standard treatments for the antecedents of suicidal behaviour should prevent such behaviour appears self-evident, but, for the reasons outlined before, the challenge is to substantiate this. Nevertheless, research has indicated that routine clinical care may be of value. For example, Hickey *et al.* (2001) reported that deliberate self-harm patients who left an accident and emergency department in Oxford without a psychiatric assessment not only had a greater past history of self-harm, but they were more likely to self-harm again in the subsequent year than a matched comparison group who had been assessed. Similarly, Kapur *et al.* (2002), in a study of six hospitals in north-west England, noted that patients who had deliberately self-poisoned and who had not received psychosocial assessment were more likely to poison themselves again. Furthermore, they calculated that only 12 patients needed to receive a psychosocial assessment to prevent one repetition of self-poisoning, and they concluded that 'if we assume that 50% of patients are assessed currently, we might prevent 7000 repeat episodes of self poisoning by complying with existing guidelines and ensuring that all patients are properly assessed'.

More specific standard treatments will now be considered under the broad headings of non-pharmacological and pharmacological approaches; following which, reference will be made to several broad programmes with demonstrated effectiveness.

Non-pharmacological approaches

Methods to enhance effective contact with those who are suicidal have been practised for the past century. Telephone crisis services were established in the USA from as early as 1895 and 1906 (Retterstol 1996), and from those beginnings suicide prevention centres emerged during the 1950s and 1960s in Europe, the USA, and in other parts of the world, sometimes under the auspices of volunteer organizations, such as Samaritans, Befrienders International, the International Federation of Telephonic Emergency Services (IFOTES), and Lifeline. Formidable methodological problems exist in demonstrating their efficacy, and inconsistent results have emerged (Bagley 1968; Barraclough *et al.* 1977). However, a review of 14 studies by Lester (1997) demonstrated a preventive effect, 'albeit small and inconsistently found'. Bearing that in mind, it is not unexpected that a recent assessment of a telephone counselling service for adolescents found significant decreases in measures of suicidality between the beginning and end of counselling sessions (King *et al.* 2003).

The effectiveness of the principles of befriending have been demonstrated in a remarkable project from Sri Lanka, initiated by Sumithrayo, a volunteer organization dedicated to suicide prevention (Marecek and Ratnayeke 2001). In response to suicidal behaviour in rural areas, ongoing emotional support was offered to a village, with another village used as a comparison. The village with the intervention had had 13 suicides and 18 other episodes of self-harm in the 6 years before the programme, but there were no examples of suicidal behaviour in the subsequent 4.5 years. That contrasted with the comparison village, which had previously had 16 suicides and 25 other episodes of self-harm, and which had a further 3 suicides and 10 other episodes of self-harm in the next 2 years, following which the investigators extended the programme to that village.

A deceptively simple form of ongoing contact with suicide attempters has been reported by Motto and Bostrom (2001). Subjects who had attempted suicide were contacted 1 month after their suicide attempt, and those who had not pursued further treatment were randomly assigned to contact and no contact groups. The contact group received correspondence each month for 4 months, then every 2 months for 8 months and then every 3 months for a further 4 years, a total of 5 years and 24 contacts per person. Over a 5-year period there was a significant decrease in death by suicide for those who had had contact when compared to the no contract group. However, a longer-term follow-up indicated that the difference became insignificant and the suicide rates were identical after 14 years. Nevertheless, the data demonstrated a difference in the first 5 years, and suggest that if further contact had been continued beyond that time, more encouraging long-term results might have eventuated.

Another example of enhancing ongoing contact is that of a service to prevent suicide in the elderly reported by De Leo et al. (2002). They used a Tele-Help and Tele-Check service for patients who had been discharged from hospital. The Tele-Help component was a portable device which allowed patients to send an alarm signal if they needed help, and the Tele-check was a regular check of patients by telephone, on average twice a week. They reported that over 10 years there were only 6 suicides, compared to an expected 20.86 for their population of 18 641 elderly persons, a highly significant result ($P < 0.001$).

More specific effective psychotherapeutic interventions date from the innovative work of Linehan, whose dialectical behaviour therapy model involving cognitive, behavioural, and supportive psychotherapies was demonstrated to reduce the number and severity of suicide attempts, and to decrease inpatient admissions for borderline patients (Linehan et al. 1991). Other variations of psychotherapeutic approaches have been effective in carefully selected groups of borderline patients. Stevenson and Meares (1992) reported that a 'coherent consistently applied' psychotherapy, based on a 'psychology of self', resulted in a significant reduction in self-harm in the year after therapy, compared to the year before; Bateman and Fonagy (1999, 2001) demonstrated the superiority of psycho-analytically oriented partial hospitalization over standard psychiatric treatment in reducing suicide attempts and acts of self-harm; Bohus *et al.* (2000), using Linehan's dialectical behaviour therapy model, reported a 'highly significant decrease in the number of parasuicidal acts'; and Verheul *et al.* (2003), also using Linehan's model in a randomized trial, found the treatment group had less self-mutilating and self-damaging behaviours than a treatment-as-usual group.

It is pertinent that these patient groups were chosen for their borderline diagnosis, rather than their suicidal behaviour *per se*. That this may be important is illustrated by the fact that a recent multi-centre randomized trial utilizing manual assisted cognitive behaviour therapy, which incorporated Linehan's (1992) concepts, found no difference in the repetition of deliberate self-harm between the experimental and treatment-as-usual groups (Tyrer *et al.* 2003). However, subjects were not chosen for their clinical diagnosis, but on the basis of them having had a previous episode of self-harm; not requiring in-patient care; and not having psychotic or bipolar disorders or substance dependence. Further comment on this study will be provided later.

Other non-pharmacological approaches include reducing media publicity and restricting access to the means of suicide. With regard to the media, Sonneck *et al.* (1994) reported that a sustained decrease of 75% in the number of subway suicides in Vienna occurred for 5 years following initiatives to abstain from reporting on such suicides. There have also been a number of studies that have indicated that restricting access to the means of suicide is an effective intervention. In Australia, Oliver and Hetzel (1972) noted that a fall in suicide in women was related to restriction on prescribing of barbiturates; Kreitman (1976) reported that there was a sustained reduction in suicide rates in England and Wales when coal gas was replaced by non-toxic North Sea gas; and, in 1983, Harvey and Solomons reported that, in the then 52 years that the Sydney Harbour Bridge had been in operation, 60 of the 92 suicide attempts, 78 of which had been fatal, occurred in the first 4 years, before a safety barrier was erected. Furthermore, using a rigorous research design, Hawton *et al.* (2001) demonstrated that legislation restricting paracetamol pack sizes had 'substantial beneficial effects on mortality and morbidity associated with self-poisoning using these drugs'.

It is evident that there are a number of non-pharmacological approaches that have used predominantly 'before and after' methodologies to demonstrate their effectiveness. It may well be that a common thread to these interventions is that they provide a sense of caring for those who are suicidal, even if it is in an anonymous restriction of means to suicide, which buys time for the suicidal crisis to dissipate. At the very least, such approaches are consistent with what has been described in the psychotherapy literature as enhancing a sense of 'connectedness to others' (Frank 1971).

Pharmacological approaches

There are several ways in which the effect of psychotropic medication can be examined in regard to suicidal behaviour. As long ago as 1972, Barraclough, in England, emphasized the importance of lithium for recurrent affective disorders when he noted that as many as a fifth of the 100 suicides he examined may have been prevented by its use. Since then, Modestin and Schwarzenbach (1992), in Switzerland, demonstrated that a significantly higher proportion of a control group, compared to 64 former psychiatric patients who had suicided, had been receiving psychotropic drugs, and a significantly higher proportion had been on lithium. Similarly, Marzuk et al. (1995), in the USA, reported that only 16.4% of 1635 subjects who had died by suicide were on psychotropic medication, and they commented: 'given the high prevalence of serious mental disorders among individuals who commit suicide, only a small proportion had used any of the more standard prescription psychotropic drugs at the time of death'. Such findings are congruent with other research from Finland (Suominen et al. 1998) and Sweden (Isacsson et al. 1999).

These general studies have been supplemented by more specific studies involving antidepressant, mood stabilizer, and antipsychotic medications.

Antidepressants

Randomized controlled trials of antidepressants versus placebo have demonstrated statistically significant reductions in suicidal ideation items of depression scales (Montgomery et al. 1995; Letizia et al. 1996) and, more recently, Szanto et al. (2003) have demonstrated a reduction of suicidal ideation during the course of antidepressant treatment of late-life depression. A 34–38-year follow-up by Angst et al. (2002) of affective disordered patients also demonstrated that 'long-term medication treatment with antidepressants alone or with a neuroleptic, or with lithium in combination with antidepressants and/ or neuroleptics significantly lowered suicide rates even though the treated were more severely ill'.

Probably the most persuasive data have come from large population studies. Rutz et al. (1992) reported that a programme to enhance the recognition and treatment of depression by general practitioners on the Swedish island of Gotland was followed by a decrease in suicide, a greater use of antidepressants, a decreased prescription of neuroleptics and hypnotics, a decrease in in-patient treatment of depression, and a reduction in sick leave due to depression. Further important work has emerged from Isacsson (2000), also in Sweden, who had predicted that a fivefold increase in antidepressant use might reduce the Swedish suicide rate by 25%. A naturalistic experiment was made possible by the fact that antidepressant prescribing did increase more than threefold, and the reduction in suicide correlated significantly with that. He also presented similar data from Finland, Norway, and Denmark, and concluded that the increased use of antidepressants was 'one of the contributing factors to the decrease in the suicide rate'. Similar findings have been reported from Australia by Hall *et al.* (2003), who noted that 'the higher the exposure to antidepressants the larger the decline in rate of suicide', and that 'their effect is most apparent in older age groups, in which rates of suicide decreased substantially in association with exposure to antidepressants'. Hall and co-workers acknowledged that it may not have simply been the antidepressants *per se*, and that increased prescribing may have been 'a proxy marker for improved overall management of depression'.

That this decrease in suicide with increased use of antidepressants is not confined to older age groups has been demonstrated recently by Olfson *et al.* (2003), who found a significant negative relationship between antidepressant treatment and suicide in different regions of the USA. They noted that a 1% increase in adolescent use of antidepressants was associated with a decrease of 0.23 suicides per 100 000 adolescents each year, and concluded that their results raised 'the possibility of a role for using antidepressant treatment in youth suicide prevention efforts'.

Such findings for the effectiveness of measures to treat depression having an impact on suicide are not unexpected in view of the earlier clinical risk findings, particularly those delineated by population attributable risk analyses. However, it has only been by large population studies, rather than randomized controlled trials, that the impact on suicide has been demonstrated.

Mood stabilizers

Following the previously noted early work of Barraclough (1972), Coppen *et al.* (1990), in the UK, reported that consistent use of lithium in patients with affective disorders resulted in their having a cumulative mortality risk similar to that of the normal population, rather than having the increased mortality traditionally associated with such illnesses. Subsequently, Ahrens *et al.* (1993) studied 512 patients in centres in Germany and Canada, and found that a 'meaningful reduction in mortality' occurred if patients were treated with lithium for longer than 2 years, when their risk of suicide was reduced to that of the general population.

Coppen (1994) extended his earlier work and noted that a number of studies without lithium had found that there are between 5.1 and 11.6 suicides per thousand patient-years in untreated unipolar and bipolar illness, whereas Nilsson (1992), Muller-Oerlinghausen et al. (1992) and Coppen (1994) demonstrated that with long-term lithium treatment there were only 1.5, 1.3 and 0.7 suicides per thousand patient-years, respectively.

More recent reviews have confirmed these earlier reports. Baldessarini et al. (2003) collated a number of studies with an aggregate of 16 221 patients with exposure to lithium of 64 233 person-years, and reported that the risk per 100 person-years for attempted suicide was 4.65 without lithium versus 0.312 with lithium, a 93% difference, and for suicide the risk was 0.942 without lithium versus 0.174 with lithium, an 82% difference. They concluded that use of lithium in bipolar and unipolar affective disorders reduced suicidal risk 'to overall levels close to general population rates'. Others, including Schou (2000) and Tondo et al. (2003), have come to similar conclusions, and Muller-Oerlinghausen et al. (2003) have also noted that although lithium probably prevents about 250 suicides per year in Germany, 'rational treatment strategies most likely would demand that prescription rates be about 10 times higher'.

The question of whether or not anticonvulsant mood stabilizers have suicide protective qualities has been addressed by Goodwin et al. (2003) in a retrospective cohort study of 20 638 health-plan members with bipolar disorder. Both suicide and suicide attempts were significantly fewer in those treated with lithium, compared to Divalproex (sodium valproate), an anticonvulsant and the most commonly prescribed mood stabilizer in the USA.

None of these studies involved randomized controlled trials, but the results are compelling.

Antipsychotic (neuroleptic) medication

It is fair to state that there had been a sense of pessimism about suicide and schizophrenia until the observations of Meltzer and Okayli (1995) that 88 neuroleptic-resistant patients treated with clozapine for between 6 months and 7 years (mean 3.5 years) had 'markedly less suicidality' than non-clozapine-treated patients. This was noted on the basis of lower scores on the Hamilton Rating Scale for depression; attempted suicide decreased from 25% to 3.5%; the lethality of the suicide attempts that did occur was reduced; the suicidal intent was reduced; and there was a significant decrease in hopelessness. Subsequently Meltzer (1996) reported that of 102 000 patients treated for schizophrenia with clozapine, there were 39 suicides, with a rate adjusted for duration of treatment of 0.1–0.2% per year, which he noted was 'one fourth of the rate that would have been expected based on the published annual incidence of completed suicide in schizophrenia'.

Reid *et al.* (1998) reported similar findings from a study of 30 000 patients with schizophrenia and schizoaffective disorder, with clozapine-treated patients having a suicide rate of 12.7 per 100 000 per year compared to the 63.1 per 100 000 per year for all patients with the disorders in the USA.

These findings led to the establishment of an ambitious randomized multicentre trial in 67 centres in 11 countries (Meltzer *et al.* 2003), comparing clozapine with olanzapine. A total of 980 patients were randomized to the treatments and non-pharmacological input was identical. Clozapine was significantly superior in reducing suicide attempts, hospitalization, and the need for emergency intervention, but the suicides were too few for statistical analysis. In a further analysis of these data, Potkin *et al.* (2003) demonstrated that clozapine was more effective than olanzapine regardless of any individual risk factor, such as substance abuse or number of previous suicide attempts. Meltzer *et al.* (2003) concluded that 'use of clozapine in this population should lead to a significant reduction in suicidal behaviour'.

When it is appreciated that clozapine is usually reserved for those with resistance to conventional antipsychotic medication, these results are particularly persuasive.

It should be emphasized that the pharmacological treatments described are not necessarily specific for the prevention of suicide. Rather, they are part of the standard care that should be provided by a modern health service.

Large population studies

A number of governments have instituted national suicide prevention programmes, but only two, one from a Western country and another from a developing country, will be considered.

In 1985 Finnish health authorities inaugurated a programme to lower the suicide rate by 20% over the next 10 years (Kerkhof 1999). In fact, suicide increased initially, but then reduced to a figure about 9% below the initial level. This was the first research-based, comprehensive, national programme in the world, and involved community education about risk factors, with guidebooks for health promotion provided for schools, the armed services, and clergy, as well as the social services sector. It was acknowledged that there were gaps 'between medical paradigms and socio-cultural paradigms in understanding and preventing suicidal behaviour' and that more attention could have been paid to reducing access to means of suicide and suicide prevention in the elderly. However, it was considered that 'the project may have contributed to the reversal in the increasing suicide rate', and that 'the achievements of the project greatly outweigh its shortcomings' (Kerkhof 1999).

A more recent national programme from a developing country, Sri Lanka (previous Ceylon), has been associated with a reduction in reported suicides (De Silva and Jayasinghe 2003). Between 1950 and 1985 the suicide rate in Sri Lanka increased sixfold, and by 1995 the total number of suicides was 8514. In 1997 a presidential committee was established to address the high rate of suicide, with a focus on the reduction of ready access to pesticides and the introduction of less toxic alternatives; the enhancement of medical services, including those for the management of serious mental illnesses; the discouragement of sensational media reporting; and the decriminalization of suicide. Although causality cannot be claimed for any specific measure, it is reassuring that the number of suicides had reduced to 5412 in 2000.

While such large population interventions can be criticized for their general nature and the lack of specific theoretical framework, two recently published studies have been more rigorous in their research design, and have produced very encouraging results.

In a cohort of over 5 million United States Air Force personnel, Knox *et al.* (2003) reported a reduction of 33% in suicide between 1990–1996 and 1997–2002, following the introduction of an 11-point community-based programme to the Air Force population as a whole. This focused on the removal of stigma from seeking help for psychosocial problems, enhancing mental health literacy, and changing administrative policies to facilitate access to intervention services. It is also pertinent that they reported 'significant risk reductions' for accidental death, homicide, and family violence.

Positive results have also been reported by Hegerl *et al.* (2003), from the Nuremberg Alliance against Depression study, where a 2-year campaign in Nuremberg, a city of about half a million, to inform the community about depression, train family doctors, encourage co-operation with community facilitators such as teachers, priests, and the media, and also support self-help groups, resulted in a statistically significant reduction in suicidal acts compared to Wuerzburg, which was utilized as a control region.

Conclusion

The majority of these studies do not fulfil the required criteria for a randomized controlled trial, which is the usual gold standard of evidence-based research. However, it bears reiteration that the very fact that suicidal behaviours have such a low base rate makes it virtually impossible, at the very least with conventionally available resources, to mount the huge studies that would be necessary to have sufficient statistical power to demonstrate differences, even if it was ethically possible to do so.

Indeed, it is pertinent to reflect on the previously noted study of Tyrer *et al.* (2003), which involved 480 patients at a number of hospitals associated with five main centres. Subjects were confined to those who had had a previous episode of self-harm; they did not require in-patient care; and they did not have a psychotic or bipolar disorder, or a primary diagnosis of substance dependence. It is also pertinent that 40% of the experimental group did not return for treatment! Bearing these factors in mind, even if there had been a difference between the manual-assisted cognitive behaviour therapy and treatment-as-usual groups, it is doubtful whether that information would have been of much value to individual clinicians. Indeed, this is a good example of the fact that 'randomised controlled trials do not necessarily reflect real-world practice or experience' (Celermajer 2001). Furthermore, when one considers the apparent initial methodological soundness of that randomized controlled research design, with a large number of subjects in many different dedicated centres, it would appear to be difficult to justify similar such studies in the future, when interventions could be implemented on the basis of other research findings.

It is now no longer acceptable to state blandly that there is no convincing evidence for the effectiveness of suicide prevention measures, or that we do not know the relative importance of certain risk factors. Considerable knowledge is available, and the enigmatic comment of T.S. Eliot, who stated 'Where is the wisdom we have lost in knowledge?' is worthy of reflection.

Consider the fact that carefully controlled longitudinal case-control studies have identified and teased out the interrelationship between risk factors (Fergusson *et al.* 2003); that twin studies have confirmed the importance of both inherited and environmental factors (Statham *et al.* 1998; Glowinski *et al.* 2001; Fu *et al.* 2002); that population-attributable risk research has placed various risk factors in perspective; and that innovative research methodologies have demonstrated the effectiveness of a number of interventions.

It is also sobering to reflect on the observation that over 20% of suicides in association with hospitalization could have been prevented (Burgess *et al.* 2000; National Confidential Inquiry 2001), and this suggests that to be seen as focusing on issues such as unemployment, with a population attributable risk of 2.8% (Qin *et al.* 2003), or the impact of the media, which may be responsible for a maximum of 1–5% of suicides, with no recognition of the potential benefits of media campaigns (Goldney 2001), could be interpreted by a critical observer as an attempt to deflect attention from our own responsibility in suicide prevention.

The way ahead is clear. Broad social services efforts to counteract childhood antecedents of suicidal behaviour are important in their own right, and may pay dividends in terms of a reduction in suicide in the future. However, for more immediate results, community approaches, such as those outlined in the United States Air Force project (Knox *et al.* 2003) and the Nuremberg Alliance against Depression study (Hegerl *et al.* 2003), are models that could be emulated elsewhere, and, at the individual level, standard assessment and management health-care practices should be implemented for all who are suicidal.

Finally, it is acknowledged that this is a selective review. Indeed, the question posed by Balon (2003), after noting that the arguments in relation to SSRIs and suicidality of Healy (2003) contained 'mechanisms of good propaganda', of: 'Is the evidence, as with beauty, in the eye of the beholder?' could well apply to the present reviewer. Nevertheless, it is suggested that, far from being pessimistic about suicide prevention, by utilizing the knowledge gained from two centuries of suicide prevention research, and by putting it into practice in a manner similar to the effective interventions described, there is every reason to believe that the optimism expressed in a previous review (Goldney 1998) has been vindicated by more recent studies, and that the unacceptable rate of suicide worldwide can be reduced.

References

Agerbo, E., Nordentoft, M., and Mortensen, P.B. (2002). Familial, psychiatric and socioeconomic risk factors for suicide in young people: nested case-control study. *British Medical Journal*, **325**, 74–8.

Ahrens, B., Muller-Oerlinghausen, B., and Graf, F. (1993). Length of lithium treatment needed to eliminate the high mortality of affective disorders. *British Journal of Psychiatry*, **163** (suppl. 21), 27–9.

Angst, F., Stassen, H.H., Clayton, P.J., and Angst, J. (2002). Mortality of patients with mood disorders: follow-up over 34–38 years. *Journal of Affective Disorders*, **68**, 167–81.

Bagley, C. (1968). The evaluation of a suicide prevention scheme by an ecological method. *Social Science and Medicine*, **2**, 1–14.

Baldessarini, R.J., Tondo, L., and Hennen, J. (2003). Lithium treatment and suicide risk in major affective disorders: update and new findings. *Journal of Clinical Psychiatry*, **64**, 44–52.

Balon, R. (2003). Selective serotonin reuptake inhibitors and suicide: Is the evidence, as with beauty, in the eye of the beholder? *Psychotherapy and Psychosomatics*, **72**, 292–9.

Barraclough, B. (1972). Suicide prevention, recurrent affective disorder and lithium. *British Journal of Psychiatry*, **121**, 391–2.

Barraclough, B.M., Jennings, C., and Moss, J.R. (1977). Suicide prevention by the Samaritans: a controlled study of effectiveness. *Lancet*, **2**, 868–70.

Bateman, A. and Fonagy, P. (1999). Effectiveness of partial hospitalization in the treatment of borderline personality disorder: a randomized controlled trial. *American Journal of Psychiatry*, **156**, 1563–9.

Bateman, A. and Fonagy, P. (2001). Treatment of borderline personality disorder with psychoanalytically oriented partial hospitalization: an 18-month follow-up. *American Journal of Psychiatry*, 158, 1932–3.

Beautrais, A.L. (1999). *Risk factors for suicide and attempted suicide amongst young people*. National Health and Medical Research Council, Canberra.

Beautrais, A.L. (2001). Suicides and serious suicide attempts: two populations or one? *Psychological Medicine*, 31, 837–45.

Beautrais, A.L., Joyce, P.R., Mulder, R.T., Fergusson, D.M., Deavoll, B.J., and Nightingale, S.K. (1996). Prevalence and comorbidity of mental disorders in persons in serious suicide attempts: a case-control study. *American Journal of Psychiatry*, 153, 1009–14.

Bille-Brahe, U., Kerkhoff, A., De Leo, D., Schmidtke, A., Crepet, P., Lonnqvist, J., *et al.* (1996). A repetition–prediction study on European parasuicide populations. *Crisis*, 17, 22–31.

Bohus, M., Haaf, B., Stiglmayr, C., Pohl, U., Bohme, R., and Linehan, M. (2000). Evaluation of inpatient dialectical–behavioral therapy for borderline personality disorder—a prospective study. *Behavioral Research and Therapy*, 38, 875–87.

Burgess, P., Pirkis, J., Morton, J., and Croke, E. (2000). Lessons from a comprehensive clinical audit of users of psychiatric services who committed suicide. *Psychiatric Services*, 51, 1555–60.

Burgess, S., Geddes, J., Hawton, K., Townsend, E., Jamison, K., and Goodwin, G. (2001). Lithium for maintenance treatment of mood disorders. *Cochrane Database Systems Review*, CD003013.

Celermajer, D.S. (2001). Evidence-based medicine: how good is the evidence? *Medical Journal of Australia*, 174, 293–5.

Cheng, A.T.A. (1995). Mental illness and suicide: a case-control study in East Taiwan. *Archives of General Psychiatry*, 52, 594–603.

Coppen, A. (1994). Depression as a lethal disease: Prevention strategies. *Journal of Clinical Psychiatry*, 55 (suppl. 4), 37–45.

Coppen, A., Standish-Barry, H., and Bailey, J. (1990). Long term lithium and mortality. *Lancet*, 335, 1347.

Cuijpers, P. (2003). Examining the effects of prevention programs on the incidence of new cases of mental disorders: the lack of statistical power. *American Journal of Psychiatry*, 160, 1385–91.

De Leo, D., Marirosa, D.B., and Dwyer, J. (2002). Suicide among the elderly: the long-term impact of a telephone support and assessment intervention in northern Italy. *British Journal of Psychiatry*, 181, 226–9.

De Silva, D. and Jayasinghe, S. (2003). Suicide in Sri Lanka. In *Suicideprevention: Meeting the challenge together*, (ed. L. Vijayakumar), pp. 178–90. Orient Longman, Chennai.

Dube, S.R., Anda, R.F., Felitti, V.J., Chapman, D.P., Williamson, D.F., and Giles, W.H. (2001). Childhood abuse, household dysfunction, and the risk of attempted suicide throughout the life span. Findings from the Adverse Childhood Experiences Study. *Journal of the American Medical Association*, 286, 3089–96.

Fergusson, D.M., Beautrais, A.L., and Horwood, L.J. (2003). Vulnerability and resiliency to suicidal behaviours in young people. *Psychological Medicine*, 33, 61–73.

Frank, J. (1971). Therapeutic factors in psychotherapy. *American Journal of Psychotherapy*, 15, 350–61.

Fu, Q., Heath, A.C., Bucholz, K.K., *et al.* (2002). A twin study of genetic and environmental influences on suicide in men. *Psychological Medicine*, 32, 11–24.

Glowinski, A.L., Bucholz, K.K., Nelson, E.C., Fu, Q., Madden, P.A., and Reich, W.A.C. (2001). Suicide attempts in an adolescent female twin sample. *Journal of the American Academy of Child and Adolescent Psychiatry*, 40, 1300–7.

Goldney, R.D. (1998). Suicide prevention is possible: a review of recent studies. *Archives of Suicide Research*, 4, 329–39.

Goldney, R.D. (2000). Prediction of suicide and attempted suicide. In *The international handbook of suicide and attempted suicide*, (ed. K. Hawton and K. van Heeringen), pp. 585–95. John Wiley and Sons, Chichester.

Goldney, R.D. (2001). The media and suicide: a cautionary view. *Crisis*, 22, 173–5.

Goldney, R.D. and Schioldann, J.A. (2002). *Pre-Durkheim suicidology: the 1892 reviews of Tuke and Savage*. Adelaide Academic Press, Burnside.

Goldney, R.D., Wilson, D., Dal Grande, E., Fisher, L.J., and McFarlane, A.C. (2000). Suicidal ideation in a random community sample: attributable risk due to depression and psychosocial and traumatic events. *Australian and New Zealand Journal of Psychiatry*, 34, 98–106.

Goldney, R.D., Fisher, L.J., Wilson, D.H., and Cheok, F. (2001). Suicidal ideation and health-related quality of life in the community. *Medical Journal of Australia*, 175, 546–9.

Goldney, R.D., Dal Grande, E., Fisher, L.J., and Wilson, D. (2003). Population attributable risk of major depression for suicidal ideation in a random and representative community sample. *Journal of Affective Disorders*, 74, 267–72.

Goodwin, F.K., Fireman, B., Simon, G.E., Hunkeler, E.M., Lee, J., and Revicki, D. (2003). Suicide risk in bipolar disorder during treatment with lithium divalproex. *Journal of the American Medical Association*, 290, 1467–73.

Gunnell, D. and Frankel, S. (1994). Prevention of suicide: aspirations and evidence. *British Medical Journal*, 308, 1227–33.

Hall, W.D., Mant, A., Mitchell, P.B., Rendle, V.A., Hickie, I.B., and McManus, P. (2003). Association between antidepressant prescribing and suicide in Australia, 1991–2000: trend analysis. *British Medical Journal*, 326, 1008–11.

Harvey, P.M. and Solomons, B.J. (1983). Survival after free falls of 59 metres into water from the Sydney Harbour Bridge, 1930–1982. *Medical Journal of Australia*, 1, 504–11.

Hawton, K. (1998). Treatment studies of deliberate self-harm patients: recommended standards of the design of randomised controlled trials. Paper presented at the International Academy for Suicide Research meeting, Gent, 9 September.

Hawton, K., Arensman, E., Townsend, E., *et al.* (1998). Deliberate self harm: systematic review of efficacy of psychosocial and pharmacological treatments in preventing repetition. *British Medical Journal*, 317, 441–7.

Hawton, K., Townsend, E., Deeks, J., *et al.* (2001). Effects of legislation restricting pack sizes of paracetamol and salicylate on self poisoning in the United Kingdom: before and after study. *British Medical Journal*, 322, 1203–7.

Healy, D. (2003). Lines of evidence on the risk of suicide with selective serotonin reuptake inhibitors. *Psychotherapy and Psychosomatics*, 72, 71–9.

Hegerl, U., Althaus, D., Niklewski, G., and Schmidtke, A. (2003). Optimierte Versorgung depressiver Patienten und Suizidpravention: Ergebnisse des, Nurnberger Bundnisses gegen Depression. *Deutsches Arzteblatt*, 42, 2137–42.

Hickey, L., Hawton, K., Fagg, J., and Weitzel, H. (2001). Deliberate self-harm patients who leave the accident and emergency department without a psychiatric assessment: a neglected population at risk of suicide. *Journal of Psychosomatic Research*, 50, 87–93.

Hulten, A. and Wasserman, D. (1998). Lack of continuity—a problem in the care of young suicides. *Acta Psychiatrica Scandinavica*, 97, 326–33.

Isacsson, G. (2000). Suicide prevention—a medical breakthrough? *Acta Psychiatrica Scandinavica*, 102, 113–17.

Isacsson, G., Holmgren, P., Druid, H., and Bergman, U. (1999). Psychotropics and suicide prevention. Implications from toxicological screening of 5281 suicides in Sweden 1992–1994. *British Journal of Psychiatry*, 174, 259–65.

Joiner, T.E. Jr, Steer, R.A., Brown, G., Beck, A.T., Pettit, J.W., and Rudd, M.D. (2003). Worst-point suicidal plans: a dimension of suicidality predictors, past suicide attempts and eventual death by suicide. *Behavioural Research and Therapy*, 41, 1469–80.

Kapur, N., House, A., Dodgson, K., May, C., and Creed, F. (2002). Effect of general hospital management on repeat episodes of deliberate self poisoning: cohort study. *British Medical Journal*, 325, 866–7.

Kerkhof, A.J.F.M. (1999). The Finnish National Suicide Prevention Program Evaluated. *Crisis*, 20, 50 and 63.

King, R., Nurcombe, B., Bickman, L., Hides, L., and Reid, W. (2003). Telephone counselling for adolescent suicide prevention: changes suicidality and mental state from beginning to end of a counselling session. *Suicide and Life Threatening Behaviour*, 33, 400–11.

Knox, K.L., Litts, D.A., Feig, J.C., and Caine, D. (2003). Risk of suicide and related adverse outcomes after exposure to a suicide prevention programme in the US Air Force: cohort study. *British Medical Journal*, 327, 1376–80.

Kreitman, N. (1976). The coal gas story. *British Journal of Preventive and Social Medicine*, 30, 86–93.

Lester, D. (1997). The effectiveness of suicide prevention centres: a review. *Suicide and Life Threatening Behaviour*, 27, 304–10.

Lester, D., Beck, A.T., and Mitchell, B. (1979). Extrapolation from attempted suicides to completed suicides: a test. *Journal of Abnormal Psychology*, 88, 78–80.

Letizia, C., Kapik, B., and Flanders, W.D. (1996). Suicidal risk during controlled clinical investigations of fluvoxamine. *Journal of Clinical Psychiatry*, 57, 415–21.

Lewis, G., Hawton, K., and Jones, P. (1997). Strategies for preventing suicides. *British Journal of Psychiatry*, 171, 351–4.

Lilienfeld, A.M. and Lilienfeld, D.E. (1980). *Foundations of epidemiology*, (2nd edn). Oxford University Press, Oxford.

Linehan, M.M. (1992). *Cognitive therapy for borderline personality disorder*. Guilford Press, New York.

Linehan, M.M., Hubert, A.E., Suarez, A., Allmon, D., and Heard, H.L. (1991). Cognitive-behavioural treatment of chronically parasuicidal borderline patients. *Archives of General Psychiatry*, 48, 1060–4.

Marecek, J. and Ratnayeke, L. (2001). Suicide in rural Sri Lanka: assessing a prevention programme. In *Suicide risk and protective factors in the new millenium*, (ed. O.T. Grad), pp. 215–19. Cankarjev dom, Ljubljana.

Marzuk, P.M., Tardiff, K., Leon, A.C., *et al.* (1995). Use of prescription psychotropic drugs among suicide victims in New York City. *American Journal of Psychiatry*, 152, 1520–2.

Meltzer, H.Y. (1996). Suicidality and clozapine. *Journal of Clinical Psychiatry*, 14, 13–14.

Meltzer, H.Y. and Okayli, G. (1995). Reduction of suicidality during clozapine treatment of neuroleptic-resistant schizophrenia: Impact on risk benefit assessment. *American Journal of Psychiatry*, 152, 183–90.

Meltzer, H.Y., Alphs, L., Green, A.I., *et al.* (2003). Clozapine treatment for suicidality in schizophrenia. International Suicide Prevention Trial (InterSePT). *Archives of General Psychiatry*, 60, 82–91.

Modestin, J. and Schwarzenbach, F. (1992). Effect of psychopharmacotherapy on suicide risk in discharge psychiatric patients. *Acta Psychiatrica Scandinavica*, 85, 173–5.

Montgomery, S.A., Dunner, D.L., and Dunbar, G.C. (1995). Reduction of suicidal thoughts with paroxetine in comparison with reference antidepressants and placebo. *European Neuropsychopharmacology*, 5, 5–13.

Morgan, H.G. and Priest, P. (1991). Suicide and other unexpected deaths among psychiatric inpatients. The Bristol Confidential Inquiry. *British Journal of Psychiatry*, 158, 368–74.

Mortensen, P.B., Agerbo, E., Erikson, T., Qin, P., and Westergaard-Nielsen, N. (2000). Psychiatric illness and risk factors for suicide in Denmark. *Lancet*, 355, 9–12.

Motto, J.A. and Bostrom, A.G. (2001). A randomized controlled trial of postcrisis suicide prevention. *Psychiatric Services*, 52, 828–33.

Muller-Oerlinghausen, B., Muser-Causemann, B., and Volk, J. (1992). Suicides and parasuicides in a high-risk group on and off lithium long-term medication. *Journal of Affective Disorders*, 25, 261–70.

Muller-Oerlinghausen, B., Berghofer, A., and Ahrens, B. (2003). The antisuicidal and mortality-reducing effect of lithium prophylaxis: consequences for guidelines in clinical psychiatry. *Canadian Journal of Psychiatry*, 48, 433–9.

National Confidential Inquiry (2001). *Safety first: Five-year report of the National Confidential Inquiry into Suicide and Homicide by People with Mental Illness*. Department of Health Publications, London.

Nilsson, A. (1992). Mortality in a lithium-treated population with mood disorders. *Clinical Neuropharmacology*, 15 (suppl. 1), 448B–448b.

Olfson, M., Shaffer, D., Marcus, S.C., and Greenberg, T. (2003). Relationship between antidepressant medication treatment and suicide in adolescents. *Archives of General Psychiatry*, 60, 978–82.

Oliver, R.G. and Hetzel, B.S. (1972). The rise and fall of suicide rates in Australia: Relation to sedative availability. *Medical Journal of Australia*, 2, 919–23.

Ottoson, J.O. (1979). The suicidal patient—can the psychiatrist prevent his suicide? In *Origin, prevention and treatment of affective disorders*, (ed. M. Schou and E. Stromgren), pp. 257–67. Academic Press, London.

Pirkis, J., Burgess, P., and Dunt, D. (2000). Suicidal ideation and suicide attempts among Australian adults. *Crisis*, 21, 16–25.

Pokorny, A.D. (1983). Prediction of suicide in psychiatric patients. *Archives of General Psychiatry*, 40, 249–57.

Potkin, S.G., Alphs, L., Hsu, C., *et al.* (2003). Predicting suicidal risk in schizophrenic and schizoaffective patients in a prospective two-year trial. *Biological Psychiatry*, 54, 444–52.

Qin, P., Agerbo, E., and Mortensen, P.B. (2003). Suicide risk in relation to socioeconomic, demographic, psychiatric, and familial factors: a national register-based study of all suicides in Denmark, 1981–1997. *American Journal of Psychiatry*, 160, 765–72.

Reid, W.H., Mason, M., and Hogan, T. (1998). Suicide prevention effects associated with clozapine therapy in schizophrenia and schizoaffective disorder. *Psychiatric Services*, 49, 1029–33.

Retterstol, N. (1996). Prevention of suicide, past and present, with special reference to national programs. Paper presented at the Sixth European Symposium on Suicide and Suicidal Behaviour, Lund.

Rosen, A. (1954). Detection of suicidal patients: an example of some limitations in the prediction of infrequent events. *Journal of Consulting Psychology*, 18, 397–403.

Rutz, W., von Knorring, L., and Walinder, J. (1992). Long-term effects of an educational program for general practitioners given by the Swedish Committee for the prevention and treatment of depression. *Acta Psychiatrica Scandinavica*, 85, 83–8.

Schou, M. (2000). Suicidal behavior and prophylactic lithium treatment of major mood disorders: a review of reviews. *Suicide and Life-Threatening Behavior*, 30, 289–93.

Schulsinger, F., Kety, S.S., Rosenthal, D. and Wender, P.H. (1979). A family study of suicide. In *Origin, prevention and treatment of affective disorders*, (ed. M. Schou and E. Stromgren), pp. 277–87. Academic Press, London.

Sokero, T.P., Melartin, T.K., Rytsala, H.J., Leskela, U.S., Lestela-Mielonen, P.S., and Isometsa, E.T. (2003). Suicidal ideation and attempts among psychiatric patients with major depressive disorder. *Journal of Clinical Psychiatry*, 64, 1094–100.

Sonneck, G., Etzersdorfer, E., and Nagel-Kuess, S. (1994). Imitative suicide on the Viennese subway. *Social Science and Medicine*, 38, 453–7.

Statham, D.J., Heath, A.C., Madden, P.A.F., *et al.* (1998). Suicidal behaviour: An epidemiological and genetic study. *Psychological Medicine*, 28, 839–55.

Stevenson, J. and Meares, R. (1992). An outcome study of psychotherapy for patients with borderline personality disorder. *American Journal of Psychiatry*, 149, 358–62.

Suominen, K.H., Isometsa, E.T., Henriksson, M.M., Ostamo, A.I., and Lonnqvist, J.K. (1998). Inadequate treatment for major depression both before and after attempted suicide. *American Journal of Psychiatry*, 155, 1778–80.

Szanto, K., Mulsant, B.H., Houck, P., Dew, M.A., and Reynolds, C.F. 3rd (2003). Occurrence and course of suicidality during short-term treatment of late-life depression. *Archives of General Psychiatry*, 60, 610–17.

Tondo, L., Isacsson, G., and Baldessarini, R. (2003). Suicidal behaviour in bipolar disorder: risk and prevention. *Central Nervous System Drugs*, 17, 491–511.

Tyrer, P., Thompson, S., Schmidt, U., *et al.* (2003). Randomized controlled trial of brief cognitive behaviour therapy versus treatment as usual in recurrent deliberate self-harm: the POPMACT study. *Psychological Medicine*, 33, 969–76.

Verheul, R., van den Bosch, L.M.C., Koeter, M.W.J., de Ridder, M.A.J., Stinjnen, T., and van den Brink, W. (2003). Dialectical behaviour therapy for women with borderline personality disorder. *British Journal of Psychiatry*, 182, 135–40.

Waern, M., Beskow, J., Runeson, B., and Skoog, I. (1999). Suicidal feelings in the last years of life in elderly people who commit suicide. *Lancet*, 354, 917–18.

Whitlock, F.A. (1977). Psychiatric epidemiology: Its uses and limitations. *Australian and New Zealand Journal of Psychiatry*, 11, 9–18.

Wilkinson, G. (1994). Can suicide be prevented? Better treatment of mental illness is more appropriate aim. *British Medical Journal*, 309, 860–1.

World Health Organisation (1993). *Guidelines for the primary prevention of mental neurological and psychosocial disorders.* WHO, Geneva.

11

The burden of suicide and clinical suggestions for prevention

Kay Redfield Jamison and Keith Hawton

The burden of suicide

Suicide is often talked about as a rare event. This is misleading. If one takes the example of death in young men, first in wartime (Vietnam War) and then in relation to a killer disease (AIDS), this is very clear (Fig. 11.1). During the whole period of the Vietnam War (1965–1973) many more lives of young American men were lost to suicide than in the war. Likewise, when deaths from AIDS were at a peak, as many young men were dying from suicide as from this disease. Figure 11.1 also shows the remarkable rise and cumulative toll of deaths by suicide in young men that has occurred over the past several decades, although the numbers have plateaued of late. The trends in suicide in

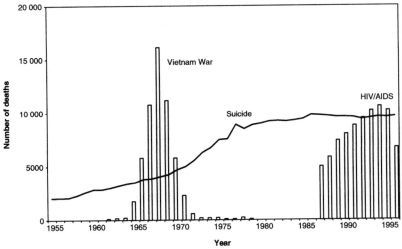

Fig. 11.1 Deaths in males (aged 35 years or younger) in the USA from suicide, the Vietnam War, and HIV/AIDS (adapted with permission from Jamison 1999).

young men shown in Fig. 11.1 are for the USA, but a similar pattern has been seen in many other developing coutries (Cantor 2000).

While men are several times more likely to kill themselves than women, in some countries, especially China, rates of suicide in young women are extremely high. As a result of this, suicide is the second most common cause of death in females aged 15–24 years worldwide (after tuberculosis).

Numerically, suicide is a leading cause of death in very young people. In students in the USA, for example, suicide is second only to accidents as a cause of death. In 15–19-year-olds in America in 1996 the number of suicides exceeded the cumulative total for cancer (including leukaemia), heart disease, lung disease, congenital abnormalities, stroke, HIV, and diabetes.

In the UK, unpublished data collected by the second author also show that, in university students, suicide is the second most frequent cause of death after accidents. This is also seen for overall suicide rates in 15–24 year-old males.

In many countries, suicide rates are higher in older than younger people. However, due to fewer people being at risk in older age groups, the numerical burden of suicide is much greater in the young. This is shown in Fig. 11.2 for males in the USA. Figure 11.2 also shows how suicide rates markedly increase at around the age of 15 years and how the maximum number of deaths occurs between the twenties and forties to fifties. In females, the numbers of suicides run more or less in parallel with rates until age 50 years, after which the numbers of suicides get steadily lower than the rate of suicide (Fig. 11.3).

Figures 11.4 and 11.5 show similar comparisons for England and Wales. Due to a decline in suicide rates in older males and a recent increase in rates in younger males, suicide rates are higher in 25–54 year-olds than in other age groups, except the oldest males. The numerical burden of suicide is also greatest in 25–64 year-olds, whereas the high rate in the oldest age group represents far fewer deaths (Fig. 11.4). The pattern is similar in women (Fig. 11.5), although the numbers and rates are much lower than in males. In females, the rate of suicide remains quite steady from age 25–34 years through to old age, reflecting a very large recent decline in suicide rates in older females.

The burden of suicide in younger adults has also been highlighted in the UK by examining the years of life expectancy (YLE) lost to suicide in younger people (Gunnell and Middleton 2003). This showed that while suicide rates have fallen, differential changes in rates within age groups, with increases in young men, have resulted in an increase in potential years of life lost through suicide.

Role of psychiatric disorder in suicide

Why does suicide become more common in the late teenage years and early twenties? There are several possible explanations. The most likely explanation

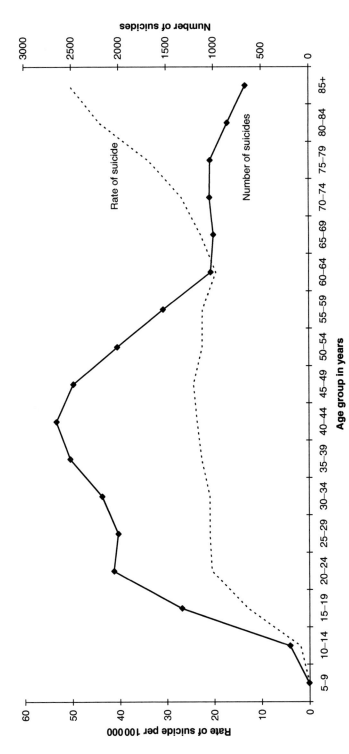

Fig. 11.2 Suicide rates and numbers of suicides, by age group, USA, 2001: males. (Data sources: NCHS Vital Statistics System for number of deaths. Bureau of Census for Population Estimates, WISQUARS Injury Mortality Report, Office of Statistics and Programming, National Center for Injury Prevention and Control, CDC.)

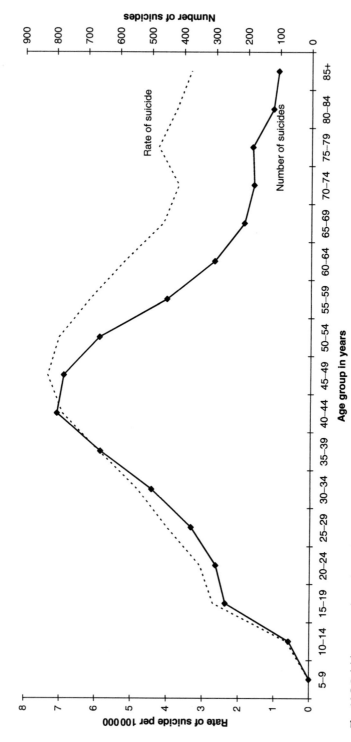

Fig. 11.3 Suicide rates and numbers of suicides, by age group, USA, 2001: females. (Data sources: NCHS Vital Statistics System for number of deaths. Bureau of Census for Population Estimates, WISQUARS Injury Mortality Report, Office of Statistics and Programming, National Center for Injury Prevention and Control, CDC.)

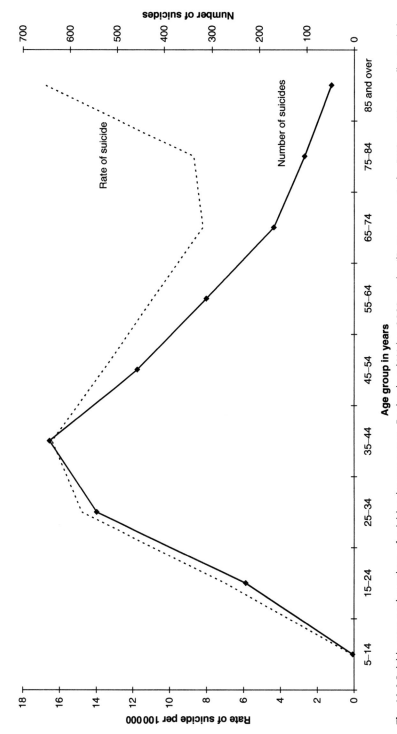

Fig. 11.4 Suicide rates and numbers of suicides, by age group, England and Wales, 2002: males. (Data source: Series DH2 no. 29, Mortality Statistics, Table 2.19 and Table 4, Office for National Statistics.)

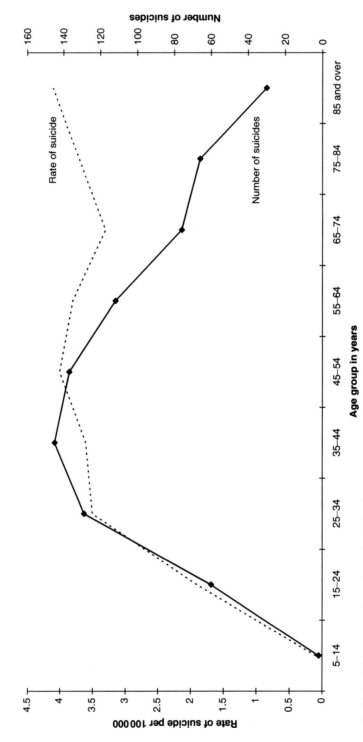

Fig. 11.5 Suicide rates and numbers of suicides, by age group, England and Wales, 2002: females. (Data source: Series DH2 no. 29, Mortality Statistics, Table 2.19 and Table 4, Office for National Statistics.)

is that this is the period of life that represents the peak time of onset for the major psychiatric disorders most implicated in suicide. For example, the average age of onset for depression is 26.5 years, bipolar disorder 18 years (bipolar 1) to 21.7 years (bipolar 2), schizophrenia 19 years, drug abuse/dependence 18 years, and alcohol abuse or dependence 21 years. So, this is the age at which first episodes of psychiatric illness are likely to occur, and it is during these initial episodes in most disorders that young people are particularly vulnerable to suicide.

Study after study of suicides worldwide has shown that the association between mental illness and suicide is extremely strong, with approximately 90% of those who commit suicide having a diagnosable mental illness (Table 11.1). The only exception is China (Phillips *et al.* 2002), but here the unusual demographic pattern of suicides (with an excess of young female suicides) might be an explanation. Unfortunately, suicide is often represented in the media as a direct response to a major life event. In reality, the causes of suicide are usually complex, but with mental illness a significant underlying factor in most cases. While life events, such as relationship break-ups, significant failures, and financial problems, may contribute to and also influence the timing of suicide, to deny the contribution of psychiatric illness is to neglect a crucial and powerful contributor to suicide. Also, these disorders are usually treatable.

Consideration of the excess risk of suicide in certain psychiatric disorders compared with the general population illustrates their importance in contributing to a suicidal outcome. For example, in their meta-analysis of studies, Harris and Barraclough (1997) showed that the number of times the rate of

Table 11.1 Suicide and psychiatric illness: results of some major psychological autopsy studies

Authors	Place	Number of suicides	Percentage with psychiatric disorder
Robins *et al.* (1959)	St Louis, USA	134	94
Barraclough *et al.* (1974)	England	100	93
Beskow (1979)	Sweden	271	97
Chynoweth *et al.* (1980)	Australia	135	88
Rich *et al.* (1986)	San Diego, USA	204	92
Cheng (1995)	Taiwan	116	97
Foster *et al.* (1997)	Northern Ireland	116	97
Vijayakumar and Rajkumar (1999)	India	100	88
Phillips *et al.* (2002)	China	519	63

suicide exceeded the expected rate in the general population was 20.4 for depression, 15.1 for manic depression, 8.4 for schizophrenia, 14 for opiate abuse, and 5.9 for alcohol abuse. There is also a particularly strong link to previous suicide attempts; the excess risk of suicide in Harris and Barraclough's meta-analysis was 40.7 for attempts by self-poisoning and 38.4 for attempts involving other methods.

An added factor that considerably increases suicide risk is co-morbidity of psychiatric with substance abuse or personality disorders. Alcohol abuse, for example, greatly elevates the risk of suicide in those with affective disorders. Unfortunately, people with affective disorders are also at greatly increased risk of abusing alcohol. In some, this may be a form of self-medication for their depressive symptoms. Genetic factors may also contribute to this co-morbidity. Alcohol and drug abuse can make a person more impulsive, and hence more likely to act on their suicidal thoughts. Furthermore, alcohol and drugs may also make things worse because of their damaging effects on sleep, and sleep disturbance is a factor that greatly increases risk of recurrence or worsening of affective episodes. Additionally, alcohol and drugs may undermine the effectiveness of psychotropic medication used to treat affective or other disorders.

Genetic influences on suicidal behaviour

While mood disorders, especially bipolar illness, are strongly influenced by genetic factors, there also appears to be a genetic influence on suicide risk, independent of the inheritance of illness. On the basis of combined data from several studies (Haberlandt 1967; Jeul-Nielsen and Videbech 1970; Zair 1981; Roy et al. 1991), in which a total of 399 twin pairs were examined, where one twin had committed suicide the other twin also died by suicide in 13.2% of twins who were monozygotic, compared with just 0.7% of those who were dizygotic ($P < 0.001$).

In patients with bipolar disorder, Roy (1983) found that 38% of those with a family history of suicide in first- or second-degree relatives, themselves made suicide attempts, compared with 14% of those without a family history of suicide ($P < 0.0001$). Thus there is a strong genetic contribution to both suicide and attempted suicide.

When are people with psychiatric disorders at risk of suicide?

One of the major problems for prevention of suicide in severe psychiatric illness is that, as noted above, suicide risk is usually highest early in the course of illness. It is certainly the case for depression (Lönnqvist 2000), bipolar disorder (Goodwin and Jamison 1990), and schizophrenia (De Hert and Peuskens 2000). This is well illustrated in bipolar disorder. In Sweden, Osby *et al.* (2001) found that, for the 15 386 patients discharged from hospital with a diagnosis of bipolar disorder between 1973 and 1995, the standardized mortality ratio for suicide in the first year of follow-up was 15.0 in males and 22.4 in females. However, in those under 30 years of age the ratio was 81.6 in males and 71.7 in females.

The important link between suicide risk and the early stages of psychiatric illness underscores the importance of trying to detect and treat these illnesses at an early stage. One reason for the elevated suicide rate early in the illness is that it is the time when accurate diagnosis is least likely. This may partly be because of patients' failure to recognize the significance of symptoms and hence to seek help, and, in those who do come to clinical attention, reluctance of clinicians to make a firm diagnosis based on a first episode of mood abnormalities. This means that to improve prevention one needs to put considerable effort into diagnosis and treatment of first episodes of illness. As noted earlier, this is likely to be when people are in their teenage years or twenties, a time when patients may be most reluctant to accept treatment. In part, this may reflect their limited understanding of the illness and hence the need for treatment. Also, young people in the early stages of illness are particularly likely to deny the fact that they have a major illness. This is easily understandable in terms of the complications that it might have for their lifestyle and future. Even if they start on medication, compliance is often poor, especially if there are side-effects which they perceive as interfering with their cognitive abilities, energy, and enthusiasm.

The well-recognized seasonal variation in suicide, with a late spring/early summer peak (Meares *et al.* 1981; Goodwin and Jamison 1990), may be particularly marked in patients with affective disorders, especially bipolar disorder. Interestingly, however, there appears to have been some flattening out of the traditional seasonal variation in suicide rates generally (Rihmer *et al.* 1998; Yip *et al.* 1998). Some people have attributed this to the fact that modern living circumstances, especially well-lit buildings and effective heating, have meant that many people today are less subject to seasonal variation in environmental influences (Aschoff 1981). Others have suggested that antidepressants may also have been a factor in this change (Rihmer *et al.* 1998).

A further important temporal pattern of suicide is that the time of risk in relation to an episode of illness may be particularly high when a person is going into or coming out of an episode of mania, depression, or psychosis. Agitation may then be a marked feature, and this can contribute to impulsiveness and suicidal thinking. In bipolar disorders the transition points between mania and depression, or the transition from depression into recovery, are periods of greatly heightened risk, as agitation may then be particularly marked.

Some implications for treatment and prevention

While antidepressants and mood stabilizers are clearly effective in treatment of depression and bipolar illness, the problems of compliance that have already been highlighted mean that other measures may need to be used in order to maximize their efficiency. Combining antidepressants with psychotherapeutic measures is likely to be the most effective option (Blackburn *et al.* 1981; Murphy *et al.* 1984; Lam *et al.* 2000). Unfortunately, limitations in access to psychotherapy may undermine the extent to which it is available. This treatment option is particularly likely to be useful for young people experiencing the early stages of illness, the time we have already highlighted as that when risk is greatest. Psychotherapeutic measures can also be used to enhance compliance with medication (Cochran 1984; Lam *et al.* 2000).

Particular attention needs to be paid to the problems of severe insomnia, anxiety, agitation, and impulsivity. Patients and relatives need to be informed that these are symptoms to look out for, especially given their link to suicide risk. This also underlines the need for there to be ease of access to clinicians for relatives and patients, particularly when such symptoms are present. Things to look out for need to be written down, especially given the cognitive problems that often accompany psychiatric illness.

Evidence is pointing strongly towards a specific anti-suicidal effect of lithium (Baldessarini *et al.* 2003). While there are considerable limitations to some of the studies that have been put forward to make this case, the sheer weight of studies pointing in the same direction supports this notion. A recent systematic review of randomized controlled trials, in which lithium therapy was compared with either placebo or comparator drugs, has provided more substantial support for the anti-suicidal effect of lithium (Cipriani *et al.* 2005). Why should lithium have this effect? It has been known for several years that, not only does lithium have benefits for mood disorder in stabilizing mood (Geddes *et al.* 2004), but it also has beneficial effects on aggression, violence, and impulsivity (Sheard *et al.* 1976), all of which are related to suicide risk (Mann *et al.* 1999). Thus the specific benefits of lithium in preventing suicide may result from its double action, first in reducing risk of relapse, and second in attenuating these potentially dangerous symptoms.

Unfortunately, lithium prescriptions for newly diagnosed bipolar disorders have steadily declined in recent years. On the other hand, those for Divalproex (sodium valproate) have markedly increased, so that it has become the most common drug used for bipolar disorder, at least in the USA (Goodwin *et al.* 2003). Such trends clearly reflect the potential financial return of drug companies, in that advertising and promotion of lithium represents a tiny fraction of that of Divalproex. Yet, there is evidence to suggest that the occurrence of suicidal behaviour in patients receiving lithium may be two or three times less than the occurrence in those on Divalproex (Goodwin *et al.* 2003).

There is also early evidence that clozapine may have anti-suicidal effects in schizophrenia. The strongest evidence for this comes from a randomized controlled study in which patients with schizophrenia or schizoaffective disorders, who were known to be at risk of suicidal behaviour, were prescribed either clozapine or olanzapine (Meltzer *et al.* 2003). There were significantly fewer subsequent suicide attempts in the patients prescribed clozapine and also a smaller number of admissions because of suicidal crises. There were significantly fewer subsequent suicide attempts in the patients prescribed clozapine and also a smaller number of admissions because of suicidal crises.

It is highly unusual for a drug trial in psychiatry to focus on patients at significant risk of suicide, as was the case in the study of clozapine versus olanzipine. Usually, such patients are excluded from trials, which partly explains why we lack definitive information on whether antidepressants have anti-suicidal effects. Indeed, there is currently much controversy about the potential role of antidepressants in the prevention of suicide. It is difficult to conclude whether or not antidepressants have anti-suicidal effects, because the evidence put forward in support of such an effect is largely indirect. This includes the reduction in suicide rates in Scandinavia that has paralleled the increase in use of antidepressants (Isacsson 2000), and a similar pattern for antidepressant use and suicide in Hungary (Rihmer *et al.* 2001).

There seems to be a large potential role for psychotherapy in the prevention of suicide in people with major psychiatric disorders. Several randomized controlled trials have been conducted, in which a psychological intervention was evaluated in the management of bipolar disorder (reviewed by Jones, 2004). These have generally shown that the patients who received the psychological treatment had fewer subsequent episodes of illness. In some studies the episodes were also shorter, and hospitalization rates were lower. These patients also tended to have improved social functioning. The possible therapeutic mechanisms of psychotherapy in bipolar disorder include close monitoring of affective symptoms, modification of environmental factors that may influence the cause of illness, enhanced compliance with medication, enhanced social support, improved family adjustment, regulation of daily routines, and improved coping strategies (Zaretsky *et al.* 1999). Unfortunately, financial factors may make it less likely that patients will receive such interventions. This is especially the case in the USA where lack of health insurance may be the reason, or, even if patients have health insurance, this might not cover psychotherapy.

One specific component of psychological management of patients is helping them to realize that recovery from episodes of illness can be particularly difficult, in that are they are likely to experience many setbacks. The key is to explain that setbacks are common, and to try and help the patient accept such setbacks without reacting catastrophically in a way that leads to relapse or interferes with recovery. Education, perhaps using daily ratings of mood, can assist patients in recognizing this.

Conclusions

Suicide is far more common than most people believe. The largest number of suicides is in males in younger adulthood, and suicide is the second most common cause of death in the very young. While suicide is a complex phenomenon in terms of the causes and processes that lead up to it, the extremely strong link to psychiatric disorders is undeniable. These disorders especially include depression, bipolar disorder, schizophrenia, and alcohol and drug abuse/dependence, and severe personality disorders. Suicide risk tends to be greatest in the early stages of affective disorders and schizophrenia. Yet these are times when these disorders may not have been diagnosed and effective treatment initiated. Also, because the onset of all the major disorders is greatest in late adolescence and early adulthood, there may be considerable reluctance to start, or to continue, taking psychotropic medication, because of fears about interference with lifestyle and a sense of being labelled. Denial is a particular problem in young patients. Yet early diagnosis and effective treat-ment are of paramount importance to prevention of the suicide risk associated with these disorders. Psychotherapy may have a significant role to play in helping people understand and accept their illness, in encouraging compliance with medication, and in facilitating coping with the often erratic recovery process.

References

Aschoff, J. (1981). Annual rhythms in man. In *Handbook of behavioural neurobiology* Vol. 4. *Biological rhythms*, (ed. J. Aschoff). Plenum, New York.

Baldessarini, R.J., Tondo, L., and Hennen, J. (2003). Lithium treatment and suicide risk in major affective disorders: update and new findings. *Journal of Clinical Psychiatry,* **64** (suppl. 5), 44–52.

Barraclough, B., Bunch, J., Nelson, B., and Sainsbury, P. (1974). A hundred cases of suicide: clinical aspects. *British Journal of Psychiatry*, 125, 355–73.

Beskow, J. (1979). Suicide and mental disorder in Swedish men. *Acta Psychiatrica Scandinavica*, 277 (Supplement), 1–138.

Blackburn, I M., Bishop, S., Glen, A.I.M., Whalley, L.J., and Christie, J.E. (1981). The efficacy of cognitive therapy and pharmacotherapy, each alone and in combination. *British Journal of Psychiatry*, 139, 181–9.

Cantor, C.H. (2000). Suicide in the Western world. In *The international handbook of suicide and attempted suicide*, (ed. K. Hawton and K. Van Heeringen). Wiley, Chichester.

Cheng, A.T. (1995). Mental illness and suicide: a case-control study in East Taiwan. *Archives of General Psychiatry*, 52, 592–603.

Chynoweth, R., Tonge, J.I., and Armstrong, J. (1980). Suicide in Brisbane: a retrospective psychosocial study. *Australian and New Zealand Journal of Psychiatry*, 14, 37–45.

Cipriani, A., Wilder, H., Hawton, K., and Geddes, J.R. (2005). Lithium in the prevention of suicidal behaviour and all-cause mortality in patients with mood disorders: a systematic review of randomised trials *American Journal of Psychiatry* (in press).

Cochran, S.D. (1984). Preventing medical noncompliance in the outpatient treatment of bipolar affective disorders. *Journal of Consulting and Clinical Psychology*, 52, 873–8.

De Hert, M. and Peuskens, J. (2000). Psychiatric aspects of suicidal behaviour: schizophrenia. In *International handbook of suicide and attempted suicide,* (ed. K. Hawton and K. Van Heeringen). Wiley, Chichester.

Foster, T., Gillespie, K., and McClelland, R. (1997). Mental disorders and suicide in Northern Ireland. *British Journal of Psychiatry*, 170, 447–52.

Geddes, J., Burgess, S., Hawton, K., Jamison, K., and Goodwin, G.M. (2004). Long-term lithium therapy for bipolar disorder: systematic review and meta-analysis of randomized controlled trials. *American Journal of Psychiatry*, 161, 217–22.

Goodwin, F. and Jamison, K.R. (1990). *Manic depressive illness.* Oxford University Press, New York.

Goodwin, F.K., Fireman, B., Simon, G.E., Hunkeler, E.M., Lee, J., and Revicki, D. (2003). Suicide risk in bipolar disorder during treatment with lithium and Divalproex. *Journal of the American Medical Association*, 290, 1467–73.

Gunnell, D. and Middleton, N. (2003). National suicide rates as an indicator of the effect of suicide on premature mortality. *Lancet*, 362, 961–2.

Haberlandt, W. (1967). Aportación a la genética del suicidio. *Filio Clinica Internacional*, 17, 319–22.

Harris, E.C. and Barraclough, B. (1997). Suicide as an outcome for mental disorders. A meta-analysis. *British Journal of Psychiatry*, 170, 205–28.

Isacsson, G. (2000). Suicide prevention – a medical breakthrough? *Acta Psychiatrica Scandinavica*, 102, 113–17.

Jamison, K.R. (1999). *Night falls fast: Understanding suicide.* Alfred A. Knopf, New York.

Jeul-Nielsen, N. and Videbech, T. (1970). A twin study of suicide. *Acta Geneticae Medicae et Gemellologiae*, 19, 307–310.

Jones, S. (2004). Psychotherapy of bipolar disorder: a review. *Journal of Affective Disorders*, 80, 101–14.

Lam, D., Bright, J., Jones, S., Hayward, P., Schuck, N., Chisholm, D., and Sham, P. (2000). Cognitive therapy for bipolar illness – a pilot study of relapse prevention. *Cognitive Research and Therapy*, 24, 503–20.

Lönnqvist, J.K. (2000). Psychiatric aspects of suicidal behaviour: depression. In *The International handbook of suicide and attempted suicide*, (ed. K. Hawton and K. Van Heeringen). Wiley, Chichester.

Mann, J.J., Waternaux, C., Haas, G.L., and Malone, K.M. (1999). Toward a clinical model of suicidal behavior in psychiatric patients. *American Journal of Psychiatry*, 156, 181–9.

Meares, R., Mendelsohn, F.A.O., and Milgrom-Friedman, J. (1981). A sex difference in the seasonal variation of suicide rate: a single cycle for men, two cycles for women. *British Journal of Psychiatry*, 138, 321–5.

Meltzer, H.Y., Alphs, L., Green, A.I., Altamura, A.C., Anand, R., Bertoldi, A., *et al.* (2003). Clozapine treatment for suicidality in schizophrenia. *Archives of General Psychiatry*, 60, 82–91.

Murphy, G.E., Simons, A.D., Wetzel, R.D., and Lustman, P.J. (1984). Cognitive therapy and pharmacotherapy: singly and together in the treatment of depression. *Archives of General Psychiatry*, 41, 33–41.

Osby, L., Brandt, L., Correia, N., Ekbom, A., and Sparen, P. (2001). Excess mortality in bipolar and unipolar disorder in Sweden. *Archives of General Psychiatry*, 58, 844–50.

Phillips, M.R., Yang, G., Zhang, Y., Wang, L., Ji, H., and Zhou, M. (2002). Risk factors for suicide in China: a national case-control psychological autopsy study. *Lancet*, 360, 1728–36.

Rich, C.L., Young, D., and Fowler, R.C. (1986). San Diego Suicide Study: young vs. old subjects. *Archives of General Psychiatry*, 43, 577–82.

Rihmer, Z., Rutz, W., Pihlgren, H., and Pestality, P. (1998). Decreasing tendency of seasonality in suicide may indicate lowering rate of depressive suicides in the population. *Psychiatry Research*, 81, 233–40.

Rihmer, Z., Belso, N., and Kalmar, S. (2001). Antidepressants and suicide prevention in Hungary. *Acta Psychiatrica Scandinavica*, 103, 238–9.

Robins, E., Murphy, G.E., Wilkinson, R.H., Gassner, S., and Kayes, J. (1989). Some clinical considerations in the prevention of suicide based on a study of 134 successful suicides. *American Journal of Public Health*, 49, 888–99.

Roy, A. (1983). Family history of suicide. *Archives of General Psychiatry*, 40, 971–4.

Roy, A., Segal, N., Centerwall, B., and Robinette, D. (1991). Suicide in twins. *Archives of General Psychiatry*, 48, 29–32.

Sheard, M.H., Marini, J.L., Bridges, C.I., and Wagner, E. (1976). The effect of lithium on impulsive aggressive behaviour in man. *American Journal of Psychiatry*, 133, 1409–13.

Vijayakumar, L. and Rajkumar, S. (1999). Are risk factors for suicide universal? A case-control study in India. *Acta Psychiatrica Scandinavica*, 99, 407–11.

Yip, P.S.F., Chao, A., and Ho, T.P. (1998). A re-examination of seasonal variation in suicides in Australia and New Zealand. *Journal of Affective Disorders*, 47, 141–50.

Zair, K. (1981). A suicidal family. *British Journal of Psychiatry*, 139, 68–9.

Zaretsky A.E., Segal Z.V., and Gemar M. (1999). Cognitive therapy for bipolar depression: a pilot study. *Canadian Journal of Psychiatry*, 44, 491–4.

12

Psychosocial treatments following attempted suicide: evidence to inform clinical practice

Keith Hawton

Introduction

Attempted suicide, more correctly termed 'deliberate self-harm' because of the often mixed motivation involved in the behaviour, is common, often repeated, and denotes a very significant risk of subsequent suicide. It represents considerable psychological distress, and is commonly associated with psychiatric disorders, especially depression, anxiety, and substance misuse. A large proportion of patients have co-morbid personality disorders. Deliberate self-harm is often linked to psychosocial problems, including long-standing adversity and also acute life events.

These facts partly explain why it has been so difficult to find effective treatments for patients following deliberate self-harm. Clearly, one single approach would be unlikely to be effective for people with such a diverse range of problems. In this chapter the characteristics and needs of these patients are first presented in more detail. Then treatment approaches that have been developed to try and meet these needs are considered, together with evidence regarding their efficacy based on the results of randomized controlled trials. General conclusions from the evidence are reached and then specific research needs and requirements for future evaluations are considered.

The chapter is mainly focused on adults, but separate sections are devoted to consideration of psychosocial treatments for adolescents and older people.

Adults

Treatments need to be based on the problems and characteristics of patients

In planning treatments for deliberate self-harm patients it is clearly crucial that these are tailored to their needs. As indicated above, these vary greatly between individuals. There are, however, certain factors that are common to many patients. These have been described in detail elsewhere (Hawton, 2001) and therefore will only be summarized here.

Life events and difficulties

Deliberate self-harm is usually a response to life events, often in the context of longer-term life problems (Paykel *et al.* 1975; Bancroft *et al.* 1977). Common problems include difficulties in the relationship with a partner or with other family members, loss of a relationship, alcohol and drug misuse, occupational problems and unemployment, social isolation, and housing and financial problems (Hawton *et al.* 2003*b*).

Psychiatric and personality disorders

Recent studies have shown that psychiatric and personality disorders are common in deliberate self-harm patients. Psychiatric disorders are found in approximately 90% of cases, with depression, anxiety disorders, and substance misuse predominating (Suominen *et al.* 1996; Haw *et al.* 2001). Personality disorders are found in at least 40% of cases, with co-morbidity of both types of disorder being frequent (Hawton *et al.* 2003*c*). While psychiatric symptoms may diminish following an act of self-harm (Newson-Smith and Hirsch 1979), in many patients psychiatric disorders persist (or recur) several months later (Suominen *et al.* 1998).

In some series of deliberate self-harm patients, personality disorders of the borderline or emotionally unstable type have been found to be particularly common. These are often associated with multiple repetition of self-harm and extreme difficulties in interpersonal relationships, both of which pose particular demands in terms of finding effective therapeutic responses.

Problem-solving difficulties

It is well-recognized that deliberate self-harm is often indicative of general difficulty in dealing with problems, especially those of an interpersonal nature (Williams and Pollock 2000). This may result in a passive approach to problem solving (Linehan *et al.* 1987). Alternatively, a person may resort to maladaptive means of dealing with problems in order to reduce stress and distress, such as through substance abuse, aggression, or some other dysfunctional strategy, which may bring immediate relief but will, at the same time, be likely to compound their problems.

As discussed by Williams and colleagues in Chapter 5, there is accumulating evidence that deficits in problem solving shown by many patients who deliberately self-harm may be the result of their having a paucity of specific examples of problem-solving strategies, due to their tendency to have overgeneralized autobiographical memory patterns. This is thought to relate to exposure to traumatic or unpleasant experiences during childhood or adolescence which results in development of non-specific memories in order to modify the emotions linked to these and other experiences. Unsurprisingly, treatment interventions aimed at modifying difficulties in problem solving have been a major focus of therapeutic initiatives for deliberate self-harm patients.

Other personality traits and characteristics

Two other personality traits that may make individuals vulnerable to suicidal behaviours are impulsivity and aggression (Mann *et al.* 1999). Deliberate self-harm often itself appears to be impulsive (although more specifically this may be related to difficulties in problem solving and the need to find some immediate way of coping with stress). Williams and colleagues have related this to the sense of entrapment that patients may face (Williams and Pollock 2000; and see Chapter 5). Some individuals who carry out suicidal acts or non-suicidal self-harm also show aggressive tendencies, as reflected in a history of violence (Nock and Marzuk 2000). Evidence points to this reflecting a trait phenomenon that may have a genetically determined biological basis, most likely hypofunction of the serotonergic system. It may also be the result of exposure to chronic stress during early life and the effects of sustained activation of the hypothalamic–pituitary–adrenal axis, resulting in overproduction of cortisol and consequent disturbed metabolism of serotonin (Van Praag 2001). However, actual manifestation of this trait may be related to low mood, further stress, and/or substance misuse.

Another well-recognized characteristic of many deliberate self-harm patients is the tendency to feel hopeless (Williams and Pollock 2000, and see Chapter 5). Hopelessness appears to mainly reflect anticipation of a lack of positive events (MacLeod *et al.* 1992). It is associated with increased risk of repetition of deliberate self-harm (Petrie *et al.* 1988) and risk of suicide (Beck *et al.* 1985).

A further common characteristic in this population is low self-esteem, that is a negative view a person holds of their self-worth, attractiveness to others, and abilities. While closely related to depressed mood, low self-esteem appears to increase the risk of suicidal ideation beyond that explained by depression and hopelessness.

Repetition of deliberate self-harm

Repetition of deliberate self-harm is very common, at least 15–25% repeating the act within a year of an earlier episode (Sakinofsky 2000; Owens *et al.* 2002). The risk of repetition is greatest in the first few weeks following an act, and repetition increases the risk of eventual suicide (Zahl and Hawton 2004).

Some people frequently self-harm, often in what is termed a self-mutilative pattern. This usually consists of self-cutting, self-burning (e.g. with cigarettes), or self-battery. The motives associated with such behaviour may involve tension relief, self-punishment, and dealing with depersonalization or feelings of inner emptiness (Favazza 1996; Rodham *et al.* 2004). Self-mutilation is particularly common in people with borderline personality disorders.

Barriers to effective treatment

It is well-recognized that engagement of deliberate self-harm patients in treatment is often difficult. This seems to reflect poor motivation, although it is important to recognize the reasons underlying this. One may be the result of repeated exposure to negative or traumatic life experiences, which establishes a low expectation of success. This may relate to low self-esteem and hopelessness. Another factor that needs highlighting is that deliberate self-harm rarely seems to result from a specific intention to seek help (Bancroft *et al.* 1976; Hjelmeland *et al.* 2002), and therefore there may be a mismatch between what a clinician thinks is an appropriate response and that of patients. Negative attitudes towards mental health services (Rotheram-Borus *et al.* 1996) may be another relevant factor. Finally, for some patients, especially males, the idea of participating in a treatment which involves examination of thoughts and feelings may be very alien. Engagement in treatment and management of apparent motivational problems should therefore be key features of the initial phases of any therapeutic approach.

Psychosocial treatment approaches

A range of psychosocial treatment approaches have been developed for deliberate self-harm patients. Broadly, the most important of these can be grouped into four main categories: (a) brief psychological therapies; (b) increased intensity of care combined with outreach; (c) intensive therapeutic approaches; and (d) use of emergency cards. In evaluating the effectiveness of these approaches, reference will be made to a systematic review of the results of randomized controlled treatment studies (Hawton *et al.* 1998, 2004) and to a recent update of this review (National Institute for Clinical Excellence 2004).

Brief psychological therapies

The most widely investigated treatment approach for deliberate self-harm patients has been problem-solving therapy. This is understandable given the characteristics of many of these patients that have already been described, including the wide range of problems they face and their difficulties in problem solving. Problem-solving therapy involves careful assessment of a patient's problems, including the links between individual problems, joint decision between patient and therapist on which problems can and should be tackled, agreement on specific goals, and then planning the steps that the patient might try in order to reach these goals. There is a major focus on homework, especially practical steps the patient will try to take. Cognitive therapy is an important aspect of the treatment, including addressing motivational issues, brain-storming of possible goals and solutions, and examining pros and cons of different approaches. There is a major focus on encouraging specificity of goals and tasks. The approach is highly collaborative, and it can be used for individual, couple or family treatment. It is usually brief, consisting of between two or three and ten sessions, is tailored in intensity to suit a patient's needs, and can be combined with other therapeutic approaches. A detailed description of problem-solving therapy is provided by Hawton and Kirk (1989).

In the systematic review mentioned above, five randomized controlled trials were identified in which repetition of deliberate self-harm was used as an outcome measure (Gibbons *et al.* 1978; Hawton *et al.* 1987; Salkovskis *et al.* 1990; McLeavey *et al.* 1994; Evans *et al.* 1999*a*). The trials compared problem-solving therapy with some form of control treatment, usually 'treatment as usual'. When the results of the five trials were combined in a meta-analysis, there appeared to be a difference in the rates of repetition between patients assigned to problem solving (15.5%) compared to those who were offered the control treatment (19.2%), but this difference was not statistically significant (odds ratio = 0.7; 95% CI 0.45–1.11).

Several other outcome measures were assessed in these trials (plus a sixth trial in which repetition of deliberate self-harm was not reported, Patsiokas and Clum 1985). Depression was assessed in four of the studies, hopelessness in three, and problem resolution in two. In meta-analyses significant differences were found for all three of these outcomes, indicating better outcome for the patients allocated to problem-solving therapy (Townsend *et al.* 2001).

Another brief form of psychotherapy was evaluated in a further treatment study (Guthrie *et al.* 2001). While the theoretical framework underpinning the treatment seemed somewhat different to that for problem-solving therapy, the aims were similar, namely addressing specific interpersonal problems. Treatment was brief (four sessions) and delivered at home by nurses. It was compared with routine care. The main outcome was repetition of deliberate self-harm, this outcome being based on self-reported episodes of any type of self-harm. There was a significantly lower repetition rate at the 6 months follow-up in the psychotherapy condition (9%) compared with that in the control group (28%; difference in proportions = 19%, 95% CI 9–30%). When the result of this study was combined with that of the five problem-solving therapy trials discussed above, the overall repetition rate across the six trials significantly favoured brief psychotherapy (14.4% versus 20.8%; odds ratio = 0.59; 95% CI 0.39–0.89).

In a further, much larger trial, another brief psychological therapy, based upon a self-help manual which was given to all patients, was also compared with routine care (Tyrer *et al.* 2003). The patients in this study were all repeaters of deliberate self-harm at the point of entry. The treatment approach included problem-solving therapy, combined with elements from dialectical behaviour therapy (see below). However, as there was a disappointingly low rate of attendance at treatment sessions (38% of patients attended no sessions), much reliance was based on patients benefiting from the self-help manual. It is not known how acceptable the manual was to the patients, nor how many actually read it or made use of it. There was no difference in outcome between patients in the two treatment groups in terms of repetition of deliberate self-harm. The usefulness or otherwise of self-help manuals for this patient population remains to be determined.

Increased intensity of care combined with outreach

Several treatment studies have been conducted in which the main therapeutic strategies have been outreach, usually combined with a relatively intensive intervention (Welu *et al.* 1977; Hawton *et al.* 1981; Allard *et al.* 1992; Van Heeringen *et al.* 1995; Van der Sande *et al.* 1997; Cedereke *et al.* 2002). The actual intervention approach has varied considerably, from general psychiatric outpatient care to brief in-patient care followed by outpatient treatment. Outreach has usually consisted of home visits or telephone contact, and has either been provided for all patients or only for those who failed to attend their initial treatment sessions. When a meta-analysis of the results of all trials of this kind, in terms of repetition of deliberate self-harm, was conducted, there was no convincing evidence of greater effectiveness compared with routine care (Hawton *et al.* 1998, 2004). However, in one study from Belgium, a single home visit by a nurse for patients who failed to attend their initial outpatient appointment, with the aim of increasing motivation to attend, resulted in a significant increase in the rate of outpatient attendance (51.2%) compared with that of patients who were not visited if they did not attend the first treatment session (39.8%). There was also a markedly lower rate of repetition of deliberate self-harm in the experimental treatment group (10.7% versus 17.4%), which only just failed to reach statistical significance after adjustment for age, marital status, and history of previous deliberate self-harm (Van Heeringen *et al.* 1995). The results of this study offer limited support for inclusion of home-based visits and/or treatment for some patients.

Intensive therapeutic approaches

Brief psychological approaches are unlikely to be of benefit for patients with major personality difficulties, especially in terms of impulse control and emotional reactivity. Therefore intensive psychotherapeutic interventions have been developed, of which dialectical behaviour therapy (Linehan 1993) is the most promising. In the initial trial in which this approach was tested, female patients with a diagnosis of borderline personality disorder and a history of multiple episodes of self-harm were provided with weekly group therapy plus individual therapy for 1 year. There was ready access to the therapists between treatment sessions. Treatment was focused on several problems, including motivational issues, emotional reactivity, and impulsivity, and also on behavioural skills, especially in relation to interpersonal difficulties. In a randomized comparison with routine care, there was a significant reduction in repetition of self-harm plus several other positive outcomes in those who received dialectical behaviour therapy (Linehan *et al.* 1991). The beneficial effect on repetition appeared to persist for the first 6 months after treatment was completed, but was lost after that (Linehan *et al.* 1993).

The results of dialectical behaviour therapy have provided considerable encouragement that people with severe personality disorders and repeated deliberate self-harm can be helped, although the intensity of this approach means that it is costly and requires considerable training.

Use of emergency cards

Because of the apparent acuteness of problems faced by many deliberate self-harm patients and the tendency for repetition to occur relatively impulsively, there has been interest in the UK in providing emergency access to care by giving patients a card which allows them to get immediate access to help at times of crisis. The aim is to prevent such crises precipitating repetition of deliberate self-harm, through taking advantage of the fact that some patients will only consider seeking help when in a crisis. In a small initial study of this approach from Bristol, provision of an emergency ('green') card combined with routine care produced encouraging results when compared with provision of routine care alone (Morgan *et al.* 1993). However, a much larger study did not provide support for the initial findings, there being no difference in the rate of repetition of deliberate self-harm between patients in the two treatment groups (Evans *et al.* 1999*b*). Moreover, on the basis of a *post-hoc* analysis, it appeared that provision of the emergency card may have been detrimental for those who were already repeaters of self-harm, in that their repetition rate was significantly greater than that of the patients who were not provided with the emergency card. A possible explanation was that some of these patients, especially those with major personality difficulties, may have become angry and frustrated when they telephoned for emergency help and found that the clinical service could not immediately solve their problems. By contrast, patients who had carried out their first act of deliberate self-harm at the time of entry to the study appeared to benefit from receiving the emergency card, showing a lower rate of repetition than first-timers in the control group. One must be cautious in interpreting results of such a *post-hoc* analysis, but it suggests that there needs to be careful selection of patients who are offered such an emergency card facility. Also, back-up of such an initiative necessitates availability of a 24-hour service that can deal with emergency calls.

Other interventions

Because of the well-developed general practitioner service in the UK and the fact that patients are often well known to their family doctors and might be more willing to visit them than a mental health service, an intervention study in Bristol focused on arranging for general practitioners to send their patients who had presented to hospital following deliberate self-harm an appointment to attend for an early consultation. The general practitioners were also given simple clinical guidelines on how to help with the common problems faced by such patients. In a randomized controlled trial, patients allocated to receive this intervention were compared to those who received routine care (Bennewith *et al.* 2002). There was no apparent effect of enhanced general practitioner care on repetition of deliberate self-harm.

The focus of this chapter is on psychosocial interventions. Nevertheless, brief mention should be made of pharmacological treatments, especially as these are often combined with psychosocial treatments. In an early trial, patients who had had multiple episodes of deliberate self-harm were treated with the depot phenothiazine flupenthixol in a dose of 20 mg for 6 months (Montgomery *et al.* 1979). Compared with patients who were given placebo injections, those receiving flupenthixol had a much lower rate of repetition of deliberate self-harm. Unfortunately, this trial has not been replicated. In a more recent study, no difference in the rate of repetition was found between similar patients receiving injections of either 12.5 mg or 1.5 mg of flupenthixol, but, as there was no placebo group, the effectiveness of the active drug could not be evaluated (Battaglia *et al.* 1999). If neuroleptics prove of benefit in this patient population, this may be due to inhibition of arousal and emotional reactivity in response to life events. Evaluation of the use of oral neuroleptics is required.

Early trials in which antidepressants were evaluated against placebo in the prevention of repetition of deliberate self-harm produced negative results (Hirsch *et al.* 1982; Montgomery and Montgomery 1982). In a subsequent study from The Netherlands, non-depressed repeaters of deliberate self-harm were randomized to receive either the SSRI antidepressant paroxetine or placebo (Verkes *et al.* 1998). No overall difference in repetition of self-harm was found between the two groups. A *post-hoc* subgroup analysis suggested that patients with a history of between two and four episodes of self-harm treated with paroxetine repeated less than those who received placebo, whereas there was no apparent benefit of the active drug in those who had a history of five or more episodes of self-harm. However, one must be cautious in interpreting the results of such a *post-hoc* analysis, especially as they appear to be somewhat contrary to expectation. Also, in a recent meta-analysis of a large number of placebo-controlled trials of SSRIs, there appeared to be no difference in rates of suicidal behaviour between patients receiving active drugs and those receiving placebo (Khan *et al.* 2000, 2003; and see Chapter 14, this volume). The role of antidepressants in the prevention of deliberate self-harm remains unclear.

Clinical implications

Unfortunately, in spite of a fairly large number of treatment studies over the past three decades, there is only limited evidence on which to base recommendations for clinical practice regarding treatments for adult deliberate self-harm patients. This may be due, in part, to the limited size of the treatment studies which have been conducted and, in part, to the heterogeneous characteristics of this patient population (National Institute for Clinical Excellence 2004). There is general agreement that a careful psychosocial assessment should be conducted with all patients presenting to clinical services. This should address psychiatric, psychological, and social factors, including risk of further deliberate self-harm and of suicide. Provision of treatment should be based on the results of this assessment. There is limited evidence to support provision of outreach for patients who fail to attend for treatment. It is unclear what are the most effective elements of treatment for deliberate self-harm patients in general. There is some evidence that brief psychological intervention is more effective than routine care. Also, there is limited support for provision of intensive intervention combined with outreach. This suggests that strong efforts should be made to follow up patients who do not attend clinic appointments. There is also encouraging evidence for the efficacy of dialectical behaviour therapy in helping patients with borderline personality disorder and a history of repeated self-harm, although the resource implications of this intensive approach may limit its applicability, at least in routine clinical settings.

Adolescents

Problems faced by adolescents who deliberately self-harm

While earlier commentators on adolescents who had presented to hospital following deliberate self-harm emphasized the social nature of their problems and placed less emphasis on their psychiatric difficulties, recent studies in the UK have shown quite clearly that many of such adolescents have psychiatric disorders. In a study of 40 adolescents who presented following overdoses in Manchester, 75% had a psychiatric disorder (compared with 10% of community controls and 70% of adolescents attending a psychiatric clinic) (Kerfoot et al. 1996). Most of the adolescents with psychiatric disorder had major depression (67% of all the adolescents). In addition 35% had oppositional disorder and 7% a substance misuse disorder. Similar findings emerged from a study of adolescents who presented to hospital with overdoses in Oxford (Burgess et al. 1998).

Over half of the Manchester adolescents (57%) came from a broken home (compared with 15% of community controls and 22% of psychiatric controls). One in five said they had no friends (compared with 27% of community controls). Half (52%) knew of someone else who had taken an overdose (compared with 25% of community controls).

An explanatory model of deliberate self-harm in adolescents should include the interaction between mental disorders (especially depression and substance misuse), chronic and acute stress (e.g. family problems), and the social milieu (e.g. deliberate self-harm by friends or family). Factors that may determine that suicidal thoughts are translated into actual self-harm include: disinhibition by substance misuse, availability of method for self-harm, exposure to suicidal behaviour in the media, and certain aspects of mental state (e.g. depressed mood, hopelessness, anger). Factors that may inhibit translation of suicidal thoughts into self-harm include: social support, lack of opportunity, and personal beliefs against self-harm and suicide. This model suggests that a variety of approaches to aftercare and prevention in adolescents are required. Mental disorders, including substance misuse, may require direct treatment, support may be necessary to tackle acute chronic stress, and specific social strategies may be required for tackling environmental influences on suicidal behaviour. Possible approaches for those with suicidal thoughts include crisis services, use of emergency cards, and telephone hotlines. Further strategies for prevention of translation of suicidal thoughts into self-harming behaviour include tackling substance misuse, limiting availability of methods for self-harm, and treatment of psychiatric disorder.

Treatments for adolescents who deliberately self-harm

The types of treatment approaches to deliberate self-harm in adolescents which have been evaluated can be divided into:

(1) interventions that are designed primarily to prevent repetition of self-harm (e.g. family problem solving, emergency cards); and

(2) interventions that target emotional or behavioural disorders of which suicidal behaviour is a part (e.g. depression, conduct disorder).

Interventions that are designed primarily to prevent repetition of self-harm in adolescents

Brief home-based family therapy after deliberate self-harm

Harrington and colleagues (1998a) in Manchester developed and evaluated a family-based treatment approach for adolescents who had presented to hospital after taking overdoses. This consisted of five treatment sessions at home with other family members and included an action-orientated approach. In summary, the initial phase included a careful assessment of the problems faced by the adolescent and the family, discussion of the episode of self-harm and its meaning for those present, encouragement of open communication about feelings and problems, problem-solving, and discussion of specific developmental issues (Kerfoot et al. 1995). Evaluations conducted 2 months after entry to treatment, and again after 6 months, showed no extra benefits for the adolescents randomly assigned to the experimental treatment compared with a control group of the adolescents who were randomly assigned to receive routine care (i.e. treatment as usual) in terms of repetition of self-harm, suicidal thinking, or depression (Harrington et al. 1998a). However, the overall costs, excluding those for the specific treatment, were lower for the group assigned to the family treatment condition, especially in terms of social services' costs (Byford et al. 1999). Also, parents were significantly more satisfied with the family treatment approach (Harrington et al. 1998a). The last finding may have been because the treatment was home-based. Finally, a subgroup of the patients in the family therapy group, who were without major depression at entry to the study, had much less suicidal ideation at both outcome points.

Group therapy for repeated self-harm

Self-harm in adolescents is often repeated (Hawton et al. 2003a), and repetition greatly increases the risk of further episodes. In another randomized controlled treatment study from the Manchester group, Wood and colleagues (2001) investigated the possible benefits for adolescents who were repeaters of self-harm from attending group treatment. While this was a pilot study, the results were encouraging. Sixty-three adolescents who had engaged in at least two episodes of deliberate self-harm in the previous year were randomized to receive either group therapy plus routine care or routine care alone. The adolescents who received group therapy attended a median of eight treatment sessions over six months. Several received additional individual sessions of cognitive behaviour therapy as necessary. The group therapy was based on a variety of techniques, including cognitive behavioural therapy and problem-solving, dialectical behaviour therapy, and psychodynamic group psychotherapy. The focus was on specific themes known to be important in adolescents who harm themselves, namely relationships, school problems and peer relationships, family problems, anger management, depression and self-harm, and hopelessness, and feelings about the future. There was an initial phase of six 'acute' treatment sessions, followed by weekly group sessions in 'a long-term group' until the person felt able to leave. This phase was focused on group processes. Both types of group ran continuously so that adolescents could join them at any time, without having to wait for treatment.

Adolescents in the group therapy condition received significantly less routine care than those in the routine care alone condition. Levels of depression, episodes of further deliberate self-harm, and other outcomes were identified through interview approximately 7 months after entry to the study. Adolescents in the group therapy condition repeated deliberate self-harm significantly less often (6%) than those in the control group (32%). They also had fewer overall episodes of self-harm. They had better school attendance and had a lower rate of behavioural disorders, but they did not differ with regard to level of depression and global outcome (based on a broad outcome measure).

Use of emergency cards

As discussed earlier in this chapter, there has been interest in the use of emergency cards for deliberate self-harm patients. Such an approach was evaluated in a small, randomized controlled trial for young adolescents who had presented with self-harm (Cotgrove et al. 1995). Adolescents in the experimental group were, in addition to receiving routine care, given an emergency card which allowed them to gain admission to hospital. Those in a control group received routine care alone. There was a lower rate of repetition of deliberate self-harm in the emergency card group (6.4% versus 12.1%), but the number of patients in the trial was far too small for this statistical significance difference to reach statistical significance.

Interventions that target emotional or behavioural disorders of which suicidal behaviour is a part

Prevention of deliberate self-harm and suicide in adolescents may also be facilitated through specific therapies focused on psychopathological phenomena related closely to suicidal behaviour. The most important of these phenomena are depression and behavioural disorders.

Depression

A wide range of treatments for depression in adolescents has been evaluated. Three of the most important are cognitive behaviour therapy, interpersonal psychotherapy, and treatment with SSRI antidepressants.

A meta-analysis of trials of cognitive behaviour therapy by Harrington and colleagues (1998*b*) provided strong evidence for a positive benefit of this treatment compared with control treatments, with 62% of adolescents who received cognitive behaviour therapy no longer reaching criteria for major depressive disorder at the end of therapy compared with 36% of controls (odds ratio = 3.2, 95% CI 1.9–5.2). The number needed to treat to get an extra recovered individual was four. Specific results for suicidal behaviour were not generally reported in the studies included in the review.

In a more recent study from the USA, depressed adolescents were randomly assigned to receive: (1) fluoxetine alone; (2) cognitive behaviour therapy alone; (3) fluoxetine and cognitive behaviour therapy; or (4) placebo medication (March *et al.* 2004). The combination of fluoxetine and cognitive behaviour therapy appeared to be most effective in terms of improvement in both depression and suicidal ideas.

The use of SSRI antidepressants to treat depression (or other disorders) in adolescents has recently taken a blow because of publication of previously unpublished data from trials which suggested that frequency of self-harm and suicidal thoughts may be increased in adolescents receiving SSRIs (except fluoxetine) or (especially) the selective serotonin reuptake inhibitor (SNRI) venlafaxine (Whittington *et al.* 2004). This has prompted guidance from the United Kingdom Committee on Safety of Medicines (2004) that these drugs (except fluoxetine) should not be used for treating adolescents, and a 'black box warning' for these drugs by the Food and Drug Administration (2004) in the USA. Earlier studies had suggested that SSRIs may be more effective than tricyclic antidepressants in the treatment of depression in adolescents (Keller *et al.* 2001). The current position clearly presents major difficulties for clinicians involved in treatment of depressed adolescents, especially those adolescents with suicidal ideas or with a history of previous deliberate self-harm. It is likely to result in greater interest in psychosocial interventions for this population.

Behavioural disorders

As already noted, behavioural disorders (especially conduct disorder) are common in adolescents who present with deliberate self-harm. A wide range of treatments for such disorders has been evaluated (Kazdin and Weisz 1998). These include interpersonal problem-solving therapy, multisystemic therapy, anger management, and family therapy. One example is the treatment of serious adolescent offenders with multisystemic therapy, which included individualized family treatment utilizing intervention strategies based on family therapy and behaviour therapy. In a randomized trial, Henggeler *et al.* (1992) found that the frequency of arrests and self-reported delinquency in such adolescents decreased significantly more than in those who received treatment from usual services.

Clinical implications of evidence regarding treatment of adolescents either following or at risk of deliberate self-harm

At present, unfortunately, the evidence base regarding interventions that are primarily designed to prevent repetition of self-harm by adolescents is weak. However, a group therapy approach for adolescent repeaters of self-harm has shown some promise and one awaits the outcome of a larger evaluation of this approach. It is well recognized that deliberate self-harm in adolescents is strongly associated with emotional and behavioural disorders. There is also evidence that these disorders can be treated effectively. In terms of prevention of suicidal behaviour by adolescents, it may therefore be appropriate to infer that comprehensive aftercare programmes for adolescents with emotional or behavioural disorders, and those specifically for adolescents who have engaged in deliberate self-harm, should include services to treat these disorders with a range of potential, but evidence-based, approaches. The specific benefits of provision of such approaches in prevention of suicidal behaviour await evaluation.

Future directions in prevention of deliberate self-harm by adolescents

Much more research on the natural history of adolescent deliberate self-harm is required. For example, it is important to know what are the most important outcomes in terms of adolescent distress and dysfunction. It tends to be assumed that further deliberate self-harm is the most relevant. Yet, low-risk self-harm, such as superficial self-cutting, may not be as important in terms of persistent psychopathology as certain other outcomes, such as depression or behavioural disorders. Also there needs to be further research on the main psychological characteristics associated with poorer or better outcome, which can then inform development of effective therapeutic interventions.

Treatment research in adolescents should focus especially on high-risk groups. These would include repeaters of deliberate self-harm and those with major mental disorders.

Finally, we need to know more about what effects interventions designed for other problems, such as depression, conduct disorder, and substance misuse, have on repetition of deliberate self-harm.

Older people

An episode of deliberate self-harm by an older person often represents a failed suicide attempt. Thus the ratio of non-fatal acts of deliberate self-harm to suicides is much lower in older people than in younger adults, suicidal intent is often high, and the eventual risk of suicide is greater than in younger persons. Psychiatric disorders, bereavement, and physical illness are common in this population (see Chapter 13).

All episodes of deliberate self-harm by older persons must be taken particularly seriously, with admission to a general hospital bed, as well as careful assessment, being mandatory. The range of problems the patients usually face will often necessitate intensive and multidisciplinary clinical interventions. Because of this and the relative infrequency of deliberate self-harm in older persons, it is perhaps not surprising that there do not appear to have been any evaluations of treatments focused specifically on this population. However, cognitive behaviour therapy has been developed for older people with depression and other psychiatric conditions (Wilkinson 2002). Also, dialectical behaviour therapy has shown promising results in older people with largely long-term depressive disorders (Lynch et al. 2003).

Research and clinical needs in relation to treatments for deliberate self-harm patients

There is clearly a need for more research on treatments for deliberate self-harm patients, especially in view of the growing extent of the problem of deliberate self-harm, evidence of increasing rates of repetition (Hawton et al. 2003b; Henriques et al. 2004), and the strong link to suicide (Hawton et al. 2003d). In our systematic review of treatments, we identified several methodological issues which need addressing in future studies (Arensman et al. 2001). There are also areas for potential therapeutic developments.

Methodological issues

Clearly, research evaluations of treatments for deliberate self-harm patients must adhere to accepted standards of research trials in general, including description of all potential participants approached for inclusion in the trial, the numbers of patients actually included, drop-outs from treatment and the reasons for withdrawal, and the numbers of patients on whom outcome data can be collected. When designing a trial, consultation of the CONSORT statement (Altman 1996), which provides a comprehensive set of guidelines for the reporting of randomized controlled trials in biomedical journals, will help improve the methodology.

One specific issue in relation to many trials is the use of a 'treatment as usual' control condition. While this is understandable, since the aim is often to improve on current practice and also to ensure that patients in the control group receive an acceptable level of care, very often the details of this condition are not provided. For example, what specific treatments were included, what was the level of compliance with treatment, and how much clinical contact was involved? Omission of such details is a major limitation, especially as the content and quality of 'treatment as usual' will vary from centre to centre within the same country, and even more between centres in different countries. Clearly, experimental treatments should also be described in full (preferably in a manual), in order to allow clinicians and other investigators to replicate the treatment. Also, researchers investigating psychosocial treatments should try to evaluate whether the interventions result in changes in the psychological or social mechanisms which are the target of treatment (e.g. improved problem solving, regulation of emotions, changes in interpersonal skills).

A major weakness of most treatment evaluations in this field to date is that too few participants have been included to ensure that clinically relevant treatment effects can be detected. As an example, to detect at a statistically significant level (with significance set at 5% and power at 80%) a difference in repetition of deliberate self-harm between, say, 20% in a control group and 14% in an experimental treatment group (i.e. a reduction of 30%), 647 patients will be required in each treatment condition. To detect smaller differences, much larger numbers will be required. While deliberate self-harm is common, such numbers present a considerable challenge to investigators. Therefore multicentre studies (e.g. Tyrer *et al.* 2003) may be required to properly evaluate treatments.

The types of outcomes investigated in treatment studies in this field so far have included a wide range of measures. This makes comparison between studies difficult. It would clearly be advantageous if certain key measures were included in future studies whenever possible. Repetition of deliberate self-harm (both non-fatal and fatal) is clearly a crucial measure. Other important measures are depression, hopelessness, suicidal ideation, and hospitalization. For repetition of deliberate self-harm, it is important that researchers report the source of the information (e.g. patient report, clinical records) and what types of behaviour were included. Also, outcome data should be analysed on an intention-to-treat basis, so that all subjects entering the trial are included, with clear indication of how missing information has been dealt with in the analyses.

Developments in treatments and groups of patients to be investigated

We also require innovative new approaches. While brief psychosocial interventions are likely to be the mainstay of treatment for many patients, not least because it is necessary that pragmatic and relatively brief approaches are available to meet the needs of the very large numbers of patients seen in clinical practice, further evaluations of this type of approach and development of more intensive therapies for certain groups of patients are required. One need is for evaluation of the therapeutic value of a thorough clinical assessment. Another is for development and evaluation of measures, such as motivational interviewing techniques, to increase motivation for treatment and hence enhanced participation in aftercare. Patients who are repeaters of deliberate self-harm, especially frequent repeaters, are clearly an important target population because of the persistent distress repetition signifies, the burden on clinical resources, and the fact that repetition increases the risk of eventual suicide (Zahl and Hawton 2004). More intensive therapies are likely to be required for this patient population, especially those showing personality traits that interfere with interpersonal relationships and make them vulnerable to substance misuse and behavioural problems. The encouraging results of dialectical behaviour therapy represent a positive step forward. It would be helpful if effective shorter variations of this approach can be developed that can then be provided for a larger number of patients. There is also a need for development of this approach for male patients.

Mindfulness training (Segal *et al.* 2002) is another treatment approach that requires evaluation in deliberate self-harm patients (Williams and Swales 2004). It was developed for people with multiple episodes of depression with the aim of preventing further episodes. Mindfulness training is described in Chapter 5. It has proven effective in reducing depressive relapses (Teasdale *et al.* 2000). Given the similarity of such relapses to repetition of deliberate self-harm in some patients in response to recurrent life events and problems, there would seem to be a good rationale for evaluating this approach in this population.

Other subgroups of patients in which treatments require development and evaluation are alcohol and drug abusers who present with deliberate self-harm. Alcohol abuse, in particular, is associated with greatly enhanced risk of suicide, as well as repetition of deliberate self-harm.

This chapter has been focused mainly on psychosocial treatments. Clearly, pharmacological therapies also have a significant potential role in the treatment of deliberate self-harm patients, especially where major psychiatric disorders are present. Combined psychosocial and pharmacological approaches also merit investigation.

Conclusions

The wide range of characteristics and difficulties of deliberate self-harm patients necessitates a range of treatment responses. While the results of evaluation of treatments by means of randomized controlled treatment studies have so far been somewhat limited, they do provide some evidence-based guidelines for treatment provision. There are clearly major challenges ahead in this important field in terms of development of new treatment approaches and the research requirements for their meaningful evaluation.

Acknowledgement

This chapter is dedicated to the memory of Professor Richard Harrington, who died during the preparation of this book. He made major contributions in the field of adolescent psychiatry, including in the field of therapeutic interventions for adolescents following deliberate self-harm. He developed new approaches for such adolescents and evaluated these in high-quality research trials. Richard was due to contribute a chapter to this book, but became ill before he could do this. The section of this chapter on treatments of adolescents with deliberate self-harm was largely based (with Richard's permission) on a presentation he gave to the 9th European Symposium on Suicidal Behaviour at Warwick University in September 2002. Richard was an innovator and an inspiration for all who came into contact with him. He is, and will continue to be, sadly missed.

References

Allard, R., Marshall, M., and Plante, M.C. (1992). Intensive follow-up does not decrease the risk of repeat suicide attempts. *Suicide and Life-Threatening Behavior,* 22, 303–14.

Altman, D.G. (1996). Better reporting of randomised controlled trials: the CONSORT statement. *British Medical Journal,* 313, 570–1.

Arensman, E., Townsend, E., Hawton, K., Bremner, S., Feldman, E., Goldney, R., *et al.* (2001). Psychosocial and pharmacological treatment of patients following deliberate self-harm: the methodological issues involved in evaluating effectiveness. *Suicide and Life-Threatening Behavior*, 31, 169–80.

Bancroft, J.H.J., Skrimshire, A.M., and Simkin, S. (1976). The reasons people give for taking overdoses. *British Journal of Psychiatry*, 128, 538–48.

Bancroft, J., Skrimshire, A., Casson, J., Harvard-Watts, O., and Reynolds, F. (1977) People who deliberately poison or injure themselves: their problems and their contacts with helping agencies. *Psychological Medicine*, 7, 289–303.

Battaglia, J., Wolff, T.K., Wagner-Johnson, D S., Rush, A J., Carmody, T.J., and Basco, M.R. (1999) Structured diagnostic assessment and depot fluphenazine treatment of multiple suicide attempters in the emergency department. *International Clinical Psychopharmacology*, 14, 361–72.

Beck, A.T., Steer, R.A., Kovacs, M., and Garrison, B. (1985). Hopelessness and eventual suicide: a 10 year prospective study of patients hospitalised with suicidal ideation. *American Journal of Psychiatry*, 145, 559–63.

Bennewith, O., Stocks, N., Gunnell, D., Peters, T.J., Evans, M.O., and Sharp, D.J. (2002). General practice based intervention to prevent repeat episodes of deliberate self harm: cluster randomised controlled trial. *British Medical Journal*, 324, 1254–7.

Burgess, S., Hawton, K., and Loveday, G. (1998). Adolescents who take overdoses: outcome in terms of changes in psychopathology and the adolescents' attitudes to their care and to their overdoses. *Journal of Adolescence*, 21, 209–18.

Byford, S., Harrington, R., Torgerson, D., Kerfoot, M., Dyer, E., Harrington, V., *et al.* (1999). Cost-effectiveness analysis of a home-based social work intervention for children and adolescents who have deliberately poisoned themselves. Results of a randomised controlled trial. *British Journal of Psychiatry*, 174, 56–62.

Cedereke, M., Monti, K., and Ojehagen, A. (2002). Telephone contact with patients in the year after a suicide attempt: does it affect treatment attendance and outcome? A randomised controlled study. *European Psychiatry*, 17, 82–91.

Committee on Safety of Medicines (2004). Selective serotonin reuptake inhibitors (SSRIs): overview of regulatory status and CSM advice relating to major depressive disorder (MDD) in children and adolescents including a summary of available safety and efficacy data. Available at website http://medicines.mhra.gov.uk/ourwork/monitorsafequalmed/safetymessages/ssrioverview%5F101203.htm (accessed 14 January 2005).

Cotgrove, A.J., Zirinsky, L., Black, D., and Weston, D. (1995). Secondary prevention of attempted suicide in adolescence. *Journal of Adolescence*, 18, 569–77.

Evans, K., Tyrer, P., Catalan, J., Schmidt, U., Davidson, K., Dent, J., *et al.* (1999*a*). Manual-assisted cognitive-behaviour therapy (MACT): a randomized controlled trial of a brief intervention with bibliotherapy in the treatment of recurrent deliberate self-harm. *Psychological Medicine*, 29, 19–25.

Evans, M.O., Morgan, H.G., Hayward, A., and Gunnell, D.J. (1999*b*). Crisis telephone consultation for deliberate self-harm patients: effects on repetition. *British Journal of Psychiatry*, 175, 23–27.

Favazza, A.R. (1996). *Bodies under siege: self-mutilation and body modification in culture and psychiatry.* The Johns Hopkins University Press, Baltimore.

Food and Drug Administration (2004). Antidepressant use in children, adolescents, and adults. Available at website http://www.fda.gov/cder/drug/antidepressants/default.htm (accessed 18 January 2005).

Gibbons, J.S., Butler, J., Urwin, P., and Gibbons, J.L. (1978). Evaluation of a social work service for self-poisoning patients. *British Journal of Psychiatry*, 133, 111–18.

Guthrie, E., Kapur, N., Mackway-Jones, K., Chew-Graham, C., Moorey, J., Mendel, E., *et al.* (2001). Randomised controlled trial of brief psychological intervention after deliberate self poisoning. *British Medical Journal*, 323, 135–7.

Harrington, R., Kerfoot, M., Dyer, E., McNiven, F., Gill, J., Harrington, V., *et al.* (1998*a*). Randomized trial of a home-based family intervention for children who have deliberately poisoned themselves. *Journal of the American Academy of Child and Adolescent Psychiatry*, 37, 512–18.

Harrington, R., Whittaker, J., Shoebridge, P., and Campbell, F. (1998*b*). Systematic review of efficacy of cognitive behaviour therapies in childhood and adolescent depressive disorder. *British Medical Journal*, 316, 1559–63.

Haw, C., Hawton, K., Houston, K., and Townsend, E. (2001). Psychiatric and personality disorders in deliberate self-harm patients. *British Journal of Psychiatry*, 178, 48–54.

Hawton, K. (2001). The treatment of suicidal behaviour in the context of the suicidal process. In *Understanding suicidal behaviour: The suicidal process approach to research, treatment and prevention*, (ed. K. Van Heeringen) pp. 212–29. Wiley, Chichester.

Hawton, K. and Kirk, J. (1989). Problem-solving. In *Cognitive behaviour therapy for psychiatric problems: A practical guide*, (ed. K. Hawton, P. Salkovskis, J. Kirk, and D.M. Clark) pp. 406–26. Oxford University Press, Oxford.

Hawton, K., Bancroft, J., Catalan, J., Kingston, B., Stedeford, A., and Welch, N. (1981). Domiciliary and out-patient treatment of self-poisoning patients by medical and non-medical staff. *Psychological Medicine*, 11, 169–77.

Hawton, K., McKeown, S., Day, A., Martin, P., O'Connor, M., and Yule, J. (1987). Evaluation of out-patient counselling compared with general practitioner care following overdoses. *Psychological Medicine*, 17, 751–61.

Hawton, K., Arensman, E., Townsend, E., Bremner, S., Feldman, E., Goldney, R., *et al.* (1998). Deliberate self-harm: systematic review of efficacy of psychosocial and pharmacological treatments in preventing repetition. *British Medical Journal*, 317, 441–7.

Hawton, K., Hall, S., Simkin, S., Bale, E., Bond, A., Codd, S., *et al.* (2003*a*). Deliberate self-harm in adolescents: a study of characteristics and trends in Oxford, 1990–2000. *Journal of Child Psychology and Psychiatry and Allied Disciplines*, 44, 1191–8.

Hawton, K., Harriss, L., Hall, S., Simkin, S., Bale, E., and Bond, A. (2003*b*). Deliberate self-harm in Oxford, 1990–2000: a time of change in patient characteristics. *Psychological Medicine*, 33, 987–96.

Hawton, K., Houston, K., Haw, C., Townsend, E., and Harriss, L. (2003*c*). Comorbidity of axis1 and axis2 disorders in patients who attempted suicide. *American Journal of Psychiatry*, 160, 1494–500.

Hawton, K., Zahl, D., and Weatherall, R. (2003*d*). Suicide following deliberate self-harm: long-term follow-up of patients who presented to a general hospital. *British Journal of Psychiatry*, 182, 537–42.

Hawton, K., Townsend, E., Arensman, E., Gunnell, D., Hazell, P., House, A., *et al.* (2004). Psychosocial and pharmacological treatments for deliberate self harm. *The Cochrane Library*, Issue 4.

Henggeler, S.W., Melton, G.B., and Smith, L.A. (1992). Family preservation using multisystemic therapy: an effective alternative to incarcerating serious juvenile offenders. *Journal of Consulting and Clinical Psychology*, 60, 953–61.

Henriques, G.R., Brown, G.K., Berk, M.S., and Beck, A.T. (2004). Marked increases in psychopathology found in a 30-year cohort comparison of suicide attempters. *Psychological Medicine*, 34, 833–41.

Hirsch, S.R., Walsh, C., and Draper, R. (1982). Parasuicide. A review of treatment interventions. *Journal of Affective Disorders*, 4, 299–311.

Hjelmeland, H., Hawton, K., Nordvik, H., Bille-Brahe, U., De Leo, D., Fekete, S., *et al.* (2002). Why people engage in parasuicide: A cross-cultural study of intentions. *Suicide and Life-Threatening Behavior*, 32, 380–93.

Kazdin, A.E. and Weisz, J.R. (1998). Identifying and developing empirically supported child and adolescent treatments. *Journal of Consulting and Clinical Psychology*, 66, 19–36.

Keller, M.B., Ryan, N.D., Strober, M., Klein, R.G., Kutcher, S.P., Birmaher, B., *et al.* (2001). Efficacy of paroxetine in the treatment of adolescent major depression: a randomized, controlled trial. *Journal of the American Academy of Child and Adolescent Psychiatry*, 40, 762–72.

Kerfoot, M., Harrington, R., and Dyer, E. (1995). Brief home-based interventions with young suicide attempters and their families. *Journal of Adolescence*, 18, 557–68.

Kerfoot, M., Dyer, E., Harrington, V., Woodham, A., and Harrington, R. (1996). Correlates and short-term course of self-poisoning in adolescents. *British Journal of Psychiatry*, 168, 38–42.

Khan, A., Warner, H.A., and Brown, W.A. (2000). Symptom reduction and suicide risk in patients treated with placebo in antidepressant clinicla trials. *Archives of General Psychiatry*, 57, 311–17.

Khan, A., Khan, S., Kolts, R., and Brown, W.A. (2003). Suicide rates in clinical trials of SSRIs, other antidepressants, and placebo: analysis of FDA reports. *American Journal of Psychiatry*, 160, 790–2.

Linehan, M.M. (1993). *Cognitive behavioral treatment for borderline personality disorder.* Guilford, New York.

Linehan, M.M., Camper, P., Chiles, J.A., Strohsahl, K., and Shearin, E. (1987). Interpersonal problem solving and parasuicide. *Cognitive Therapy and Research*, 11, 1–12.

Linehan, M., Armstrong, H.E., Suarez, A., Allmari, D., and Heard, H.L. (1991). Cognitive behavioral treatment of chronically parasuicidal borderline patients. *Archives of General Psychiatry*, 48, 1060–4.

Linehan, M.M., Heard, H.L., and Armstrong, H.E. (1993). Naturalistic follow-up of a behavioral treatment for chronically parasuicidal borderline patients. *Archives of General Psychiatry*, 50, 971–4.

Lynch, T.R., Morse, J.Q., Mendelson, T., and Robins, C.J. (2003). Dialectical behavior therapy for depressed older adults: a randomized pilot study. *American Journal of Geriatriatric Psychiatry*, 11, 33–45.

MacLeod, A.K., Williams, J.M.G., and Linehan, M.M. (1992). New developments in the understanding and treatment of suicidal behaviour. *Behavioural Psychotherapy*, 20, 193–218.

Mann, J.J., Waternaux, C., Haas, G.L., and Malone, K.M. (1999). Toward a clinical model of suicidal behavior in psychiatric patients. *American Journal of Psychiatry*, 156, 181–9.

March, J., Silva, S., Petrycki, S., Curry, J., Wells, K., Fairbank, J., *et al.* (2004). Fluoxetine, cognitive-behavioral therapy, and their combination for adolescents with depression: Treatment for Adolescents With Depression Study (TADS) randomized controlled trial. *Journal of the American Medical Association*, 292, 807–20.

McLeavey, B.C., Daly, R.J., Ludgate, J.W., and Murray, C.M. (1994). Interpersonal problem-solving skill training in the treatment of self-poisoning patients. *Suicide and Life-Threatening Behavior*, 24, 382–94.

Montgomery, S.A. and Montgomery, D. (1982). Pharmacological prevention of suicidal behaviour. *Journal of Affective Disorders*, 4, 291–8.

Montgomery, S.A., Montgomery, D.B., Jayanthi-Rani, S., Roy, D.H., Shaw, P.J., and McAuley, R. (1979). Maintenance therapy in repeat suicidal behaviour: A placebo controlled trial. In *Proceedings of the 10th International Congress for Suicide Prevention and Crisis Intervention*, pp. 227–9. International Association for Suicide Prevention, Ottawa, Canada.

Morgan, H.G., Jones, E.M., and Owen, J.H. (1993). Secondary prevention of non-fatal deliberate self-harm. The green card study. *British Journal of Psychiatry*, 163, 111–12.

National Institute for Clinical Excellence (2004). *Clinical Guideline 16. Self-harm: the short-term physical and psychological management and secondary prevention of self-harm in primary and secondary care*. National Institute for Clinical Excellence, London.

Newson-Smith, J.G. and Hirsch, S.R. (1979). Psychiatric symptoms in self-poisoning patients. *Psychological Medicine*, 9, 493–500.

Nock, M.K. and Marzuk, P.M. (2000). Suicide and violence. In *The international handbook of suicide and attempted suicide*, (ed. K. Hawton and K. Van Heeringen) pp. 437–56. Wiley, Chichester.

Owens, D., Horrocks, J., and House, A. (2002). Fatal and non-fatal repetition of self-harm. *British Journal of Psychiatry*, 181, 193–9.

Patsiokas, A.T. and Clum, G.A. (1985). Effects of psychotherapeutic strategies in the treatment of suicide. *Psychotherapy*, 22, 281–90.

Paykel, E.S., Prusoff, B.A., and Myers, J.K. (1975). Suicide attempts and recent life events: a controlled comparison. *Archives of General Psychiatry*, 32, 327–33.

Petrie, K., Chamberlain, K., and Clarke, D. (1988). Psychological predictors of future suicidal behavior in hospitalized suicide attempters. *British Journal of Clinical Psychology*, 27, 247–57.

Rodham, K., Hawton, K., and Evans, E. (2004). Reasons for deliberate self-harm: comparison of self-poisoners and self-cutters in a community sample of adolescents. *Journal of the American Academy of Child and Adolescent Psychiatry*, 43, 80–7.

Rotheram-Borus, M.J., Piacentini, J., Van Rossem, R., Graae, F., Cantwell, C., Castro-Blanco, D., *et al.* (1996). Enhancing treatment adherence with a specialized emergency room program for adolescent suicide attempters. *Journal of the American Academy of Child and Adolescent Psychiatry*, 35, 654–63.

Sakinofsky, I. (2000). Repetition of suicidal behaviour. In *The international handbook of suicide and attempted suicide*, (ed. K. Hawton and K. Van Heeringen) pp. 385–404. Wiley, Chichester.

Salkovskis, P.M., Atha, C., and Storer, D. (1990). Cognitive-behavioural problem solving in the treatment of patients who repeatedly attempt suicide. A controlled trial. *British Journal of Psychiatry*, 157, 871–6.

Segal, Z.V., Williams, J.M.G., and Teasdale, J.D. (2002). *Mindfulness-based cognitive therapy for depression: A new approach to preventing relapse*. Guilford, New York.

Suominen, K., Henriksson, M., Suokas, J., Isometsä, E., Ostamo, A., and Lönnqvist, J. (1996). Mental disorders and comorbidity in attempted suicide. *Acta Psychiatrica Scandinavica*, 94, 234–40.

Suominen, K., Isometsä, E.T., Henriksson, M., Ostamo, A., and Lönnqvist, J. (1998). Inadequate treatment for major depression both before and after attempted suicide. *American Journal of Psychiatry*, 155, 1778–80.

Teasdale, J.D., Segal, Z.V., Williams, J.M.G., Ridgeway, V.A., Soulsby, J.M., and Lau, M.A. (2000). Prevention of relapse/recurrence in major depression by mindfulness-based cognitive therapy. *Journal of Consulting and Clinical Psychology*, 68, 615–23.

Townsend, E., Hawton, K., Altman, D.G., Arensman, E., Gunnell, D., Hazell, P., *et al.* (2001). The efficacy of problem-solving treatments after deliberate self-harm: meta-analysis of randomised controlled trials with respect to depression, hopelessness and improvement in problems. *Psychological Medicine*, 31, 979–88.

Tyrer, P., Thompson, S., Schmidt, U., Jones, V., Knapp, M., Davidson, K., *et al.* (2003). Randomized controlled trial of brief cognitive behaviour therapy versus treatment as usual in recurrent deliberate self-harm: the POPMACT study. *Psychological Medicine*, 33, 969–76.

van der Sande, R., van Rooijen, L., Buskens, E., Allart, E., Hawton, K., van der Graaf, Y., *et al.* (1997). Intensive inpatient and community intervention versus routine care after attempted suicide. *British Journal of Psychiatry*, 171, 35–41.

Van Heeringen, C., Jannes, S., Buylaert, W., Henderick, H., De Bacquer, D., and Van Remoortel, J. (1995). The management of non-compliance with referral to out-patient after-care among attempted suicide patients: a controlled intervention study. *Psychological Medicine*, 25, 963–70.

van Praag, H.M. (2001). About the biological interface between psychotraumatic experiences and affective dysregulation. In *Understanding suicidal behaviour: the suicidal process approach to research, treatment and prevention*, (ed. K. Van Heeringen) pp. 54–75. Wiley, Chichester.

Verkes, R.J., Van der Mast, R.C., Hengeveld, M.W., Tuyl, J.P., Zwinderman, A.H., and Van Kempen, G.M.J. (1998). Reduction by paroxetine of suicidal behavior in patients with repeated suicide attempts but not major depression. *American Journal of Psychiatry*, 155, 543–7.

Welu, T.C. (1977). A follow-up program for suicide attempters: evaluation of effectiveness. *Suicide and Life-Threatening Behavior*, 7, 17–20.

Whittington, C.J., Kendall, T., Fonagy, P., Cottrell, D., Cotgrove, A., and Boddington, E. (2004). Selective serotonin reuptake inhibitors in childhood depression: systematic review of published versus unpublished data. *Lancet*, 363, 1341–5.

Wilkinson, P. (2002). Cognitive behaviour therapy. In *Psychological therapies with older people: developing treatments for effective practice*, (ed. J. Hepple, J. Pearce, and P. Wilkinson) pp. 45–75. Brunner-Routledge, Hove.

Williams, J.M.G. and Pollock, L.R. (2000). The psychology of suicidal behaviour. In *The international handbook of suicide and attempted suicide*, (ed. K. Hawton and K. Van Heeringen) pp. 79–93. Wiley, Chichester.

Williams, J.M.G. and Swales, M. (2004). The use of mindfulness-based approaches for suicidal patients. *Archives of Suicide Research*, 8, 315–29.

Wood, A., Trainor, G., Rothwell, J., Moore A., and Harrington, R. (2001). Randomized trial of group therapy for repeated deliberate self-harm in adolescents. *Journal of the American Academy of Child and Adolescent Psychiatry*, 40, 1246–53.

Zahl, D. and Hawton, K. (2004). Repetition of deliberate self-harm and subsequent suicide risk: long-term follow-up study in 11,583 patients. *British Journal of Psychiatry*, 185, 70–5.

13

Suicide in older adults: determinants of risk and opportunities for prevention

Yeates Conwell and Paul Duberstein

Introduction

In recent years suicide has been recognized as a major public health problem in countries throughout the world. Less commonly recognized, however, is that in most countries older adults are at greater risk for taking their own lives than people at any other point in the life course. With increased recognition of the public health significance of suicide in later life has come greater appreciation of the need for prevention strategies tailored to the particular needs and circumstances of senior citizens. The design of these strategies hinges, therefore, on the definition of risk factors for suicide in later life. In this chapter we provide a brief overview of the epidemiology of suicidal behaviours in later life, followed by a review of current knowledge concerning factors in biological, psychological, and social domains that place senior citizens at risk for suicide.

The epidemiology of suicidal ideation and behaviours in older adults

Suicidal ideation is less common in seniors than in younger populations. Table 13.1 lists results from general population studies of older adults. Prevalence estimates for suicidal ideation range from 1% to 36%. This variation is due to a number of factors. Some studies distinguished suicidal ideation (thoughts of taking one's own life) from death ideation (thoughts of death without specification of suicidal intent), whereas others did not. Rates of suicidal ideation and death ideation tend to be far higher in clinical samples (either psychiatric or medical) than in samples of elders drawn from the general population. Finally, the time frame for prevalence estimates ranged from the past week to lifetime, with results varying accordingly.

Table 13.1 Suicidal and death ideation in community-based studies of older adults

Study[a]	Location	Sample size	Age	Prevalence[b]	(time frame)	Clinical correlates
Forsell et al. (1997)	Kungsholmen, Sweden	969	≥75	SI: 10.1 fleeting, 2.5% frequent	(2 weeks)	Major depression, institutionalization, functional disability, visual problems
Crosby et al. (1999)	USA (nationwide telephone survey)	760	≥65	SI: 1.0%	(1 year)	Older age
Rao et al. (1997)	Cambridge, UK	125	≥81	SI: 7%; DI: 20%	(2 years)	Female gender, depression symptoms and diagnosis, dementia
Linden and Barnow (1997)	Berlin, Germany	516	≥70	SI: 1%; DI:21.1%	(1 week)	Major depressive disorder.
Jorm et al. (1995)	Canberra, Australia	923	≥70	SI/DI: 2.3%	(2 weeks)	Depressive disorder, poor health, disability, vision and hearing impairments, unmarried, in residential care
Skoog et al. (1996)	Gothenberg, Sweden	345	≥85	SI/DI: 15.9%	(1 mth)	Major depression, psychotic disorders, heart and peptic ulcer disease, anxiolytics, neuroleptics
Paykel et al. (1974)	Connecticut, USA	156	≥60	SI/DI: 9.0%	(1 year)	(Analysed for all subjects ≥ 18) Psychiatric symptoms, social isolation, more life events
Scocco et al. (2001)	Padua, Italy	611	≥65	SI/DI: 6.5%; 9.2%; 17.0%	(1 mth); (1 year); (lifetime)	Depression, anxiety, hostility, hypnotic use
Yip et al. (2003)	Hong Kong SAR	917	≥60	SI/DI/SA: 5.5%	(lifetime)	Poor physical health, vision and hearing impairments, depression, financial and relationship problems; passive coping styles

[a] All studies utilized in-person interviews, except Crosby et al. (2001), which used a telephone survey.
[b] SI, suicidal ideation; DI, death ideation; AS, attempted suicide.

Like suicidal ideation, attempted suicide is less common in later life than among younger age groups (Gallo *et al.* 1994). However, because there is no systematic surveillance mechanism for attempted suicide, fewer estimates are available. In the group of seniors interviewed for the Epidemiological Catchment Area study in the United States, 1.1% reported having made a suicide attempt (Moscicki *et al.* 1988). Estimates of the ratio of attempted to completed suicides in the general population range from 8:1 to 36:1 (Crosby *et al.* 1999). In contrast, studies estimate that there are four or fewer attempts for each completed suicide in later life (McIntosh *et al.* 1994). These figures reflect the greater lethality of self-destructive acts by senior citizens, which in turn results from at least three distinctive features. Older adults carry a higher burden of physical illness and physical frailty that render them, in general, less likely to survive the insult. They are more likely to live alone than younger people, and so are less likely to be discovered in time for their lives to be saved. As well, older adults act on suicidal intent with greater planning and determination to die (Conwell *et al.* 1998). They give fewer warnings to others of their suicidal plans, implement their self-destructive acts with greater forethought, and use more lethal means. These characteristics of suicidal elders underscore the importance of strategies that promote detection of seniors at risk before the development of acute suicidal states.

Suicide rates in most nations rise progressively throughout the life course, to a peak for both men and women in the 75 and over age group (World Health Organization 2001), the most rapidly growing segment of the population worldwide. The World Health Organization estimates, for example, that there are now approximately 600 million people aged 60 years and over. By 2020 that figure will rise to over 1 billion, more than 70% of whom will live in developing countries (World Health Organization 2003), which are among those with the highest suicide rates. This demographic shift will inevitably result in far greater absolute numbers of seniors taking their own lives. We have a pressing need, therefore, for the development, testing, and wide dissemination of late-life suicide prevention strategies in anticipation of these changes.

Risk factors for suicide in later life

The progressive rise in suicide rates by age in both men and women in most cultures suggests that ageing-related biological and/or psychological processes may contribute to increased risk for suicide in older adults. However, prevalence rates for suicide in older adulthood differ dramatically across cultures, and in some countries (e.g. Australia and the UK) peak rates for men and women occur in young adulthood. Therefore, socio-cultural factors must also play an important role in determining risk. The following sections review evidence in psychiatric, medical, psychological, and social domains. We first note correlative and descriptive data, followed by reference to studies in which sufficiently rigorous methodologies were used and control samples included to enable quantification of suicide risk.

Our focus is on completed rather than attempted suicide, for several reasons. First, prevention programmes should be designed based on best evidence concerning the highest risk behaviour. Given the characteristics of late-life suicidal behaviour noted above—physical frailty, living alone, and high lethality of intent—it is likely that those elders who survive a suicide attempt represent, to some significant extent, a separate population from those who die by their own hand. Finally, research on attempted suicide is most often conducted with clinical samples. Yet a small minority of elders who take their own lives have a prior history of psychiatric treatment, again suggesting that these samples may not be representative of the population that represents the highest priority for late-life suicide preventive interventions.

Psychiatric symptoms and syndromes associated with completed suicide in later life

Uncontrolled studies

Psychological autopsy studies indicate that from 71 to 95% of persons aged 65 years and over who took their own lives had a diagnosable major psychiatric disorder at the time of death (Table 13.2).

Mood disorders are most common, present in a larger proportion of late-life suicides than in younger cohorts. Furthermore, our group observed that the affective illnesses associated with later-life suicide are typically of moderate severity and infrequently associated with co-morbid substance use disorders. These clinical characteristics suggest the likelihood of response to standard therapies, a reason for therapeutic optimism (Conwell *et al.* 1996).

Primary psychotic illnesses (schizophrenia, schizoaffective illness, and delusional disorder), personality and anxiety disorders are less common than affective illness among older adults who take their own lives, and less prevalent in late-life suicides than in people who die by suicide at younger ages. Alcoholism and other drug-use disorders, present in from 3 to 43% of late-life suicides, are also less common than in suicides at earlier points in the life course.

Controlled studies

Five psychological autopsy studies have been reported recently that included control samples, thus enabling quantification of risk for suicide associated

Table 13.2 Axis I diagnoses made by psychological autopsy in studies of late-life suicide

Study	Country	Sample size	Age	Diagnosis: % with					
				Major depression	Other mood disorder	Alcohol use disorder	Other drug use disorder	Non-affective psychosis	No diagnosis[a]
Barraclough (1971)	UK	30	≥65	87	3	0	13		
Clark (1991)	USA	54	≥65	54	11	19	0	24	
Conwell et al. (1991)	USA	18	≥50	67	17	42	0	11	
Carney et al. (1994)	USA	49	≥60	54	22	–	14		
Henriksson et al. (1995)	Finland	43	≥60	44	21	25	5	12	9
Conwell et al. (1996)	USA	36	55–74	47	17	43	3	6	8
		14	75–92	57	21	27	7	0	29
Beautrais (2002)	New Zealand	31	≥55	86	14	–	9		
Conwell et al. (2001)	USA	73	≥50	71	18	7	12		
Harwood et al. (2001)	UK	100	≥60	63	5	5	4	23	
Waern et al. (2002)	Sweden	85	≥65	46	36	27	8	5	

[a] Includes cases with insufficient data to allow diagnosis.

with specific late-life disorders. All five found that the presence of any axis I mental disorder is associated with elevated risk for suicide in older adults (Conwell et al. 2000, 2001; Harwood et al. 2001; Beautrais 2002; Waern et al. 2002), with odds ratios ranging from 27.4 to 113.1. Mood disorders were particularly prominent in each study. Waern and colleagues further subdivided the illness, finding that recurrent major depressive disorder was associated with the greatest relative risk in multivariate analyses, although single episodes of depression, dysthymia, and minor depression were also significant predictors of suicide (Waern et al. 2002).

Three studies found no significant difference between suicides and controls in the proportions with dementia (Conwell et al. 2000, 2001; Waern et al. 2002), and none found that anxiety disorders were associated with elevated risk after controlling for depression in multivariate analyses. Three of the five studies reported that substance-use disorders placed subjects at statistically increased risk for suicide, with odds ratios (ORs) ranging from 4.4 to 43.1 (Conwell et al. 2000; Beautrais 2002; Waern et al. 2002).

In addition to these psychological autopsy studies, two prospective non-clinical cohort studies have used a nested case-control design to investigate risk factors for completed suicide in older adults, focusing on symptoms and behaviours rather than diagnoses. Ross and colleagues followed almost 12 000 retirement community residents for 5 years, 19 of whom died by suicide (Ross et al. 1990). They found that subjects with the greatest depressive symptomatology were 23 times more likely to take their own lives than asymptomatic subjects. In addition, in a multivariate analysis, drinking three or more alcoholic beverages and sleeping nine or more hours per night were independently associated with significantly increased risk for suicide (OR = 3.5 and OR = 4.6, respectively).

Turvey and colleagues used data from the Established Populations for Epidemiological Studies of the Elderly (EPESE) database in a similar manner (Turvey et al. 2002). Of almost 14 500 elderly subjects followed for 10 years, 21 died by suicide. Significantly greater depressive symptoms, poorer perceived health status and sleep quality, and absence of a relative or friend in whom to confide distinguished cases from controls. The finding that sleep disturbance is a risk factor for suicide in later life supports Barraclough's early observation (Barraclough 1971). In a descriptive study of 30 seniors who took their own lives, 26 (87%) had diagnosable affective disorders. Among these 26 cases, insomnia was present in 23 (90%), the most prevalent symptom in the sample other than mood change. Weight loss and reduction in activities were present in 75%, while hypochondriasis, guilt, anxiety, and difficulty concentrating were present in 50% of cases.

The association between suicide and hopelessness in general adult clinical samples has been the subject of intensive study (Beck *et al.* 1985, 1990), but hopelessness has been less thoroughly examined in older adults. Hill and colleagues reported that hopelessness was associated with suicidal ideation in older outpatient depressives (Hill *et al.* 1988). In Ross and colleagues' prospective cohort study, a single hopelessness item was significantly associated with suicide (Ross *et al.* 1990). Szanto and colleagues found that hopelessness remains significantly higher, even after treatment to resolution of a depressive syndrome, in elderly patients with major depression and a lifetime history of suicide attempts, than among either persons with suicidal ideation only or non-suicidal elderly patients (Szanto *et al.* 1998). They interpreted these findings to mean that hopelessness may represent a trait as well as state vulnerability to suicide.

Finally, studies have demonstrated a clear and powerful association between a past history of suicide attempt and completed suicide in older people. Between 19 and 53% of elders who took their own lives had made prior attempts (Conwell *et al.* 2000; Beautrais 2002). In her comparison of elder suicides and near lethal suicide attempts with matched normal controls, Beautrais calculated that the cases were over 36 times more likely to have made one or more previous suicide attempts (Beautrais 2002).

Personality traits

Relatively fewer investigators have systematically examined the role of personality in late-life suicide. In their study of suicides aged 60 years or more, Harwood *et al.* (2001) determined that 16% had personality disorder diagnoses, a figure similar to the 14% prevalence of axis II diagnoses found by Henriksson and colleagues among elderly Finnish suicides (Henriksson *et al.* 1995). When Harwood and co-workers compared their suicide cases with age- and sex-matched controls who died in hospital, suicides were significantly more likely to have a personality disorder.

Both descriptive studies and more recent controlled research investigations have linked elder suicide with a range of personality *traits* as well. In an early, classic description, Batchelor and Napier (1953) characterized elders who took their own lives as timid, shy, and seclusive, subject to hypochondriasis and hostility, and with a rigid, independent style. Other investigators observed many of those same traits in subsequent studies (Farberow and Shneidman 1970; Clark 1993).

Guided by the five-factor model of personality, Duberstein and colleagues were the first to use validated measures in a case-control design to study personality traits of older suicides (Duberstein, et al. 1994). They demonstrated that high Neuroticism (N) and lower scores on the Openness to Experience (OTE) factor of the NEO Personality Inventory (Costa and McCrae 1992) distinguished suicides over age 50 years from a comparison group of normal, community-dwelling adults. People low in OTE may be characterized as having muted affective and hedonic responsiveness, a constricted range of interests, and comfort with the familiar. In addition to their finding concerning personality disorder diagnosis, Harwood and colleagues reported that accentuation of anankastic and anxious personality traits distinguished elder suicides from controls (Harwood et al. 2001). They further noted the similarity between the constructs of low OTE and anankastic traits. Duberstein has hypothesized that these qualities place elders at risk by making them less well equipped socially and psychologically to manage the challenges of ageing (Duberstein 1995), especially the need to adapt to changes (e.g. in lifestyle, physical and functional capacity, and living circumstances). Furthermore, seniors low in OTE have smaller social networks and are less likely to experience or express suicidal ideation. Consequently, they are likely to escape detection and lifesaving interventions (Duberstein 2001). Additional research is needed in order to establish the relationships of these traits to the depressive conditions so common in older suicide victims, and to determine whether they serve as moderators of other putative risk and protective factors present, such as stressful events and social supports.

Physical health and functioning

Suicide is often ascribed to physical illness, yet the evidence to support a causal association in older adulthood is limited. Harris and Barraclough demonstrated in a comprehensive review of over 60 medical disorders and their treatments that the illnesses for which there was evidence of increased suicide risk were disorders relatively more closely associated with middle age than later life: HIV/AIDS, Huntington's disease, multiple sclerosis, renal disease, peptic ulcer disease, spinal cord injury, and systemic lupus erythematosis (Harris and Barraclough 1994). Record linkage studies have convincingly demonstrated that malignant neoplasms of all sorts (with the exception of skin cancer) are associated with increased risk (Quan et al. 2002). Seizure disorders, other CNS conditions, cardiopulmonary complications, and urogenital diseases in men have been implicated as well (Whitlock 1986, Mackenzie and Popkin 1987). However, few studies have focused specifically on older adult samples, in which the base rate of physical illness is much higher. Furthermore, few studies to date have examined the role that mood disorders, which are closely associated with both suicide and physical illness, may play as mediators of the relationship. That is, do seniors with physical illness become suicidal because they first become depressed?

Brown and colleagues reported that among 44 terminally ill patients, 10 were suicidal or desired an early death (Brown *et al.* 1986). All 10 had depressive illness; none were suicidal in the absence of clinically significant mood disorder. Chochinov and colleagues interviewed 200 medical/surgical in-patients with terminal illness (Chochinov *et al.* 1995). They found that while wishes for an early death were present in 44.5% of subjects, suicidal thoughts were uncommon (8.5%). The desire for death was significantly associated with measures of depression.

Several investigators have examined the prevalence of physical illness and functional impairment in completed suicides and controls in later life, with mixed results. Our group found that physical illness burden and the presence of one or more serious physical conditions significantly distinguished suicides aged 60 years and over, who died within 30 days of contact with their primary-care provider, from a demographically matched sample of living primary-care patients (Conwell *et al.* 2000). However, after controlling for mood disorders, physical health and functional measures were no longer associated with suicide. Beautrais found that neither serious physical illness nor the likelihood of a visit to a primary-care provider in the past month was associated with increased risk for suicide in her case-control study conducted in New Zealand elders (Beautrais 2002), findings that are hard to interpret with confidence, due to sample size considerations and the inclusion of both attempted and completed suicides. In contrast, Waern and colleagues reported that serious physical illness in any organ category was an independent risk factor for suicide in seniors, even after controlling for psychiatric diagnosis (Waern *et al.* 2002). However, when the sexes were analysed separately, illness represented a risk factor only in elderly men. This important observation may help explain the interaction between age and gender in determining suicide risk: with increasing age in most countries, risk for men rises at a faster rate than for women. While physical illness is clearly an important factor in determining risk for suicide in later life, the mediating influence of depressive disorders, and moderators such as sex, warrant further study.

Neurobiological factors

Many investigators and studies have noted an association between low cerebrospinal fluid (CSF) levels of the primary serotonin metabolite, 5-hydroxyindoleacetic acid (5-HIAA), and aggressive, impulsive behaviour, including suicide (for a representative review, see Stoff and Mann 1997). Post-mortem studies of brain tissue from suicides and controls yield results consistent with the hypothesis that suicidal people have a presynaptic serotonergic deficit and postsynaptic compensatory response. Observations include low brain concentrations of serotonin and 5-HIAA, increased postsynaptic 5-HT receptor binding, and decreased presynaptic binding at $5-HT_1$ receptor sites and the serotonin transporter. Mann and colleagues have posited a stress-diathesis model in which those individuals with low serotonergic activity, either on a genetic or environmental basis, are more prone to act impulsively and aggressively in the face of dysphoria, hopelessness, and emergent suicidal ideation in the depressed state (Mann et al. 1999). Noradrenergic, dopaminergic, and other neuroendocrine and neurochemical systems have also been implicated.

The dramatic rise in suicide rates across the life course in most countries suggests that, in addition to psychiatric and psychological factors, ageing in neurobiological systems may contribute to suicide risk in older adults. In one of the few studies to examine neurobiological correlates of suicidal behaviour in seniors, Jones and colleagues demonstrated that CSF levels of 5-HIAA in elderly depressed patients who had attempted suicide were significantly lower than in elderly depressed controls (Jones et al. 1990). Mann and colleagues have further reported that age-related effects on serotonergic and other monoamine systems may be more pronounced in men than women (Mann and Stoff 1997). Preliminary evidence, therefore, supports the need for further investigation of neurochemical abnormalities in late-life suicide.

Structural and functional abnormalities in the ageing brain have been associated with suicidal behaviours in seniors as well. Two studies of neuropsychological testing performance have found abnormalities in executive function of subjects who attempted suicide compared with controls (Keilp et al. 2001), including in older adults (King et al. 2000). In analysis of brain tissue obtained post-mortem, we reported significantly greater Alzheimer's-type neurofibrillary pathology in the hippocampi of elders who died by suicide than in controls (Rubio et al. 2001); other brain regions have not yet been examined. Ahearn and colleagues found that elderly depressives with lifetime histories of suicide attempt had significantly more subcortical grey matter hyperintensities on magnetic resonance imaging (MRI) than did carefully matched depressives with no previous suicide attempt (Ahearn et al. 2001).

This amalgam of neurobiological findings reinforces the conception that suicide in later life may be associated with destruction of neural pathways critical to the regulation of mood, cognition, and behaviour. Additional research is necessary to confirm and extend these functional and neuroanatomical findings, define their neurochemical correlates, and establish whether they represent early, subtle presentations of vascular or other degenerative neuropathology. However, at this stage, there remains no clinical useful neurobiological marker of suicide risk in older or younger adults.

Social/cultural factors

The socio-cultural factors pertinent to suicide in later life likely differ from those at earlier ages. For example, suicides in young and middle adulthood typically occur in the context of interpersonal discord, legal, financial, and occupational problems. Suicides among seniors are more often associated with physical illness and other losses (Conwell *et al.* 1990; Carney *et al.* 1994; Heikkinen *et al.* 1995), including bereavement (Duberstein *et al.* 1998). Of course, these observations may only reflect the differing base rates of stressful events across the life course. Studies that utilize control samples are needed to determine whether they constitute risk factors for suicide.

Three psychological autopsy studies have compared seniors who died by suicide and matched controls with regard to the prevalence of specific stressors. Financial difficulties, relationship problems, and family discord distinguished the groups in all studies when examined with univariate analyses (Rubenowitz *et al.* 2001; Beautrais 2002; Duberstein *et al.* 2004). When other factors, including depression, were controlled for in multivariate analyses, however, family discord remained predictive in one study (Rubenowitz *et al.* 2001) but not another (Duberstein *et al.* 2004).

Social isolation and social support may serve as risk and protective factors, respectively, for late-life suicide. Barraclough, comparing elder suicides with census data, concluded that cases were more likely to live alone than their peers in the community (Barraclough 1971). Three of the case-control psychological autopsy studies previously mentioned have examined this question, but only one found that elder suicides were more likely than controls to live alone (unadjusted OR = 5.1) (Conwell *et al.* 2001). In their analyses of the EPESE database, Turvey and colleagues reported that having a greater number of friends and relatives in whom to confide was associated with significantly reduced suicide risk for seniors (Turvey *et al.* 2002), and in his 1978 psychological autopsy study of men in Arizona, Miller also reported that matched community controls were significantly more likely than elder male suicides to have had a confidante (Miller 1978). Beautrais reported in her New Zealand sample of late-life suicides and near fatal suicide attempts that lack of social interaction was a significant risk factor (OR = 4.5), even after adjustment for physical and mental health variables (Beautrais 2002). Similar findings were reported in the Rochester study; low levels of social interaction amplified suicide risk, even after adjusting for the presence of active mood and substance disorders (Duberstein *et al.* 2004).

Access to means

The means used by older adults to take their own lives vary by location. Harwood and colleagues reported, for example, that in Great Britain the most common methods were hanging in older men and drug overdose in elderly women (Harwood *et al.* 2000), while in Hong Kong most elder suicides result from jumping (Yip *et al.* 1998). In the United Sates 57% of all suicides are by firearm (McIntosh 2002). However, among older adults who take their own lives, that figure is 73%. Both men and women are more likely to use a firearm as a means of suicide in later life than at younger ages, although older men remain far more likely to take their lives with a gun than are women (McIntosh 2002). Miller found no difference between male suicides and controls in the proportion that owned a firearm (Miller 1978). However, a significantly greater proportion of suicides than controls had acquired the weapon within the past year. We recently reported that the presence of a handgun in the home significantly increased risk for suicide in elderly men, but not women (Conwell *et al.* 2002). Among those subjects who kept a gun in the home, storing the weapon loaded and unlocked were also independent predictors of suicide.

Implications for prevention

Knowledge of risk factors from well-conducted and controlled studies informs the design of suicide-prevention strategies. The complex, multidetermined nature of suicide suggests numerous potential targets for intervention that may result in reduced suicide rates among older people.

For example, there is no doubt that affective illnesses—primarily major depression but also other less severe forms of the illness—may play a prominent role in most late-life suicides. Beautrais (2002) calculated that if mood disorders could be eliminated from the elderly population, almost three-quarters of suicides by older adults could be prevented (population attributable risk for mood disorder in the last month = 73.6%). Prevention efforts, therefore, must target the detection and treatment of late-life affective illness (Bruce 1999), an approach that preliminary studies indicate may indeed have benefit.

Rutz and colleagues demonstrated that an education programme for primary-care providers on the Swedish island of Gotland resulted in a transient decrease in the suicide rate of women, both in comparison to rates on Gotland before the intervention as well as in comparison to contemporaneous rates in other parts of the country (Rutz *et al.* 1989, 1995). Although an uncontrolled study, it reinforces the need for further investigation into the effect that supplementing the resources and skills of health-care providers in diagnosis and treatment of late-life affective illness may have on suicide morbidity and mortality. Not only physicians, but also nurses, aides, and others who provide health care to seniors in the community and long-term care facilities should be included.

The independent contribution of social isolation to late-life suicide risk suggests a different set of preventive strategies that includes community outreach and provision of supportive services. As one example, DeLeo and colleagues have described the Telehelp/Telecheck service in Padua, Italy, in which functionally impaired, isolated, and at-risk elders are provided with access to a telephone-based response network for ongoing monitoring and emotional support via short and informal telephone contacts and additional interventions as indicated (DeLeo *et al.* 2002). Over 10 years significantly fewer suicide deaths occurred among almost 19 000 service users than were expected in the elderly population of that region. The effect was particularly strong among women, for whom the observed suicide rate was six times lower than among other such women in the community.

Finally, knowledge that access to specific means for suicide places elders at increased risk suggests the need to consider strategies that restrict access to those means. For example, the Brady Handgun Violence Prevention Act of 1994 established a nationwide requirement in the USA that licensed firearms dealers initiate a background check for individuals seeking to purchase a handgun, and observe a waiting period between application and delivery of the weapon. Ludwig and colleagues examined firearm homicide and suicide rates before and after enactment of the legislation, comparing 18 states that already had such laws in place ('control' states) with 32 in which the requirements were newly enacted (Ludwig and Cook 2000). They found that changes in homicide and suicide rates for intervention and control states were not significantly different, *except* for firearm suicides among persons aged 55 years or older, which decreased following the intervention. Although not specific to the elderly, similar reductions were observed in the UK following restriction of access to paracetamol (Hawton *et al.* 2001).

Conclusions

Over time, both descriptive and controlled, hypothesis-testing studies have helped to generate a more detailed picture of the factors that place seniors at risk for suicide. While the mechanisms that underlie the behaviour are complex, their implications are clear. Suicide in older adults results from factors in psychological, medical/psychiatric, social, and probably neurobiological domains, for which treatments and preventive interventions are, or can be made, available. With a creative approach and firm commitment by society to the health and well being of its elders, we should expect to reduce substantially the number of senior citizens who die by their own hands.

Acknowledgements

This chapter was prepared with support of the National Institute of Mental Health (K24 MH01759; Y.C.).

References

Ahearn, E.P., Jamison, K.R., Steffens, D.C., Cassidy, F., Provenzale, J.M., Lehman, A., *et al.* (2001). MRI correlates of suicide attempt history in unipolar depression. *Biological Psychiatry*, 50, 266–70.

Barraclough, B.M. (1971). Suicide in the elderly: recent developments in psychogeriatrics. *British Journal of Psychiatry*, **spec. suppl.** 6, 87–97.

Batchelor, I.R.C. and Napier, M.B. (1953). Attempted suicide in old age. *British Medical Journal*, 2, 1186–90.

Beautrais, A.L. (2002). A case control study of suicide and attempted suicide in older adults. *Suicide and Life-Threatening Behavior*, 32, 1–9.

Beck, A.T., Steer, R.A., Kovacs, M., and Garrison, B. (1985). Hopelessness and eventual suicide: a 10-year prospective study of patients hospitalized with suicidal ideation. *American Journal of Psychiatry*, 142, 559–63.

Beck, A.T., Brown, G., Berchick, R.J., Stewart, B.L., and Steer, R.A. (1990). Relationship between hopelessness and ultimate suicide: a replication with psychiatric outpatients. *American Journal of Psychiatry*, 147, 190–5.

Brown, J.H., Henteleff, P., Barakat, S., and Rowe, C.J. (1986). Is it normal for terminally ill patients to desire death? *American Journal of Psychiatry*, 143, 208–11.

Bruce, M.L. (1999). Designing an intervention to prevent suicide: PROSPECT (Prevention of Suicide in Primary Care Elderly: Collaborative Trial). *Dialogues in Clinical Neuroscience*, 1, 100–10.

Carney, S.S., Rich, C.L., Burke, P.A., and Fowler, R.C. (1994). Suicide over 60: the San Diego study. *Journal of the American Geriatrics Society*, 42, 174–80.

Chochinov, H.M., Wilson, K.G., Enns, M., Mowchun, N., Lander, S., Levitt, M., *et al.* (1995). Desire for death in the terminally ill. *American Journal of Psychiatry*, 152, 1185–91.

Clark, D.C. (1991). Suicide among the elderly. Final report to the AARP Andrus Foundation.

Clark, D.C. (1993). Narcissistic crises of aging and suicidal despair. *Suicide and Life-Threatening Behavior*, 23, 21–6.

Conwell, Y., Rotenberg, M., and Caine, E.D. (1990). Completed suicide at age 50 and over. *Journal of the American Geriatrics Society*, 38, 640–4.

Conwell, Y., Olsen, K., Caine, E.D., and Flannery, C. (1991). Suicide in later life: psychological autopsy findings. *International Psychogeriatrics*, 3, 59–66.

Conwell, Y., Duberstein, P.R., Cox, C., Herrmann, J.H., Forbes, N.T., and Caine, E.D. (1996). Relationships of age and axis I diagnoses in victims of completed suicide: a psychological autopsy study. *American Journal of Psychiatry*, 153, 1001–8.

Conwell, Y., Duberstein, P.R., Cox, C., Herrmann, J., Forbes, N., and Caine, E.D. (1998).
Age differences in behaviors leading to completed suicide. *American Journal of Geriatric Psychiatry*, 6, 122–6.

Conwell, Y., Lyness, J.M., Duberstein, P., Cox, C., Seidlitz, L., DiGiorgio, A., *et al.* (2000).
Completed suicide among older patients in primary care practices: a controlled study.
Journal of the American Geriatrics Society, 48, 23–9.

Conwell, Y., Duberstein, P., DiGiorgio, A., Cox, C., Forbes, N.T., and Caine, E.D. (2001).
Risk factors for suicide in later life. International Psychogeriatric Association Lorne,
Australia [abstract].

Conwell, Y., Duberstein, P.R., Connor, K., Eberly, S., Cox, C., and Caine, E.D. (2002). Access
to firearms and risk for suicide in middle-aged and older adults. *American Journal of Geriatric Psychiatry*, 10, 407–16.

Costa, P.T. and McCrae, R.R. (1992). *Revised NEO Personality Inventory and NEO Five Factor Inventory: professional manual.* PAR, Odessa, FL.

Crosby, A.E., Cheltenham, M.P., and Sacks, J.J. (1999). Incidence of suicidal ideation and
behavior in the United States, 1994. *Suicide and Life-Threatening Behavior*, 29, 131–40.

De Leo, D., Dello, B.M., and Dwyer, J. (2002). Suicide among the elderly: the long-term
impact of a telephone support and assessment intervention in northern Italy. *British Journal of Psychiatry*, 181, 226–9.

Duberstein, P.R. (1995). Openness to experience and completed suicide across the second
half of life. *International Psychogeriatrics*, 7, 183–98.

Duberstein, P.R. (2001). Are closed-minded people more open to the idea of killing
themselves? *Suicide and Life-Threatening Behavior*, 31, 9–14.

Duberstein, P.R., Conwell, Y., and Caine, E.D. (1994). Age differences in the personality
characteristics of suicide completers: preliminary findings from a psychological autopsy
study. *Psychiatry*, 57, 213–24.

Duberstein, P.R., Conwell, Y., and Cox, C. (1998). Suicide in widowed persons.
A psychological autopsy comparison of recently and remotely bereaved older subjects.
American Journal of Geriatric Psychiatry, 6, 328–34.

Duberstein, P.R., Conwell, Y., Conner, K.R., Eberly, S., and Caine, E.D. (2004). Suicide at 50
years of age and older: Perceived physical illness, family discord, and financial strain.
Psychological Medicine, 44, 137–46.

Duberstein, P.R., Conwell, Y., Conner, K.R., Eberly, S., Evinger, J.S., Caine, E.D. (2004).
Poor social integration and suicide risk: fact or artifact? A case-control study.
Psychological Medicine, 34, 1331–7.

Farberow, N.L. and Shneidman, E.S. (1970). Suicide among patients with malignant
neoplasms. In *The psychology of suicide*, (ed. E.S. Shneidman, N.L. Farberow, and
R.E. Litman), pp. 324–44. Science House, New York.

Forsell, Y., Jorm, A.F., and Winblad, B. (1997). Suicidal thoughts and associated factors in
an elderly population. *Acta Psychiatrica Scandinavica*, 95, 108–11.

Gallo, J.J., Anthony, J.C., and Muthen, B.O. (1994). Age differences in the symptoms of
depression: a latent trait analysis. *Journal of Gerontology*, 49, 251–64.

Harris, E.C. and Barraclough, B.M. (1994). Suicide as an outcome for medical disorders.
Medicine, 73, 281–96.

Harwood, D.M., Hawton, K., Hope, T., and Jacoby, R. (2000). Suicide in older people: mode
of death, demographic factors, and medical contact before death. *International Journal of Geriatric Psychiatry*, 15, 736–43.

Harwood, D., Hawton, K., Hope, T., and Jacoby, R. (2001). Psychiatric disorder and
personality factors associated with suicide in older people: a descriptive and case-control
study. *International Journal of Geriatric Psychiatry*, 16, 155–65.

Hawton, K., Townsend, E., Deeks, J., Appleby, L., Gunnell, D., Bennewith, O., *et al.* (2001). Effects of legislation restricting pack sizes of paracetamol and salicylate on self poisoning in the United Kingdom: before and after study. *British Medical Journal*, 322, 1203–7.

Heikkinen, M.E., Isometsä, E.T., Aro, H.M., Sarna, S.J., and Lönnqvist, J.K. (1995). Age-related variation in recent life events preceding suicide. *Journal of Nervous and Mental Disease*, 183, 325–31.

Henriksson, M.M., Marttunen, M.J., Isometsa, E.T., Heikkinen, M.E., Aro, H.M., Kuoppasalmi, K.I., *et al.* (1995). Mental disorders in elderly suicide. *International Psychogeriatrics*, 7, 275–86.

Hill, R.D., Gallagher, D., Thompson, L.W., and Ishida, T. (1988). Hopelessness as a measure of suicide intent in the depressed elderly. *Psychology and Aging*, 3, 230–2.

Jones, J.S., Stanley, B., Mann, J.J., Frances, A.J., Guido, J.R., Traskman-Bendz, L., *et al.* (1990). CSF 5-HIAA and HVA concentrations in elderly depressed patients who attempted suicide. *American Journal of Psychiatry*, 147, 1225–7.

Jorm, A.F., Henderson, A.S., Scott, R., Korten, A.E., Christensen, H., and Mackinnon, A.J. (1995). Factors associated with the wish to die in elderly people. *Age and Ageing*, 24, 389–92.

Keilp, J.G., Sackeim, H.A., Brodsky, B.S., Oquendo, M.A., Malone, K.M., and Mann, J.J. (2001). Neuropsychological dysfunction in depressed suicide attempters. *American Journal of Psychiatry*, 158, 735–41.

King, D.A., Conwell, Y., Cox, C., Henderson, R.E., Denning, D.G., and Caine, E.D. (2000). A neuropsychological comparison of depressed suicide attempters and nonattempters. *Journal of Neuropsychiatry and Clinical Neurosciences*, 12, 64–70.

Linden, M. and Barnow, S. (1997). The wish to die in very old persons near the end of life: a psychiatric problem? Results from the Berlin Aging Study. *International Psychogeriatrics*, 9, 291–307.

Ludwig, J. and Cook, P.J. (2000). Homicide and suicide rates associated with implementation of the Brady Handgun Violence Prevention Act. *Journal of the American Medical Association*, 284, 585–91.

Mackenzie, T.B. and Popkin, M.K. (1987). Suicide in the medical patient. *International Journal of Psychiatry in Medicine*, 17, 3–22.

Mann, J.J. and Stoff, D.M. (1997). A synthesis of current findings regarding neurobiological correlates and treatment of suicidal behavior. *Annals of the New York Academy of Sciences*, 836, 352–63.

Mann, J.J., Waternaux, C., Haas, G.L., and Malone, K.M. (1999). Toward a clinical model of suicidal behavior in psychiatric patients. *American Journal of Psychiatry*, 156, 181–9.

McIntosh, J.L. (2002). *U.S.A Suicide: 1999 Official Final Statistics*. NCHS/CDC. Available at website http://www.iusb.edu/~jmcintos/SuicideStats.html (accessed June 25, 2005).

McIntosh, J.L., Santos, J.F., Hubbard, R.W., and Overholser, J.C. (1994). *Elder suicide: Research, theory, and treatment*. American Psychological Association, Washington, DC.

Miller, M. (1978). Geriatric suicide: the Arizona study. *Gerontologist*, 18, 488–95.

Moscicki, E.K., O'Carroll, P., Rae, D.S., Locke, B.Z., Roy, A., and Regier, D.A. (1988). Suicide attempts in the Epidemiologic Catchment Area Study. *Yale Journal of Biology and Medicine*, 61, 259–68.

Paykel, E.S., Myers, J.K., Lindenthal, J.J., and Tanner, J. (1974). Suicidal feelings in the general population: a prevalence study. *British Journal of Psychiatry*, 124, 460–9.

Quan, H., Arboleda-Florez, J., Fick, G.H., Stuart, H.L., and Love, E.J. (2002). Association between physical illness and suicide among the elderly. *Social Psychiatry and Psychiatric Epidemiology,* 37, 190–7.

Rao, R., Dening, T., Brayne, C., and Huppert, F.A. (1997). Suicidal thinking in community residents over eighty. *International Journal of Geriatric Psychiatry,* 12, 337–43.

Ross, R.K., Bernstein, L., Trent, L., Henderson, B.E., and Paganini-Hill, A. (1990). A prospective study of risk factors for traumatic death in the retirement community. *Preventive Medicine,* 19, 323–34.

Rubenowitz, E., Waern, M., Wilhelmsson, K., and Allebeck, P. (2001). Life events and psychosocial factors in elderly suicides – a case control study. *Psychological Medicine,* 31, 1193–202.

Rubio, A., Vestner, A.L., Stewart, J.M., Forbes, N.T., Conwell, Y., and Cox, C. (2001). Suicide and Alzheimer's pathology in the elderly: a case-control study. *Biological Psychiatry,* 49, 137–45.

Rutz, W., von Knorring, L., and Walinder, J. (1989). Frequency of suicide on Gotland after systematic postgraduate education of general practitioners. *Acta Psychiatrica Scandinavica,* 80, 151–4.

Rutz, W., von Knorring, L., Pihlgren, H., Rihmer, Z., and Walinder, J. (1995). Prevention of male suicides: lessons from Gotland study [letter]. *Lancet,* 345, 524.

Scocco, P., Meneghel, G., Caon, F., Dello, B.M., and De Leo, D. (2001), Death ideation and its correlates: survey of an over-65-year-old population. *Journal of Nervous and Mental Disease,* 189, 210–18.

Skoog, I., Aevarsson, O., Beskow, J., Larsson, L., Palsson, S., Waern, M., *et al.* (1996). Suicidal feelings in a population sample of nondemented 85-year-olds. *American Journal of Psychiatry,* 153, 1015–20.

Stoff, D.M. and Mann, J.J. (1997). The neurobiology of suicide: from the bench to the clinic. *Annals of the New York Academy of Sciences,* 836, 1–365.

Szanto, K., Reynolds, C.F., III, Conwell, Y., Begley, A.E., and Houck, P. (1998). High levels of hopelessness persist in geriatric patients with remitted depression and a history of attempted suicide. *Journal of the American Geriatrics Society,* 46, 1401–6.

Turvey, C.L., Conwell, Y., Jones, M.P., Phillips, C., Simonsick, E., Pearson, J.L., *et al.* (2002). Risk factors for late-life suicide: a prospective, community-based study. *American Journal of Geriatric Psychiatry,* 10, 398–406.

Waern, M., Runeson, B., Allebeck, P., Beskow, J., Rubenowitz, E., Skoog, I., *et al.* (2002). Mental disorder in elderly suicides. *American Journal of Psychiatry,* 159, 450–5.

Whitlock, F.A. (1986). Suicide and physical illness. In *Suicide,* (ed. A. Roy), pp. 151–70. Williams and Wilkins, Baltimore.

World Health Organization (2001). Suicide rates per 100,000. Available at website http://www.who.int/mental_health/Topic_Suicide/suicide_rates.html (accessed 24 October 2003).

World Health Organization (2003). Population Ageing—A Public Health Challenge. Available at website http://www.who.int/inf-fs/en/fact135.html (accessed 22 October 2003).

Yip, P.S., Chi, I., and Yu, K.K. (1998). An epidemiological profile of elderly suicides in Hong Kong. *International Journal of Geriatric Psychiatry,* 13, 631–7.

Yip, P.S.F., Chi, I., Chiu, H., Wai, K.C., Conwell, Y., and Caine, E. (2003). A prevalence study of suicide ideation among older adults in Hong Kong SAR. *International Journal of Geriatric Psychiatry,* 18, 1056–62.

14

The resistance of suicide: why haven't antidepressants reduced suicide rates?

Herman M. van Praag

No reduction of suicide rates in the era of the antidepressants

Depression is considered to be a major precursor of both attempted and completed suicide. Psychological autopsy studies show that approximately 90% of consecutive suicide victims qualified for an axis I diagnosis at the time of suicide, 60–90% suffered from a subtype of depression, 8–10% from schizophrenia, and/or a similar proportion from a substance-related disorder (Wasserman 2000; Cavanagh *et al.* 2003). An estimated 50% of those who die through suicide have suffered from depression (Isometsä and Lönnqvist 1998). The percentage of patients that will die by suicide is estimated to be 15–19% in those ever hospitalized for depression (Guze and Robbins 1970; Goodwin and Jamison 1990). Lower figures are reported for depressed outpatient populations (Bostwick and Pankratz 2000). The rate of attempted suicide in depression, though not exactly known, is even higher (Beautrais *et al.* 1996). The strongest risk factor for suicide, moreover, is a previous suicide attempt. In the UK, 1% of a sample of patients who had attempted suicide had died by suicide within a year (Hawton and Fagg 1988). A recent study showed that attempters had a 66 times greater suicide risk than the general population, and that suicide risk remains increased even many years later (Hawton *et al.* 2003).

A major strategy in the treatment of depression, both major depression and dysthymia, is prescription of antidepressant drugs. The use of those drugs has risen substantially over the years. In The Netherlands, for instance, the increase has totalled 12% yearly over the past 4 years. Of course, antidepressants are also used in other conditions, but depression still remains the main reason for their prescription.

A paper of similar tenor appeared in the *World Journal of Biological Psychiatry*.

Since depression and suicide are postulated to be causally related, and antidepressants are considered to be an effective treatment in depression, one may rightly expect suicide rates to have gone down in proportion to prescription increases. However, this has not happened. Suicide rates differ considerably from country to country and from region to region (Diekstra 1995). Allowing for that, in most countries the rates of completed suicide seem to be quite stable (Table 14.1). In The Netherlands, for instance, the number has been approximately 1500 per year for many years. Worldwide, for men the trend is slightly upward, for women the rates have remained fairly steady (Fig. 14.1). In some countries the rise in suicide has been particularly pronounced in males between 15 and 24 years of age (Lester and Yang 1998). In Iceland the sharp increase in the sales of antidepressants since the early nineties (introduction of the SSRIs) was not accompanied by a drop in suicide rates (Helgason *et al.* 2004). Overall rates of suicide attempts are not known, but in certain delineated areas they have tended to rise rather than decrease (Hawton *et al.* 1997).

Can the latter observation be generalized? An international study comparing rates of suicide attempt in 16 different European regions showed that the figures varied from year to year and from region to region (Kerkhof 2000). In some regions the frequency increased slightly between 1989 and 1992, in others a likewise small reduction was observed. However, a robust and overall decline in the rate of attempted suicide could not be demonstrated.

Furthermore, and rather alarmingly, Khan *et al.* (2000) reported that rates of suicide and attempted suicide did not significantly differ in depressed

Table 14.1 Suicide rates per 100 000 inhabitants in selected countries (source: World Health Organization 1996)

	1980–1984	1985–1989	1995
France	20.6	20.8	20.4
Spain	5.5	7.1	8.1
Italy	7.3	7.3	7.9
Germany	20.8	16.5	15.8
Sweden	18.8	17.5	15.3
Poland	13.0	13.4	14.3
Portugal	8.7	8.7	8.2
England and Wales	8.7	7.9	6.9
Australia	11.6	12.8	12.8
USA	12.2	12.4	12.0

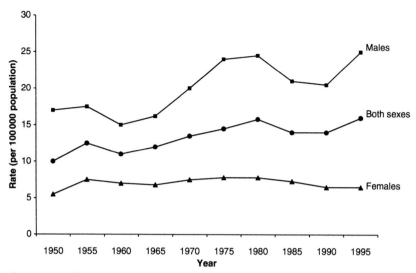

Fig. 14.1 Worldwide suicide rates by gender, 1950–1995 (data from World Health Organization 1999; De Leo and Evans 2002).

patients treated with either placebo or an antidepressant. They analysed short-term studies with seven new antidepressant drugs (i.e. fluoxetine, sertraline, paroxetine, venlafaxine, nefazadone, mirtazapine, and bupropion) using the USA Food and Drug Administration database. The study encompassed 19 639 patients. Annual rates of suicide and attempted suicide were 0.4% and 2.7% with placebo, 0.7% and 3.4% with active competitors (i.e. imipramine, amitriptyline, and trazadone) and 0.8% and 2.8% with the investigational drugs. Analysis of results of studies carried out with venlafaxine and citalopram, in which 23 201 patients had participated, showed comparable findings (Khan *et al.* 2001).

In analyses of 77 studies with antidepressants, carried out in The Netherlands between 1983 and 1997, encompassing 12 246 depressed patients, similar conclusions were reached: suicide attempt rates did not differ significantly between placebo and experimental groups. These studies were part of a registration dossier of the Medicines Evaluation Board, which is the regulatory authority in The Netherlands (Storosum *et al.* 2001).

Or did antidepressants reduce suicide rates after all?

Controlled prospective studies into the impact of antidepressants on suicide risk are scarce, but some have reported positive effects (Beasly *et al.* 1991; Leon *et al.* 1999; Roy 2001). Some data suggest that selective serotonin reuptake inhibitors (SSRIs) are superior in this respect to 'broad-spectrum antidepressants' (Montgomery *et al.* 1995; Kasper *et al.* 1996). However, this difference disappeared after 6 weeks of treatment (Mann and Kapur 1991), and other studies failed to find a specific anti-suicidal effect of SSRIs (Malone and Moran, 2001).

The relevant positive studies are unconvincing. They do not allow conclusions about possible beneficial effects of antidepressants on suicide rates. This is for several reasons. The studies have generally been short-term and with a limited number of patients. To demonstrate statistically that antidepressants produce an anti-suicidal effect, Isacsson *et al.* (1996) calculated that one needs at least 20 000 depressed patients randomly treated with either antidepressants or placebo. The studies reporting positive effects, however, were relatively small and not placebo-controlled. Nor did they control for help-seeking behaviour or for concomitant psychotherapeutic treatment. Hence it is conceivable that the positive results in the antidepressant groups, relative to the control patient groups, is due to a greater propensity to seek professional help in times of mounting stress, or to the impact of psychotherapeutic interventions.

Finally, one has to keep in mind that serious suicidality is usually an exclusion criterion in placebo-controlled therapeutic studies with antidepressants. This makes it hard to draw conclusions on the impact they might exert on suicidality.

Some larger-scale epidemiological studies also conclude that antidepressants have reduced suicide rates. Based on data for the entire population of Sweden, Isacsson and colleagues (1996) concluded that the prescription of antidepressants had reduced the risk of completed suicide 1.8 times, relative to depressed patients not using antidepressants. However, the study contained no placebo-treated group. It is unclear, moreover, whether non-pharmacological, particularly psychological interventions, had been received by the patients, what the nature of these treatments was, and whether the groups differed in this respect. Hence the conclusions drawn by Isacsson *et al.* (1997) seem to me premature. They consider that their conclusion is strengthened by the observation that the suicide rate has decreased in parallel to the increase in prescription rate of antidepressants since the 1970s. However, in past decades both doctors and patients became increasingly more aware of what depression is and how to treat it. This has led to earlier diagnosis and more intensive treatment. In this period, moreover, new and effective psychological intervention techniques have been developed. They are employed with or without antidepressants. Therefore it is not justified to attribute the observed reduction in suicide rates simply to antidepressants.

The well-known Gotland study showed that after intensive postgraduate training of GPs on recognition and treatment of depression, suicide mortality showed a marked reduction (Rutz *et al.* 1989; Pihlgren 1995). In the same period the prescription of antidepressants increased. The two phenomena were assumed to be causally related. However, this conclusion is also premature. One may presume that, due to professional education, the doctor–patient relationship was strengthened, attention for, and time spent with, patients increased, and more attention was paid to attitude and to development of a supportive and connecting demeanour. Since these effects were not accounted for, these results, too, are not conclusive.

Four years after the educational programme ended, moreover, suicide rates had again returned to baseline values, whereas the prescription of antidepressants did not, but had stabilized (Rihmer *et al.* 1995). This indicates, it seems to me, that the initial decrease in suicide rate cannot be simply attributed to the increased prescription of antidepressants.

Studies from Hungary have also reported suicide rates dropping hand in hand with increasing prescription of antidepressants (Rihmer *et al.* 1993; Rhimer 2001). In these studies, too, the possible impact of non-pharmacological factors—increasing interest in depression, leading to increased interest in the depressed—was not evaluated.

Hall and colleagues (2003) reported that in Australia between 1991 and 2000 the incidence of completed suicide in older men decreased (but increased in younger adults—this was the reason why the overall national rates of suicide did not fall significantly in that period). At the same time the use of antidepressants increased sharply (probably due to the introduction of the selective serotonin reuptake inhibitors, widely used by GPs). Increased prescribing of antidepressants and reduced suicide rate were positively correlated. The authors assumed a causal relationship. However, this conjecture is premature. In Australia, suicide rates in people over the age of 40 have gradually diminished since 1961–1965. This was the case for each 5-year group from age 40 and over (Draper 2003). In the USA, a decline in the suicide rate started in the 1940s, well before the introduction of antidepressants (Verberne 2003). The reasons for the decline are not known. Improvement of living standards of older people, increased social security, and better psychosocial care for the distressed and depressed, might all have played a role.

Between 1990 and 1997 the suicide rate in England and Wales decreased (McClure 2000). However, there are indications that this change is related to improvement in the national economy and resulting reduction in socio-economic deprivation, a known risk factor for suicide (Hawton *et al.* 2001).

Olfson *et al.* (2003) recently reported that in the USA, between 1990 and 2000, the suicide rate among adolescents decreased, while the use of antidepressants in that period had increased. The negative correlation, however, applied only to non-tricyclic antidepressants, to older and male adolescents, and to adolescents residing in low-income regions. Factors such as psychotherapeutic interventions and substance abuse were not controlled for, and diagnostic data indicating why the antidepressants had been prescribed were not available. The conclusion that the drop in suicide rate and the increased use of antidepressants hang together would thus be premature.

Finally, it should be emphasized that none of the large-scale studies referred to was placebo controlled. Depression is highly placebo responsive. Placebo response can reach levels of up to 30–35%. Even if antidepressants were the main cause of declining suicide rates, it remains to be clarified to what extent the drug acted as a placebo or as a true pharmacological agent.

The data regarding lithium are more encouraging. Administered as a mood stabilizer in bipolar and recurrent unipolar depression, it has been found to reduce suicide risk substantially, relative to depressed patients not treated with lithium (Tondo *et al.* 1997). This has not been demonstrated with other mood stabilizers. Some data suggest that lithium can exert anti-suicidal effects even if it fails to effect mood stabilization (Müller-Oerlinghausen *et al.* 1992). The observation that suicidality can be pharmacologically influenced independently from mood regulation/normalization will be discussed below.

One has to keep in mind, however, that lithium clinics/programmes generally do not rely on lithium alone, but in addition offer psycho-educational and other group-oriented programmes. Most of the long-term lithium studies have not controlled for this. Definitive conclusions about the anti-suicidal potency of lithium have to await prospective, double-blind, placebo-controlled studies, in which the groups are treated in similar fashion, pharmacologically *and* psychologically.

Patients with personality disorders, in particular those categorized as having borderline disorder, constitute another patient group with an increased suicide risk for whom antidepressants are a therapeutic option. A few placebo-controlled studies have been published on the effect of antidepressants on suicidality and aggression regulation in this group of patients. They concern particularly the SSRIs. According to Coccaro and Kavoussi (1997), outward directed aggression responds favourably. Verkes *et al.* (1998) studied the effect of paroxetine versus placebo in 91 suicidal, non-depressed patients with personality disorders, mainly of the borderline type. The study extended over a period of 1 year. In the group as a whole, paroxetine had no effect on the rate of suicide attempts. In the subgroup of patients who had attempted suicide five times or more in the previous years, paroxetine did reduce the number of suicide attempts significantly. These data await confirmation and further exploration.

Taking all these data together, I arrive at the conclusion that one can advance only few and rather weak arguments against the thesis that suicide remained stubbornly present in the era of antidepressants. Rihmer (2001) disagrees. He stated that the antidepressant era has shown a reduction in suicide rates and said: 'The sometimes presented statement ("increasing use of antidepressants did not reduce suicide rates") is counterproductive, rather than a counterargument'. Overall, however, the available facts do not support this notion. Facts are just facts. They cannot (and should not) be qualified as productive or counter-productive. Points of view can be. Facts can be introduced or produced to support or repudiate a notion. If such a notion pertains to a desirable situation (e.g. antidepressants have reduced suicide rates) but the facts are non-support-ive, the reasons why should be traced and ways explored to abolish them.

In the following sections I carry out the first exercise. Thus I address the question of what might be the reasons why the suicide problem has proved so obstinate. Some possible explanations are then discussed.

Coincidence

One possible explanation is that depression and suicidality are unrelated states, and that their co-occurrence is a matter of coincidence; and hence it is not to be expected that suicide rates will be affected by treatment of depression.

This is not a likely explanation, for two reasons First, because if this were the case, one would expect suicidality to occur as frequently in the depressed as in the remitted state, and this is not so. Suicide risk is, to a high degree, state-dependent and at its greatest by far during a depressive episode (Roy 2001). Secondly, experiential data are contradictory. Depressed patients themselves generally experience a strong connection between feelings of hopelessness and suicidal tendencies.

Experiential data have substantial evidential power in psychiatry. The ob-servation that suicide risk correlates stronger with feelings of hopelessness, as measured with the Beck Hopelessness scale, than with depression as such is a case in point. Hopelessness, moreover, may occur independently of depres-sion, or to a degree discrepant with depression severity (Mann et al. 1999).

As an aside, experiential (i.e. purely subjective data) are not highly regarded in research circles these days, the main preoccupation being with assessment of behavioural data that can be established with a fair degree of objectivity. Subjective data are conceived as 'soft', because it is alleged that they are not measurable reliably and reproducibly. I believe that this view is prejudiced (Van Praag 1992*a*). Methods are available to measure and to follow up, prospectively and in a systematic and careful way, individual mood states and related cognitions. I am alluding to the experience sampling method. Although, regrettably, so far only sparingly used, the results obtained underscore the diagnostic importance of subjective psychopathology (Van Eck *et al.* 1998; Myin-Germeys *et al.* 2001). There is no convincing justification for neglecting substantial domains of psychopathology because they are subjective (van Praag 1992*a*, 1997).

Continuity of treatment

Continuity of treatment is often not well maintained in patients with recurrent unipolar depression, even if their history includes suicide attempts (Isacsson *et al.* 1997; Lecrubier 1998; Oquendo *et al.* 1999, 2002; Druss *et al.* 2000). A majority of individuals who die by suicide do so without having made contact with primary-care providers (Luoma *et al.* 2002), yet in a Finnish study only 17% of a group of patients with major depression who presented to a hospital following a suicide attempt had been prescribed antidepressant medication 1 month later (Suominen *et al.* 1998). In a study from England, the corresponding figures were more favourable, 56% of patients having been prescribed antidepressant medication in adequate dosages 1 month after the attempt (Haw *et al.* 2002). For many patients with recurrent depression it appears to be difficult to continue taking medication over long periods of time, particularly if their symptoms have vanished.

It is thus conceivable that the small effect antidepressants may have had on suicide rates is due to discontinuity of treatment. This may be the result of either misconceptions on the part of the doctor, or lack of perseverance on the part of the patient. This explanation shifts responsibility from the remedy to the consumer and/or prescriber. If correct, educational measures for both parties should receive top priority.

However, it is improbable that this conjecture holds good for the data of Khan *et al.* (2000, 2001) and Storosum *et al.* (2001) referred to earlier, since these data were derived from controlled trials in which medication intake was generally under strict control.

Efficacy of antidepressants

Antidepressants may be less effective than is generally accepted. If so, one cannot expect antidepressant treatment to have a major impact on suicidality being a frequent complication of the depressed state. This is not an unreal proposition. The response to antidepressants is quite often partial, in that residual symptoms persist (see below). Moreover, re-emergence or worsening of depressive symptoms during maintenance treatment with antidepressants is a common occurrence. It was found to occur in 9–57% of patients in published studies (Byrne and Rothschild 1998). Many studies over the past 20 years have shown generally modest effect sizes when comparing antidepressant drugs with placebo. A case in point is the study of Khan *et al.* (2000) cited above, which reported symptom reduction of 40.7% of patients treated with investigational drugs, 41.7% in those on active comparators, and 30.9 % in those assigned to receive placebo. The data of Storosum *et al.* (2001) are comparable. They analysed 32 placebo-controlled studies ($N = 4314$) and found 46% responders in the antidepressant group versus 31% in the placebo group. In a meta-analysis of 33 antidepressant trials, Bollini and colleagues (1999) found an average improvement of 53% versus 35% in the placebo arms. The initial findings with antidepressants in the 1960s and 1970s were much more encouraging, reporting at least 30–35% placebo/drug differences (Van Praag 1978). It now looks as if those data were misleading. However, there may be other explanations other than that they were wrong.

Blurring of syndrome

Before the introduction of DSM III and ICD 8, diagnosis in psychiatry was not standardized but it was detailed, at least in the USA and Western Europe. Two philosophies were dominant at the time: phenomenology and psychoanalysis. The first required precise accounting of symptomatological and experiential data; the second a detailed analysis of developmental factors possibly, or supposedly, involved in the aetiology of the disorder.

With the introduction of specific diagnostic systems, syndromal differentiation became a thing of the past. Symptomatologically, a person qualifies for a particular diagnosis if x out of a series of y symptoms are demonstrable, irrespective of which ones. One diagnostic category, for example major depression or dysthymia, therefore covers a variety of syndromes. This approach has severely compromised diagnostic acuity. It is currently impossible to establish whether a particular antidepressant is preferentially effective in a particular depressive syndrome. There are, however, strong indications that such differences exist. Tricyclic antidepressants, for instance, were shown to be more helpful in endogenous than in non-endogenous depression (van Praag 1962; Heiligenstein *et al.* 1994; Roth 2001).

Monoamine oxidase inhibitors are considered by some investigators (Quitkin *et al.* 1989)—though not all (Pande *et al.* 1996)—to be particularly efficacious in atypical depression. Another example of the therapeutic importance of precise phenomenological characterization of mood disorders is anxiety/aggression-driven depression, a construct that we introduced some years ago (Van Praag 1992b, 1994, 1996, 1998) but which remains hypothetical. Important features of this subtype of depression are:

- the depression is heralded by anxiety and increased outward by directed aggression, manifesting itself in short-temperedness, irritability, and anger outbursts with little provocation; while
- mood lowering is a late-occurring phenomenon, if it appears at all. Some episodes remain restricted to signs of increased anxiety and aggression and do not develop into a full-blown depression. It was hypothesized that anxiety/aggression are pacemakers of the depression.

Disturbances in the 5-hydroxytryptamine (5-HT, serotonin) system accumulate in this type of depression, particularly a trait-related diminution of 5-hydroxyindoleacetic acid (5-HIAA), the major metabolite of 5-HT in cerebrospinal fluid (CSF). The level of CSF 5-HIAA is a crude indicator of 5-HT metabolism in certain parts of the central nervous system.

Another trait-related phenomenon that may occur in depression is decreased binding capacity of the 5-HT_{1A} receptor, both pre- and postsynaptically. It is not yet known whether this phenomenon occurs preferentially in anxiety/aggression-driven depression.

Decreased 5-HT activity, particularly in the 5-HT_{1A} receptor-mediated systems, is associated with an increase in anxiety and aggression (reviewed by Van Praag et al. 2004) .

Based on these data, selective, full, postsynaptic 5-HT_{1A} receptor agonists, in combination with cortisol or corticotrophin-releasing hormone (CRH) antagonists, preferably administered in the pre-depression stage, are hypothesized to be the treatment of choice in this subtype of depression. Both types of drugs are presently in development, which will soon make it possible to put these suppositions to the test.

If, in the study of antidepressants, patients presumably responsive to a particular antidepressant and those probably less- or non-responsive are lumped together, the effect size of the drug will drop and approach the placebo response. This particularly holds for drugs with high biological specificity.

Boundary problems

In recent years more and more individuals with depressive symptoms have been marked as candidates for treatment with antidepressants. The borderline between distress and depression, between worrying and a true mood disorder, is, however, ill-defined (Van Praag 2000). Distressed people and worriers cannot be expected to respond to antidepressant drugs. If an experimental group is made up of depressed and distressed individuals, the response rate obtained with an antidepressant will be low and presumably lower than if only people with 'case-depression' had participated. As an analogy, if one aspired to explore the efficacy of antibiotics in pneumonia one would guard against inclusion of patients with a common cold in the experimental group as this would result in underestimation of their therapeutic potential.

Neglect of psychogenesis and its consequences

In the DSM classification the concept of psychogenesis has all but disappeared. Psychiatric diagnoses have become 'flat'. Psychological development, which was a prime focus of attention until the 1970s, was marginalized. It is true that personality deviations and psycho-traumatic events are registered in the classification, but the question of their possible relationship with axis I diagnoses is no longer addressed. I still consider this question fundamental to psychiatric diagnosis. More often than not the answer will be merely a hypothesis, but it is an essential one.

The life of an individual remains largely a closed book if diagnosis is dissociated from the person's past. The past—the wealth of bygone experiences and recollections one carries along—determines to a considerable degree the way in which the present is lived and experienced. The 'apparatus' that perceives and registers this information and accords it meaning is one's personality. Of course, personality exists by the grace of a functioning brain, but it cannot be identified with the brain. It is an entity in its own right, to be studied in its own right.

Neglect of the past as a possible aetiological factor in today's psychopathology, or analysis of the past without counting in personality structure, amounts to diagnostic malpractice. Official diagnostic guidelines in psychiatry have authorized these simplifications. Indeed, axis II pathology *is* recorded (categorically; not, unfortunately, dimensionally), but the diagnostician is not requested to indicate, or hypothesize, whether he or she deems it likely that axis II pathology has contributed to axis I pathology. In the heyday of psychoanalysis, this was considered to be a key diagnostic question. While psychoanalysis has lost much ground, this question has not. In terms of treatment planning it is still crucial. The objection that the DSM system is just a taxonomy and not a diagnostic system does not cut ice. This taxonomy rules psychiatric diagnostic practice. Concepts not mentioned in the DSM tend to be regarded as irrelevant.

Lack of interest in psychological make-up and psychological development, and their possible contributions to current psychopathology, led many psychiatrists to lose interest in psychotherapy, particularly in psychodynamic psychotherapy (i.e. in psychotherapeutic interventions geared towards the dismantling of past events and situations suspected of having undermined psychic endurance). A recent review by Hirschfeld *et al.* (2002) poignantly illuminates this state of affairs. They discuss treatment of depressed patients who have not responded, or only partially responded, to standard antidepressants. Their conclusion was to institute a treatment targeting both the 5-HT system and the noradrenergic system. Psychological interventions were not even mentioned. Granted, research in the field of dynamic psychotherapy lagged behind due to the resistance of practitioners. However, this fact calls for active research in insight-providing interventions, not for cold-shouldering them.

The excessive confidence in the therapeutic power of psychological methods in treating depression, which prevailed in the 1960s and 1970s, has been offset by a heavy reliance on antidepressant drugs as monotherapy. Mood disorders frequently occur in subjects with personality disorders or deviant personality traits (Van Praag *et al.* 2004). Personality frailties may play an important role in the aetiology of mood disorders. Personality imperfections do not generally respond to antidepressants but require psychological interventions. It is known, moreover, that personality disorders diminish the efficacy of antidepressants in depression (O'Leary and Costello 2001). Exclusive reliance on antidepressants alone might have reduced their therapeutic return.

Worrying rather than depression is the main precursor of suicide

As mentioned in earlier, psychiatry has so far failed to clearly define in detail the border between distress and depression, between worrying and a true mood disorder. We do not even know what the relevant criteria are: number of symptoms, kind of symptoms, their severity or duration, social and professional incapacity, or degree of subjective suffering.

Many people worry—worry about real issues. They feel low, sleep badly, have little appetite, decreased libido, and lack lust for life. This may occur once in a while, quite often, or over longer stretches of time. Only a minority of those suffer from 'case-depression'. Sub-syndromal depression would be a misnomer. Someone complaining about headache, but with no objective neurological signs, does not suffer from a subsyndromal brain tumour. Medical terms should not be used to give a name to problems of living.

Worriers who suffer from a true depression have a fair chance to improve on antidepressants, worriers without depression probably not. I use the term 'probably', because it is not known what the response to antidepressants is in this group. Neither do we know what the suicidal risk is in these individuals.

If worriers, like depressives, are at increased risk of suicide, one cannot expect antidepressants to reduce overall suicide rates significantly in this group.

Residual symptoms

In a substantial proportion of depressed patients, treatment with antidepressants does not result in full recovery, and residual symptoms persist (Faravelli et al. 1986; Agosti et al. 1993; Fava 1999; Sonino and Fava 2002). These can be true remnants of the depressive syndrome or manifestations of disappointment that treatment has been less successful than was hoped for. In this way, suicidal tendencies might be maintained or triggered. I am not aware of any data to substantiate or refute this possibility. The association between residual symptoms and suicidality has not been studied systematically .

Personality traits

Depression and personality deviations often occur together (Hirschfeld et al. 1983; Clayton et al. 1994; Haw et al. 2001; Overholser et al. 2002). Stress, produced by traumatic events or situations together with inadequate coping skills, is probably an important aetiological factor in many cases of depression (Van Praag et al. 2004). Thus suicidality might be not so much a feature of depression as such, but rather a consequence of pre-existing personality traits. Personality pathology shows generally little or no response to antidepressants, and hence, in this case, one cannot expect antidepressants to be of much benefit for suicidality.

Suicidal behaviour does indeed occur in non-depressed, personality-disordered individuals. This speaks in favour of this hypothesis. On the other hand, if personality pathology is the major cause of suicidality in depression, one would expect suicidal behaviour to occur as frequently in depressive episodes as in states of remission, but this is not what actually happens. This matter is pursued further in the next section.

Suicide proneness, a possible trait factor in its own right

Several sets of clinical data suggest that suicide proneness—that is, preoccupation with death, and considering death as a genuine option to resolve problems—might be a trait-factor, intensifying in certain psychiatric conditions such as depression, but not disappearing in remission (Mann et al. 1999).

Lithium, for instance, although a weak antidepressant, appears to diminish suicide risk. This is even true in those in whom the episode-preventive effect of lithium is unsatisfactory (Müller-Oerlinghausen et al. 1992; Müller-Oerlinghausen and Berghöfer 1999). The notion of suicidality as a possible trait factor is further supported by recent studies of late-life depression. Treatment with antidepressants significantly reduced overall depression and suicidal ideas. The antidepressant response, however, was smaller in patients in the high suicide risk group (suicidal ideation or recent suicide attempt) and moderate risk group (thoughts about death) than in the low-risk group (no such symptoms) (Szanto *et al.* 2003). Moreover, half of the patients with suicidal ideation at the beginning still reported thoughts of death in the 12th week of treatment (Szanto *et al.* 2003). Some elderly persons seem to remain hopeless even when their depression is resolved (Szanto *et al.* 1998).

Some genetic data point in the same direction. Genes do contribute to suicide risk (Roy *et al.* 1997) and several 5-hydroxytryptamine (5-HT)-related genes seem to be involved, most notably those expressing tryptophan hydroxylase (TPH), the 5-HT transporter (5-HTT) protein, and monoamineoxidase A (Preisig *et al.* 2000; Abbar *et al.* 2001; Courtet *et al.* 2001). Some evidence suggests that the 'suicide-vulnerability genes' operate independently from genes transmitting psychiatric disorders in which suicide risk is increased, such as depression.

Joiner and colleagues (2003), for instance, demonstrated that the short allele variant of the 5-HTT gene confers increased risk for depression and independently increased risk for suicidality. With regard to the same 5-HTT polymorphism, furthermore, no difference was found between non-suicide attempters with and without a history of major depression. Hence major depression cannot account for the difference observed between suicide attempters and controls (Courtet *et al.* 2001). The fact that the highest odds ratios were obtained for (violent) suicide attempters with a history of major depression, compared to individuals with a history of major depression who had never attempted suicide, suggests that this polymorphism is most common in subjects with a history of major depression and (violent) suicide attempt (Courtet *et al.* 2001). Similar conclusions were drawn from studies with a TPH polymorphism found to be associated with suicide (Abbar *et al.* 2001), and possibly also with outwardly directed aggression (Manuck *et al.* 1999).

If, indeed, suicidality and depression, though interrelated, are to a certain extent independent variables, each requiring a separate therapeutic approach, this could explain why successful treatment of depression is not necessarily accompanied by a significant and sustained drop in suicidality.

Social factors

Suicide rates may have dropped due to antidepressants, but this effect could have been counterbalanced by the impact of social factors. This is a conceivable explanation. The socio-economic environment and prevalence of depression and suicidality are clearly associated (Hawton and Fagg 1988; Gunnell *et al.* 1999). Among the unemployed, the risk of suicide is increased and an inverse relationship has been established between social class and suicide risk (Platt and Hawton 2000). Social circumstances, too, influence suicide risk. In a small geographic area in Bristol, for instance, Gunnell *et al.* (2000) found that over a period of 30 years social deprivation had risen and so had suicidal behaviour, the association reaching a statistically significant level. The social deprivation index was based on the sum of Z-scores of four variables: unemployment, car ownership, household overcrowding, and house ownership. Hence it is conceivable that social factors have overridden the beneficial effects of antidepressants on suicide rates. Conversely, improvement in the national economy might have contributed to the decrease in suicides in England and Wales between 1960 and 1997 (McClure 2000).

It is, however, implausible that social deprivation has occurred on such a large scale in the developed world that it has overshadowed the beneficial effects of antidepressants, hence explaining why these drugs have had such meagre effects on suicidal behaviour.

Have antidepressants increased suicide rates?

Antidepressants might have boosted suicidal impulses, cancelling out possible positive effects on depression *per se*. First, they might energize an anergic patient before mood elevation has commenced, and thus advance, temporarily, the drive to self-harm or destruction. This happens sometimes in the early phases of electroconvulsive treatment. The same could happen with antidepressants, particularly if they exert a pronounced stimulating effect on motor behaviour and level of initiative. Some evidence supports this notion (Damluji and Ferguson 1988; Montgomery 1997).

Another possibility is that antidepressants enhance the suicidal drive directly. A decade ago, a stir was caused by a publication claiming that fluoxetine, a selective serotonin re-uptake inhibitor (SSRI), might increase suicidality in depression (Teicher *et al.* 1990). However, meta-analysis of a large number of studies could not confirm those conclusions (for reviews see Beasly *et al.* 1991; Fava and Rosenbaum 1991; Healy 1994; Walsh and Dinan 2001). Yet, this notion recently re-emerged, when Healy (2000) reported that suicidal tendencies had occurred acutely in a few normal subjects during treatment with the SSRI antidepressant sertraline.

Theoretically, an influence of SSRI antidepressants on the regulation of (auto) aggression is certainly conceivable. Serotonin (5-hydroxytryptamine,

5-HT) systems are associated with the regulation of (auto)aggression in both animals and humans. The $5\text{-}HT_{1A}$ and $5\text{-}HT_{1D}$ receptor-mediated systems are most notably involved. Increased activity in those neuronal systems will inhibit, and decreased activity will enhance, (certain forms of) aggression (Olivier and Mos 1992). These 5-HT receptors are located both pre-and postsynaptically. Activation of the postsynaptic receptor leads to activation of the system, and activation of the pre-synaptic counterpart leads to reduced activity.

The immediate effect of an SSRI is to increase availability of 5-HT in the synapse and stimulation of both pre- and postsynaptic $5\text{-}HT_{1A}$ and $5\text{-}HT_{1D}$ receptors. The net-effect on 5-HT-ergic activity will thus be small because pre- and postsynaptic effects will generally cancel each other out. After some time (weeks) SSRIs will desensitize the presynaptic $5\text{-}HT_{1A}$ receptor (it is not known whether this is also the case with the $5\text{-}HT_{1D}$ receptor). This does not happen with the postsynaptic counterpart (Blier and De Montigny 1994). In this way the $5\text{-}HT_{1A}$ system is activated and this effect is considered to be crucial for antidepressant activity. As already said, this is also associated with reduced aggressivity.

If, for whatever reason, during a certain phase, activation of the presynaptic $5\text{-}HT_{1A}$ (and/or the $5\text{-}HT_{1D}$) receptor should outstrip activation of the post-synaptically located $5\text{-}HT_{1A}$ receptor, causing reduction of neuronal activity in the $5\text{-}HT_{1A}$ system, theoretically, depressive behaviour might be intensified and (auto) aggressive impulses accentuated, with suicidality as a possible result. However, for the time being, this possibility is speculative. It has not been demonstrated and indeed will be hard to study in humans.

Conclusions

Over the past decades the rate of completed suicide has remained quite stable, and that of suicide attempts seems to have even increased. These are puzzling observations, since depression is the major precursor of suicide and antide-pressants have been increasingly used in the treatment of depression. These observations have not attracted sufficient attention, possibly because they do not accord with consensus opinions about depression treatment in psychiatry today. A number of possible explanations have been discussed in this chapter. They warrant systematic investigation. Knowledge arising from such investi-gations might help to both improve treatment of depression itself and reduce suicidal behaviour in this and related conditions.

References

Abbar, M., Courtet, P., Bellivier, F., Leboyer, M., Boulenger, J.P., Castelhau, D., *et al.* (2001). Suicide attempts and the tryptophan hydroxylase gene. *Molecular Psychiatry*, 6, 268–73.

Agosti, V., Steward, J.W., Quitkin, F.M., and Ocepek-Welikson, K. (1993). How symptomatic do depressed patients remain after benefiting from medication treatment? *Comprehensive Psychiatry*, 34, 182–6.

Beasly, C.M., Dornseif, B.E., Bosomworth, J.C., Sayler, M.E., and Rampey, A.H. (1991). Fluoxetine and suicide: a meta-analysis of controlled trials of treatment for depression. *British Medical Journal*, 303, 685–92.

Beautrais, A., Joyce, P., Mulder, R., Furgusson, D.M., Denvoll, B.J., and Nightingale, S.K. (1996). Prevalence and comorbidity of mental disorders in persons making serious suicide attempts: a case control study. *American Journal of Psychiatry*, 153, 1009–14.

Blier, P. and De Montigny, C. (1994). Current advances and trends in the treatment of depression. *Trends in Pharmalogical Sciences*, 15, 220–6.

Bollini, P., Pampallona, S., Tibaldi, G., Kupelnick, B., and Munizza, C. (1999). Effectiveness of antidepressants. Meta-analysis of dose–effect relationships in randomised clinical trials. *British Journal of Psychiatry*, 174, 297–303.

Bostwick, J.M. and Pankratz, V.S. (2000). Affective disorders and suicide risk: a reexamination. *American Journal of Psychiatry*, 157, 1925–32.

Byrne, S.E. and Rothschild, A.J. (1998). Loss of antidepressant efficacy during maintenance therapy. *Journal of Clinical Psychiatry*, 59, 279–88.

Cavanagh, J.T.O., Carson, A.J., Sharpe, M., and Lawrie, S.M. (2003). Psychological autopsy studies of suicide: a systematic review. *Psychological Medicine*, 33, 395–405.

Clayton, P.J., Trust, C., and Angst, J. (1994). Premorbid personality traits of men who develop unipolar or bipolar disorders. *European Archives of Psychiatry and Clinical Neuroscience*, 243, 340–6.

Coccaro, E.F. and Kavoussi, R.Y. (1997). Fluoxetine and impulsive agressive behavior in personality – disordered subjects. *Archives of General Psychiatry*, 54, 1081–8.

Courtet, P., Baud, P., Abbar, M., Boulenger, J.P., Castelnau, D., Mouthon, D., *et al.* (2001). Association between violent suicidal behavior and the low activity allele of the serotonin transporter gene. *Molecular Psychiatry*, 6, 338–41.

Damluji, N.F. and Ferguson, J.M. (1988). Paradoxical worsening of depressive symptomatology caused by antidepressants. *Journal of Clinical Psychopharmacology*, 8, 347–9.

De Leo, D. and Evans, R. (2002). *Suicide in Queensland 1996–1998: mortality rates and related data*. Australian Institute of Suicide Research and Prevention (AISRAP), Griffith University.

Diekstra, R.F.W. (1995). The epidemiology of suicide and parasuicide. In *Preventive strategies on suicide*, (ed. W. Gulbinat, I. Kienhorst, D. DeLeo). EYJ Brill, Leiden.

Draper, B.M. (2003). Associations attribute possible causality inappropriately [letter]. *British Medical Journal*, 327, 288.

Druss, B.G., Hoff, R.A., and Rosenheck, R.A. (2000). Underuse of antidepressants in major depression: prevalence and correlates in a national sample of young adults. *Journal of Clinical Psychiatry*, 61, 234–7.

Faravelli, C., Ambonetti, A., Pallanti, S., and Pazzagli, A. (1986). Depressive relapse and incomplete recovery from index episode. *American Journal of Psychiatry*, 143, 888–91.

Fava, G.A. (1999). Subclinical symptoms in mood disorders: pathophysiological and therapeutic implications. *Psychological Medicine*, 29, 47–61.

Fava, M. and Rosenbaum, J.F. (1991). Suicidality and fluoxetine: is there a relationship? *Journal of Clinical Psychiatry*, 52, 108–11.

Goodwin, F.K. and Jamison, K.R. (1990). *Manic-depressive illness*. Oxford University Press, New York.

Gunnell, D., Lopatatzidis, A., Dorling, D., Wehner, H., Southall, H., and Frankel, S. (1999). Suicide, unemployment and gender – an analysis of trends in England and Wales 1921–1995. *British Journal of Psychiatry*, 175, 263–70.

Gunnell, D., Shepherd, M., and Evans, M. (2000). Are recent increases in deliberate self-harm associated with changes in socio-economic conditions? An ecological analysis of patterns of deliberate self-harm in Bristol 1972–3 and 1995–6. *Psychological Medicine*, 30, 1197–203.

Guze, S.B. and Robins, E. (1970). Suicide and primary affective disorders. *British Journal of Psychiatry*, 117, 437–8.

Hall, W.D., Mant, A., Mitchell, P.B., Rendle, V.A., Hickie, I.B., and McManus, P. (2003). Association between antidepressant prescribing and suicide in Australia, 1991–2000: trend analysis. *British Medical Journal*, 326, 1008–11.

Haw, C., Hawton, K., Houston, K., and Townsend, E. (2001). Psychiatric and personality disorders in deliberate self-harm patients. *British Journal of Psychiatry*, 178, 48–54.

Haw, C., Houston, K., Townsend, E., and Hawton, K. (2002). Deliberate self harm patients with depressive disorders: treatment and outcome. *Journal of Affective Disorders*, 70, 57–65.

Hawton, K. and Fagg, J. (1988). Suicide, and other causes of death following attempted suicide. *British Journal of Psyhiatry*, 152, 359–66.

Hawton, K., Fagg, J., Simkin, S., and Bale, E. (1997). Trends in deliberate self-harm in Oxford, 1985–1995. Implications for clinical services and the prevention of suicide. *British Journal of Psychiatry*, 171, 556–60.

Hawton, K., Harriss, L., Hodder, K., Simkin, S., and Gunnell, D. (2001). The influence of the economic and social environment on deliberate self-harm and suicide: an ecological and person-based study. *Psychological Medicine*, 31, 827–36.

Hawton, K., Zahl, D., and Weatherall, R. (2003). Suicide following deliberate self-harm: long term follow-up of patients who presented to a general hospital. *British Journal of Psychiatry*, 182, 537–42.

Healy, D. (1994). The fluoxetine and suicide controversy. *CNS Drugs*, 1, 223–31.

Healy, D. (2000). Antidepressant induced suicidality. *Primary Care Psychiatry*, 6, 23–8.

Heiligenstein, J.H., Tollefson, G.D., and Faries, D.E. (1994). Response patterns of depressed outpatients with and without melancholia: a double-blind, placebo-controlled trial of fluoxetine versus placebo. *Journal of Affective Disorders*, 30, 163–73.

Helgason, T., Tomasson, H., and Zoëga, T. (2004). Antidepressants and public health in Iceland. *British Journal of Psychiatry*, 184, 157–62.

Hirschfeld, R.M., Klerman, G.L., Clayton, P.J., and Keller, M.B. (1983). Personality and depression. Empirical findings. *Archives of General Psychiatry*, 40, 993–8.

Hirschfeld, R.M., Montgomery, S.A., and Aguglia, E. (2002). Partial response and non-response to antidepressant therapy: current approaches and treatment options. *Journal of Clinical Pyschiatry*, 63, 826–37.

Isacsson, J., Bergman, U., and Rich, C.L. (1996). Epidemiological data suggest antidepressants reduce suicide risk among depressives. *Journal of Affective Disorders*, 41, 1–8.

Isacsson, J., Holmgren, P., Druid, H., and Bergman, U. (1997). The utilization of antidepressants: a key issue in the prevention of suicide. *Acta Psychiatrica Scandinavica*, 96, 94–100.

Isometsä, E.T. and Lönnqvist, J.K. (1998). Suicide attempts preceding completed suicide. *British Journal of Psychiatry*, 173, 531–5.

Joiner, T.E., Johnson, F., Soderstrom, K., and Brown, J.S. (2003). Is there an association between serotonin transporter gene polymorphism and family history of depression? *Journal of Affective Disorders*, 77, 273–5.

Kasper, S., Schindler, S., and Neumeister, A. (1996). A risk of suicide in depression and its implication for psychopharmacological treatment. *International Clinical Psychopharmacology*, 11, 71–9.

Kerkhof, A.J.F.M. (2000). Attempted suicide: patterns and trends. In *The international handbook of suicide and attempted suicide*, (ed. K. Hawton and K. Van Heeringen). John Wiley, Chichester.

Khan, A., Warner, H.A., and Brown, W.A. (2000). Symptom reduction and suicide risk in patients treated with placebo in antidepressant clinical trials: an analysis of the Food and Drug Administration Database. *Archives of General Psychiatry*, 57, 311–17.

Khan, A., Khan, S.R., Leventhal, R.M., and Brown, W.A. (2001). Symptom reduction and suicide risk in patients treated with placebo in antidepressant clinical trials: a replication analysis of the Food and Drug Administration Database. *International Journal of Neuropsychopharmacology*, 4, 113–18.

Lecrubier, Y. (1998). Is depression under-recognised and undertreated? *International Clinical Psychopharmacology*, 13, 3S–6S.

Leon, A.C., Keller, M.B., Warshaw, M.G., Mueller, T.I., Solomon, D.A., Coryell, W., et al. (1999). Prospective study of fluoxetine treatment and suicidal behavior in affectively ill subjects. *American Journal of Psychiatry*, 156, 195–201.

Lester, D. and Yang, B. (1998). *Suicide and homocide in the twentieth century; changes over time*. Nova Science, Commack, New York.

Luoma, J.B., Martin, C.E., and Pearson, J.L. (2002). Contact with mental health and primary care providers before suicide: a review of the evidence. *American Journal of Psychiatry*, 159, 909–16.

Malone, K.M. and Moran, M. (2001). Psychopharmacological approaches to the suicidal process. In *Understanding suicidal behavior. The suicidal process. Approach to research, treatment and prevention*, (ed. K. Van Heeringen). John Wiley, Chichester, UK.

Mann, J.J. and Kapur, S. (1991). The emergence of suicidal ideation and behaviour during antidepressant pharmacotherapy. *Archives of General Psychiatry*, 48, 1027–33.

Mann, J.J., Waternaux, C., Haas, G.L., and Maone, K.M. (1999). Toward a clinical model of suicidal behavior in psychiatric patients. *American Journal of Psychiatry*, 156, 181–9.

Manuck, S.B., Flory, J.D., Ferell, R.E., Dent, K.M., Mann, J.J., and Muldoon, M.F. (1999). Aggression and anger-related traits associated with a polymorphism of the tryptophan hydroxylase gene. *Biological Psychiatry*, 45, 603–14.

McClure, G.M.G. (2000). Changes in suicide in England and Wales, 1960–1997. *British Journal of Psychiatry*, 176, 64–7.

Montgomery, S.A. (1997). Suicide and antidepressants. *Annals of the New York Academy of Sciences*, 836, 329–38.

Montgomery, S.A., Dunner, D.L., and Dunbar, G.C. (1995). Reduction of suicidal thoughts with paroxetine in comparison with reference antidepressants and placebo. *European Neuropsychopharmology*, 5, 5–13.

Müller-Oerlinghausen, B. and Berghöfer, A. (1999). Antidepressants and suicidal risk. *Journal of Clinical Psychiatry*, 60, 94–9.

Müller-Oerlinghausen, B., Müser-Causemann, B., and Volk, J. (1992). Suicides and parasuicides in a high-risk patient group on and off lithium long-term medication. *Journal of Affective Disorders*, 25, 261–70.

Myin-Germeys, I., Van Os, J., Schwartz, J.E., Stone, A.A., and Delespaul, Ph. A. (2001). Emotional reactivity to daily life stress in psychosis. *Archives of General Psychiatry*, 58, 1137–44.

O'Leary, D. and Costello, F. (2001). Personality and outcome in depression: an 18-month prospective follow-up study. *Journal of Affective Disorders*, 63, 67–78.

Olfson, M., Shaffer, D., Marcus, S.C., and Greenberg, T. (2003). Relationship between antidepressant medication treatment and suicide in adolescents. *Archives of General Psychiatry*, 60, 978–82.

Olivier, B. and Mos, J. (1992). Rodent models of agressive behaviour and serotonergic drugs. *Progress in Neuropsychopharmacology and Biological Psychiatry*, 16, 847–70.

Oquendo, M.A., Malone, K.M., Ellis, S.P., Sackeim, H.A., and Mann, J.J. (1999). Inadequacy of antidepressant treatment for patients with major depression who are at risk for suicidal behavior. *American Journal of Psychiatry*, 156, 190–4.

Oquendo, M.A., Kamali, M., Ellis, S.P., Grunebaum, M.F., Malone, K.M., Brodsky, B.S., *et al.* (2002). Adequacy of antidepressant treatment after discharge and the occurrence of suicidal acts in major depression: a prospective study. *American Journal of Psychiatry*, 159, 1746–51.

Overholser, J.C., Stockmeier, C., Dilley, G., and Freiheit, S. (2002). Personality disorders in suicide attempters and completers: preliminary findings. *Archives of Suicide Research*, 6, 123–33.

Pande, A.C., Birkett, M., Fechner-Bates, S., Haskett, R.F., and Greden, J.F. (1996). Fluoxetine versus phenelzine in atypical depression. *Biological Psychiatry*, 40, 1017–20.

Pihlgren, H. (1995). Depression and suicide on Gotland. An intensive study of all suicides before and after a depression-training programme for general practitioners. *Journal of Affective Disorders*, 35, 147–52.

Platt, S. and Hawton, K. (2000). Suicidal behaviour and the labour market. In *The international handbook of suicide and attempted suicide*, (ed. K. Hawton and K. Van Heeringen). John Wiley, Chichester.

Preisig, M., Bellivier, F., Fenton, B.T., Baud, P., Berney, A., Courtet, P., *et al.* (2000). Association between bipolar disorder and monoamine oxidase a gene polymorphisms: results of a multi-center study. *American Journal of Psychiatry*, 157, 948–55.

Quitkin, F.M., McGrath, P.J., Stewart, J.W., Harrison, W., Wager, S.G., Nunes, E., *et al.* (1989). Phenelzine and imipramine in mood reactive depressives. Further delineation of the syndrome of atypical depression. *Archives of General Psychiatry*, 46, 787–93.

Rihmer, Z. (2001). Can better recognition and treatment of depression reduce suicide rates? A brief review. *European Psychiatry*, 16, 406–9.

Rihmer, Z., Rutz, W., and Barsi, J. (1993). Suicide rate, prevalence of diagnosed depression and prevalence of working physicians in Hungary. *Acta Psychiatrica Scandinavica*, 88, 391–4.

Rihmer, Z., Rutz, W., and Pihlgren, H. (1995). Depression and suicide on Gotland. An intensive study of all suicides before and after a depression-training programme for general practitioners. *Journal of Affective Disorders*, 35, 147–52.

Roth, U. (2001). Unitary or binary nature of classification of depressive illness and its implications for the scope of manic depressive disorder. *Journal of Affective Disorders*, 64, 1–18.

Roy, A. (2001). Psychiatric treatment and suicide prevention. In *Suicide prevention. Resources for the millenium*, (ed. D. Lester). Brunner-Routledge, Philadelphia.

Roy, A., Rylander, G., and Sarchiapone, M. (1997). Genetic studies of suicidal behavior. *The Psychiatric Clinics of North America*, 20, 595–611.

Rutz, W., Walinder, J., Eberhard, G., Holmberg, G., von Knorring, A.L., von Knorring, L., *et al.* (1989). An educational program on depressive disorders for general practitioners on Gotland: background and evaluation. *Acta Psychiatrica Scandinavica*, 79, 19–26.

Sonino, N. and Fava, G.A. (2002). Residual symptoms in depression: an emerging therapeutic concept. *Progress in Neuro-Psychopharmacology and Biological Psychiatry*, 26, 763–70.

Storosum, J.G., Van Zwieten, B.J., Van den Brink, W., Gersons, B.P.R., and Broekmans, A.W. (2001). Suicide risk in placebo-controlled studies of major depression. *American Journal of Psychiatry*, 158, 1271–5.

Suominen, K.H., Isometsa, E.T., Hendriksson, M.M., Ostamo, A.I., and Lonnqvist, J.K. (1998). Inadequate treatment for major depression both before and after attempted suicide. *American Journal of Psychiatry*, 155, 1778–80.

Szanto, K., Reynolds, C.F., Conwell, Y., Begley, A.E., and Houck, P.R. (1998). High levels of hopelessness persist in geriatric patients with remitted depression and a history of suicide attempt. *Journal of American Geriatric Society*, 46, 1401–6.

Szanto, K., Mulsant, B.H., Houck, P., Dew, M.A., and Reynolds, C.F. (2003). Occurrence and course of suicidality during short-term treatment of late-life depression. *Archives of General Psyhiatry*, 60, 610–17.

Teicher, M.H., Glod, C., and Cole, J.O. (1990). Emergence of intense suicidal preoccupation during fluoxetine treatment. *American Journal of Psychiatry*, 147, 207–10.

Tondo, L., Jamison, K.R., and Baldessarini, R.J. (1997). Effect of lithium maintenance on suicidal behavior in major mood disorders. *Annals of the New York Academy of Sciences*, 836, 339–51.

Van Eck, M., Nicolson, N.A., and Berkhof, J. (1998). Effects of stressful daily events on mood states: relationship to global perceived stress. *Journal of Personality and social Psychology*, 75, 1572–85.

Van Praag, H.M. (1962). A critical investigation into the significance of monoamineoxydase inhibition as a therapeutic priciple in the treatment of depression. Thesis, Utrecht.

Van Praag, H.M. (1978). *Psychotropic drugs. A guide for the practitioner.* Brunner/Mazel, New York.

Van Praag, H.M. (1992a). Reconquest of the subjective. Against the waning of psychiatric diagnosing. *British Journal of Psychiatry*, 160, 266–71.

Van Praag, H.M. (1992b). About the centrality of mood lowering in mood disorders. *European Neuropsychopharmacology*, 2, 393–402.

Van Praag, H.M. (1994). 5-HT related, anxiety- and/or aggression driven depression. *International Clinical Psychopharmacology*, 9, 5–6.

Van Praag, H.M. (1996). Faulty cortisol/serotonin interplay. Psychopathological and biological characterisation of a new hypothetical depression subtype (SeCa depression). *Psychiatry Research*, 65, 143–57.

Van Praag, H.M. (1997). Over the mainstream: diagnostic requirements for biological psychiatric research. *Psychiatry Research*, 72, 201–12.

Van Praag, H.M. (1998). Anxiety and increased aggression as pacemakers of depression. *Acta Psychiatrica Scandinavica*, 98, 81–8.

Van Praag, H.M. (2000). Nosologomania: a disorder of psychiatry. *World Journal of Biological Psychiatry*, 2, 151–8.

Van Praag, H.M., Van Os, J., and De Kloet, D. (2004). *Stress, the brain and depression.* Cambridge University Press, Cambridge UK.

Verberne, T.J. (2003). Antidepressant prescribing and suicide: Decline in suicide rate among older people predates 1991.*British Medical Journal,* 327, 288 [author reply 289].

Verkes, R.J., Van der Mast, R.C., Hengeveld, W., Tuyl, J.P., Zwinderman, A.H., and Van Kempen, G.M. (1998). Reduction by paroxetine of suicidal behavior in patients with repeated suicide attempts but not major depression. *American Journal of Psychiatry,* 155, 543–7.

Walsh, M.-T. and Dinan, T.G. (2001). Selective serotonin reuptake inhibitors and violence: a 3review of the available evidence. *Acta Psychiatrica Scandinavica,* 104, 84–91.

Wasserman, D. (ed.) (2000). *Suicide. An unnecessary death.* Martin Dunitz, London.

World Health Organisation (1996). *World Health Statistics Annual.* World Health Organisation, Geneva.

World Health Organisation (1999). *World Health Statistics Annual.* World Health Organisation, Geneva.

15

Substance use and suicidal behaviour

Ingeborg Rossow

The international research literature consistently shows a significant association between substance use and suicidal behaviour, as is well documented in a number of previous reviews (see for instance Lester 1992; Murphy 1992; Berglund and Öjehagen 1998; Murphy 2000; Rossow 2000; Stack 2000; Hufford 2001; Darke and Ross 2002). In addition to adding recent empirical studies to the previous reviews, this chapter will focus on various measures of associations, present possible explanations for the observed associations, discuss how the associations between substance use and suicidal behaviour may vary according to gender and social and cultural conditions, and, finally, present some implications for prevention and treatment. The term 'substance use' will in this review refer to both alcohol and illegal drug use and cover a wide range of behaviours and problem severity.

Estimates of associations between substance use and suicidal behaviour

Alcohol and suicide

A large number of studies have demonstrated a significant co-occurrence between alcohol abuse and suicide. In most of these studies 'alcohol abuse' is generally assessed in terms of treatment for alcohol problems in prospective studies, or identified through interviews with relatives and other informants after suicide has occurred. In studies of suicides, a substantial proportion of the suicides are considered to have been alcohol abusers, generally in the range of 25–50% (for a review, see Berglund and Öjehagen 1998). In line with this, it has also been shown in follow-up studies of cohorts of alcohol abusers that their risk of suicide is significantly higher compared to the general population of same age and gender, the standardized mortality ratios being reported as mostly in the range from 5 to 10 among males (Rossow 2000). Values given in earlier reports, suggesting that around 11–15% of alcohol abusers would die from suicide (Roy and Linnoila 1986), now seem too high. More recent studies have estimated the lifetime risk of suicide in alcohol abusers to be some 2–5% (Murphy and Wetzel 1990; Duffy and Kreitman 1993; Rossow and Amundsen 1995). In a meta-analysis of several studies (Inskip *et al.* 1998), the figure was 7%.

Apart from the large number of studies demonstrating an association between alcohol abuse and suicide, there are also studies indicating an association between both alcohol intoxication and total alcohol consumption, and suicide. In a recent large-scale study of suicides in Finland, 40% had a blood alcohol concentration above 0.05%, the majority of these being above 0.1% (Pirkola *et al.* 2000). Moreover, among the alcohol abusers in this study 70% were intoxicated by alcohol at the time of death. Data from a comprehensive follow-up study of Swedish military conscripts demonstrated an increasing risk of suicide with increasing alcohol intake at baseline (Andreasson *et al.* 1988, 1991). These data imply a straight-linear relationship between alcohol intake and suicide risk.

During the past 10–15 years several studies have demonstrated an association between alcohol consumption and suicide rates at the aggregate level (Rossow 2000). Most of these studies have estimated the relative change in suicide rates given a one-litre increase in per capita consumption of alcohol. Generally, a positive and statistically significant association is reported from these studies, the estimates implying that an increase in total consumption of alcohol of 1 litre/capita in a population tends to be followed by a 2–15% increase in suicide rates (Rossow 2000).

Alcohol and attempted suicide

In studies of attempted suicide, it is generally reported that a significant proportion of the patients were alcohol abusers. For instance, 23% of a Norwegian sample of suicide attempters were alcohol abusers (Hjelmeland 1996a); 19% of an English sample of patients with deliberate self-harm were alcohol misusers (Hawton *et al.* 1997); and one-third of Swedish males admitted to hospital with attempted suicide were alcohol abusers (Rossow *et al.* 1999). Not many studies have reported the relative risk of attempted suicide in alcohol abusers. Preuss and co-workers (2002) found that alcohol abusers in the USA were three times more likely to report attempted suicide compared to the general population (of the same age and sex), whereas Rossow *et al.* (1999) found that the relative risk of hospital admission for attempted suicide was 27 times higher among male alcohol abusers compared to other men of the same age. Among alcohol abusers the lifetime prevalence of attempted suicide is rather high; around 20–30% according to a review by

Berglund and Öjehagen (1998) and slightly lower (16%) in a study in the USA by Preuss *et al.* (2002). It is also noteworthy that alcohol abusers often report repeated suicide attempts (Swift *et al.* 1996), and that repeated attempts occur more frequently among alcohol abusers than among other patients with deliberate self-harm (Hjelmeland 1996*b*; Hawton *et al.* 1997). So far no studies have explored whether changes in alcohol consumption at the population level have an impact on rates of attempted suicide within that population. However, a study by Fombonne (1998) of suicidal behaviour in young people referred to psychiatric services in London over a 21-year period showed that an increase in suicidal behaviour among males was strongly associated with alcohol misuse.

A large number of studies, particularly of young people, have shown a higher prevalence of self-reported attempted suicide among those who report frequent alcohol intake or alcohol intoxication than in those who do not abuse alcohol (e.g. Vega *et al.* 1993; Rossow and Wichstrom 1994; Dawson 1997). The latter two studies also indicate a straight-linear relationship between alcohol intoxication and risk of attempted suicide. It has also been shown that alcohol intoxication is a prominent feature of attempted suicide, particularly among younger people. Suokas and Lönnqvist (1995) found that 62% of Finnish suicide attempters were intoxicated by alcohol at the time of the event, and they also noted that this was more common among young or lonely men with previous suicide attempts. In a study of suicide attempters in a Swedish county, 37% were intoxicated at the time of the event (Salander-Renberg and Jacobsson 1994), and a similar figure (35%) was reported from a Norwegian county (Hjelmeland, 1996*a*). Furthermore, Borges and Rosovsky (1996) found that suicide attempters in emergency rooms in Mexico City were significantly more likely than controls to have been drinking prior to their attempts.

Drug abuse and suicide and attempted suicide

There are no direct measures of lifetime risk of suicide in drug addicts, due to follow-up periods being restricted to young and middle age. An excellent review by Darke and Ross (2002) presents a summary of follow-up studies, mainly of patients in treatment for drug addiction, demonstrating that among persons who died during follow-up, between 3 and 35% committed suicide. The proportion tends to be higher in Scandinavian countries, i.e. 10–35% (Tunving 1988; Engstrom *et al.* 1991; Eskild *et al.* 1993; Rossow 1994; Andersen 1996; Andersen *et al.* 1996; Fugelstad *et al.* 1997), compared to some 5–8% in Italy (Perucci *et al.* 1991; Quaglio *et al.* 2001), Switzerland (Marx *et al.* 1994), and Australia (Zador and Sunjic 2000). This is much in line with the assumption that suicide risk among substance abusers is higher in countries or cultures where suicide rates are high (see Murphy and Wetzel 1990). However, the huge variation in proportion of deaths due to suicide among drug addicts within the UK (varying between 3 and 23% in nine follow-up studies) (see Darke and Ross 2002) implies that various methodological factors probably account for more of the variation across studies than varying levels of suicide rates and suicide proneness across countries.

Given the high mortality rates among drug addicts and the significant proportions of suicides among those who die, it is clear that drug addicts have a much higher risk of suicide compared to the general population. Harris and Barraclough (1997) estimated, on the basis of a review of previous studies, that heroin users had a 14 times higher risk of suicide compared to age- and sex-matched peers, although the relative risk of suicide among drug addicts is also found to vary significantly. Such variation is seen not only across countries and studies (Darke and Ross 2002), but also over time within the same country (Rossow 1994; Oyefeso *et al.* 1999), suggesting that variation in suicide risk among substance abusers may reflect period effects, cohort effects, or both.

In studies of drug abusers, it is reported that a significant proportion have experienced suicide attempts. It is clear that lifetime prevalence of attempted suicide is high among drug addicts, usually around 20–40%, and thus far higher than levels generally found in community samples (Darke and Ross 2002). The proportion of drug addicts who report past suicide attempts is also high, and many report multiple attempts (Darke and Ross 2002).

Although suicidal behaviour is common among drug addicts, most studies indicate that drug abusers do not constitute a large proportion of suicides and attempted suicides. In a French study it was found that 10% of young suicides were heroin users (Lecomte and Fornes 1998). Hawton *et al.* (1997) reported that 8% of patients with deliberate self-harm were drug misusers, and Hjelmeland (1996*a*) found that 6% of patients with suicide attempts were illicit drug abusers. A probable explanation for the relatively low proportion of drug misusers, as compared to alcohol misusers, among suicides and attempted suicides, is that drug addicts constitute a minority of substance abusers and a very small fraction of the general population in most societies.

Survey studies, particularly school surveys, have found a significantly higher lifetime prevalence of self-reported suicide attempts among those who reported experience with illegal drugs than in those who did not (Vega *et al.* 1993; Rossow and Wichstrom 1994; Burge *et al.* 1995; Windle and Windle 1997; Borges *et al.* 2000; Wichstrom 2000).

Table 15.1 Types of associations and magnitude of associations between substance use and suicidal behaviour

	Suicide	Attempted suicide
Alcohol		
Proportion of cases with abuse	25–50%	20–30%
Proportion of cases with intoxication	40%	35–60%
Lifetime risk among abusers	2–7%	16–30%
Relative risk among abusers	5–10	3–27
Individual risk curves		Straight-linear: increasing risk with increasing consumption
Straight-linear: increasing risk with increasing consumption		
Aggregate associations		Increase in rates (2–15%) with increase in per capita consumption (by 1 litre)
Illicit drugs		
Proportion of cases with abuse	<10%	6–8%
Lifetime risk among abusers		20–40%
Relative risk among abusers	14	
Individual risk curves		Higher risk among students who have used drugs

Table 15.1 summarizes the data discussed in this section.

Risk factors for suicide and attempted suicide in substance abusers

A number of studies have addressed risk factors for suicidal behaviour within samples of substance abusers. It is generally found that depression and other psychiatric co-morbidity is a significant risk factor for both completed and attempted suicide among both alcohol abusers and drug abusers (Berglund and Öjehagen 1998; Darke and Ross 2002; Preuss *et al.* 2002). Psychiatric co-morbidity is highly prevalent among substance abusers (Berglund and Öjehagen 1998; Darke and Ross 2002) and, in line with this, Cavanagh *et al.* (2003) concluded, on the basis of a review of 76 autopsy studies of suicides, that co-morbid mental disorder and substance abuse were found in a large proportion of the cases (varying from 19% to 57%).

Other significant risk factors for suicidal behaviour among substance abusers include recent interpersonal loss or conflict, social isolation, unemployment, financial trouble, serious medical illness, adverse childhood events (e.g. physical or sexual abuse), family history of suicidal behaviour, impulsivity and conduct disorder (Lester 1992; Berglund and Öjehagen 1998; Murphy 2000; Darke and Ross 2002; Preuss *et al.* 2002; Roy 2002; Conner *et al.* 2003). These factors are all associated with increased risk of suicidal behaviour in the general population, and they all occur more frequently among substance abusers compared to the general population. Risk factors specific for substance abusers are reported in some studies. Hence, poly-drug use and addiction severity are factors associated with higher risk of attempted suicide among substance abusers (Darke and Ross, 2002).

A few studies have addressed the risk of eventual suicide among substance abusers who present with suicide attempts, reporting conflicting results. Thus, Cullberg *et al.* (1988) in Sweden, Beck and Steer (1989) in the USA and Hawton *et al.* (1993) in the UK found that among suicide attempters, substance abusers were at higher risk of committing suicide compared to other attempters, whereas two studies from Sweden (Ettlinger 1975; Rossow *et al.* 1999) found that alcohol abusers were less likely to commit suicide following a suicide attempt. It is possible that the conflicting results may be due to differences in criteria for substance abuse, and in sample characteristics such as age range and proportion of men.

Explaining the associations

The associations between substance use and abuse and suicidal behaviour are probably due to several underlying mechanisms. First, it is likely that substance abuse or frequent substance use serves as a *causal factor*, by increasing an individual's vulnerability for suicidal behaviour. This may be explained in terms of several pathways derived from various disciplines and theoretical foundations. Clinical studies have shown that depression or a depressive state often occurs secondary to substance abuse or heavy substance intake (Davidson and Ritson 1993). From a more sociological point of view, suicide proneness in substance abusers may be due to the social disintegrative effect of alcohol or drug abuse (Skog 1991), in the sense that marriage, family relations, and other social relations are often ruined during the course of substance addiction. Other consequences of substance abuse, such as unemployment and severe somatic disease, may also increase the individual's vulnerability for attempted or completed suicide. Besides the effects of chronic abuse, it is also likely that a state of acute intoxication (by alcohol) may serve as a causal factor by triggering the suicidal act in vulnerable individuals (whether they have a substance abuse problem or not) (Hufford 2001). It has been shown that a state of acute intoxication may increase impulsiveness and thus trigger impulsive acts, enhance depressive thoughts and suicidal ideation, limit cognitive functions and ability to see alternative coping strategies, and finally reduce barriers for self-inflicted harm (Hufford 2001).

Secondly, it is likely that the co-occurrence of substance abuse and suicidal behaviour is, to some extent, due to shared common underlying risk factors. It has been shown that primary depression and other psychiatric disorders are risk factors for developing substance abuse as well as suicidal behaviours (Beautrais *et al.* 1996; Hanna and Grant 1997). It also seems that personality traits, such as impulsiveness, are risk factors for both substance abuse and suicidal behaviour (Putnins 1995; Suominen *et al.* 1997; Darke and Ross 2002). And, finally, traumatic or adverse childhood experiences and family dysfunction also seem to be common risk factors for substance abuse as well as suicidal behaviour (Beautrais *et al.* 1996; Fergusson *et al.* 1996; Thatcher *et al.* 2002). To further complicate this picture, it is also likely that substance use and abuse may enhance vulnerability to suicidal behaviour due to primary psychiatric disorder, personality traits, or adverse childhood experiences.

Thirdly, it is likely that, in some cases, alcohol or other intoxicating substances are used as part of the suicidal act; to get the courage to fulfil one's plans and/or to reduce pain, consciousness, or fear.

Finally, it is also likely that substance abuse may cause vulnerability for suicidal behaviour in other persons than the abuser themselves; for instance, in children or the partner of the abuser. Little attention has been paid to this aspect of the substance abuse–suicide association in the literature so far. Yet, the issue of 'externalities', or costs borne by third parties, is central in alcohol research, and particularly in relation to alcohol policy (Skog 1999*a*). A few studies have demonstrated that children of substance abusers have a higher risk of attempted suicide compared to their peers (Fergusson *et al.* 2000; Cornelius *et al.* 2001; Dube *et al.* 2001). It is possible that the higher risk of suicidality in this group is due to higher levels of depression and poor parent–child attachments (Fergusson *et al.* 2000), yet it may also be mediated by the child's own substance abuse, which is common among children of substance abusers (Dawson *et al.* 1992; Dube *et al.* 2001).

Gender differences in suicidal behaviour among substance abusers

There are generally significant gender differences in risk of suicidal behaviour: rates for completed suicides tend to be 2–3 times higher among males than among females, whereas rates of attempted suicide tend to higher among females than among males (Cantor 2000; Kerkhof 2000). Also, rates of self-reported self-harm in general population surveys tend to be higher among females than in their male counterparts. Surveys of drinking habits have demonstrated a higher alcohol intake, more frequent intoxication, and a larger proportion of alcohol abusers among men than among women (Nelson *et al.* 1998; Babor *et al.* 2003). Also, with respect to illicit drug use, generally a somewhat higher proportion of males than females report experience with illicit drug use (Morgan *et al.* 1999; Calafat *et al.* 2001), and there is a significantly higher proportion of men than women among clients in treatment (Schildhaus *et al.* 2000). Thus there are fewer women than men with substance abuse in the general population. Since we also find a larger proportion of males than females with substance abuse among both suicides and suicide attempters (Hjelmeland 1996*a*; Hawton *et al.* 1997; Berglund and Öjehagen 1998), the male preponderance of substance abusers in the general population seems to be reflected in the subpopulation of people with suicidal behaviour.

However, if we compare the risk of suicidal behaviours between male and female substance abusers, the picture tends to be more complex. Although the risk of suicide is generally higher among males, several large-scale follow-up studies have reported the risk of completed suicide to be of the same magnitude for men and women among both alcohol abusers (Lindberg and Ågren 1988) and drug abusers (Engström *et al.* 1991; Rossow 1994; Sørensen *et al.* 1996). Studies of the lifetime prevalence of attempted suicide in substance abusers have, in part, reported a higher prevalence among women than among men (see Darke and Ross 2002), whereas other studies have reported very small or no differences between men and women (Hasin *et al.* 1988; Lester 1992; Rossow and Lauritzen 2001). Thus it seems that there are aspects of substance abuse that not only elevate the risk of suicidal behaviour but also, to some extent, tend to reduce or eliminate the gender differences in risk of both attempted and completed suicide. Given that female substance abusers are more burdened with psychiatric co-morbidity (Helzer and Pryzbeck 1988; Davidson and Ritson 1993; Zilberman *et al.* 2003), social disapproval and stigmatization, and a faster progression to alcohol or drug dependence (see Lynch *et al.* 2002), one might have assumed that there would be a higher risk of suicidal behaviour among female substance abusers compared to male abusers.

Social or cultural differences in the association between substance use and suicidal behaviour

Although there is no doubt that the risk of suicidal behaviour increases with substance use and abuse, there is clearly a large variation in the magnitude of the association between substance use and suicidal behaviour. It is likely that some of this variation is due to methodological differences across studies, such as different study designs, including types of samples, criteria, and measurement. On the other hand, assuming that suicidal behaviours also reflect social and cultural conditions, comparative studies not only of the level of suicidal behaviour, but also cross-cultural studies of the associations between these behaviours and significant risk factors, are of interest. There are some comparative studies suggesting that the magnitude of the substance use–suicide associations differ across different cultures. Norström (1988, 1995*a*) showed that the associations between alcohol consumption and male suicide rates were higher in Norway and Sweden than in Denmark and France, and ascribed this to the different drinking cultures in these countries. In Norway and Sweden, alcohol consumption is more often accompanied by acute intoxication compared to that of France (and to some extent Denmark). A series of studies applying the same methods as used by Norström have further demonstrated that a rather strong association between alcohol consumption and male suicide rates is found in the most northern European countries, where intoxication is a prominent feature of the drinking culture, whereas more modest associations have been demonstrated in southern European countries, where a moderate drinking pattern with less intoxication is the norm (for a review, see Rossow 2000). Thus it has been shown that a one litre increase in alcohol consumption tends to be associated with a larger increase in suicide rates in countries where intoxication is a prominent feature of the drinking culture, compared to countries with moderate drinking patterns. In their review of follow-up studies, Murphy and Wetzel (1990) showed that lifetime risk of suicide among alcohol abusers tended to be higher in countries with high suicide rates compared to countries with lower suicide rates. Hence, it appears that associations between heavy drinking and suicide may depend on the drinking culture as well as the 'social availability' of suicide in a society.

Prevention and treatment

Given the high risk of both attempted suicide and suicide in substance abusers, there is clearly a need to consider how these significant health risks can be curbed by preventive strategies and treatment. Since substance abuse is clearly a causal factor in suicidal behaviour, there is the potential to prevent non-fatal and fatal suicidal behaviour in the population by substance abuse treatment and by prevention of substance abuse. But, what kinds of strategies or efforts are likely to work, or to work better than other efforts?

Lewis *et al.* (1997) argued, on a more general basis, that high-risk group strategies aimed at reducing suicide among patients with deliberate self-harm, even when effective, would only have a modest effect on population suicide rates. Hence, they suggested population-based strategies, such as reducing availability of methods used for suicide. Norström (1995*b*), on the other hand, argued that, in the case of alcohol abuse and suicide, both high-risk group strategies and population-based strategies could have an impact on population suicide rates. There are some empirical studies to support this view.

From the literature on prevention of alcohol-related harm, it is generally found that harm that is closely related to acute intoxication (such as aggressive behaviour) tends to show a straight-linear relationship with alcohol intake and frequency of intoxication, and in such cases the majority of the alcohol-related incidents are found among the large majority of light or moderate drinkers and not among the small fraction of heavy drinkers (Skog 1999*b*). This implies that more harm may be prevented by targeting the whole population (of drinkers) rather than the small fraction of heavy drinkers. This is often referred to as the prevention paradox. Consequently, given the straight-linear associations between alcohol intake and intoxication frequency, on the one hand, and suicidal behaviour on the other, one may argue that suicidal behaviour due to acute intoxication may be prevented by effective popula-tion-targeted strategies.

Recent literature reviews on policy measures to prevent alcohol and drug abuse and related problems, may, however, make the reader somewhat less optimistic and enthusiastic. In the alcohol field, a particularly wide range of strategies and interventions has been evaluated. The effectiveness of these measures has recently been summarized by Babor *et al.* (2003). It is clear that control policy measures, such as excise duties on alcohol and restricted availability, are effective in limiting drinking and drinking problems, whereas information campaigns and school interventions have no detectable effect. The extent to which alcohol control measures have an impact on suicidal behaviour is well demonstrated in a number of studies from the former Soviet Union on changes in alcohol consumption and mortality rates before, during, and after President Gorbachev's anti-alcohol campaign (Reitan 2000). This campaign lasted from 1985 to 1987/88 and comprised an increase in alcohol prices and restrictions on alcohol availability, as well as penalties for public drunkenness, drinking at work, and drunk driving. During the campaign, the significant decrease in recorded alcohol sales was in part compensated for by an increase in unrecorded consumption (home-distilled spirits), yet there was a net reduction in total alcohol consumption. In line with this, all-cause mortality, particularly among males, decreased from 1984 to 1987. Following the cessation of the campaign, all-cause mortality increased dramatically in Russia and the Baltic states (Babor *et al.* 2003). During the campaign, suicide rates decreased by 42% in males and by 20% in females, but after the campaign the rates increased again (Varnik *et al.* 1998; Wasserman *et al.* 1998; Pridemore and Spivak 2003). A similar substantial drop in suicide rates was also observed in Denmark in 1917 following a huge increase in alcohol taxes and consequent reduction in alcohol consumption (Skog 1993).

Relatively few studies have addressed the possible impact of treatment of substance abuse on suicide. Some studies have examined the extent to which suicide attempters with substance abuse are offered treatment for their alcohol or drug problems, and whether they actually receive treatment. Merrill and co-workers (1992) reported that 1 in 5 suicide attempters with alcohol problems in Birmingham in England received alcohol treatment or advice. On the other hand, in Oxford, Hawton *et al.* (1997) found that among 200 deliberate self-harm patients with substance abuse, the majority were offered substance abuse treatment. However, 28% did not accept the treatment they were offered. Suominen *et al.* (1999) reported that in a small sample of Finnish alcohol-dependent suicide attempters the majority had a history of substance abuse treatment, whereas less than a quarter received alcohol treatment during the 1 month after their attempts. A few studies have reported on changes in suicidal behaviour as a treatment outcome in clients who received treatment for substance abuse. Magruder-Habib *et al.* (1992) found that self-reported suicidal thoughts and attempts (as well as depression) declined significantly after 1 month in treatment, and that even at 12 months follow-up almost half of those who were suicidal at entry to treatment were asymptomatic, whereas the other half remained suicidal. Schildhaus *et al.* (2000) reported on various behavioural changes from a large study of clients in substance abuse treatment, and stated (only in the abstract of the article) that suicide attempts decreased by more than one-third after treatment.

For the clinical worker dealing with substance-abusing patients, the question is how therapeutic sessions may help prevent suicidal events. Benjaminsen (1998) has provided a guide on assessment, referral, and treatment of suicidal alcohol abusers. He emphasizes the need to first evaluate suicidal risk at admission to treatment by obtaining a history of suicidal thoughts, suicide attempts, and suicidal intent. If a patient is considered to be currently at risk of suicidal behaviour, this is indicative of the need for immediate admission to in-patient psychiatric treatment or referral to a psychiatric ward for further evaluation of suicidal risk. A particular problem with substance abusers may be that they make suicide threats in order to obtain admission for treatment, without having any motivation for treatment but rather as a means of escaping from an unpleasant situation (Benjaminsen 1998). Moreover, the high rates of both psychiatric co-morbidity and inclination to reject or avoid treatment among substance-abusing patients with deliberate self-harm (Hawton *et al.* 1997) imply that it may be more difficult to provide the patient with suitable and effective treatment.

Conclusions

It is clear that substance abusers have an elevated risk of suicide and attempted suicide. Moreover, intoxication (by alcohol) also elevates the risk of suicidal behaviour in people who are not considered to be substance abusers, and at the aggregate level an increase in total alcohol consumption tends to be accompanied by an increase in suicide rates. Correspondingly, a significant proportion of suicides and attempted suicides are substance abusers and/or intoxicated (by alcohol) at the time of the event (Table 15.1).

These observed associations between substance use and abuse, on the one hand, and suicidal behaviour, on the other, may be explained by several possible underlying mechanisms. These are that substance abuse may enhance vulnerability through depression and social disintegration, intoxication may trigger suicidal impulses in vulnerable individuals, and use of intoxicants may serve as part of the act. Some of the co-occurrence may, however, be due to shared risk factors, and, finally, substance abuse may also cause vulnerability for suicidal behaviour in children or the partner of the abuser. Substance abusers at risk of suicidal behaviour may be difficult to reach with suitable and effective treatment. However, some of the suicides and attempted suicides related to substance use may probably be prevented by effective alcohol policy measures.

References

Andersen, B.B. (1996). Dødelighed blant 174 narkomaner i Vejle Amt 1980–1995 [Mortality among 174 drug addicts in the county of Vejle 1980–1995]. In *Dødsfall blant stofmisbrugere 1970 1995 – stigning, stagnation, forandring!* [Deaths among drug addicts 1970–1995 – increase, stagnation, change!], pp. 25–29. National Directorate of Health Denmark, Copenhagen.

Andersen, S., Berg, J.E., Bjerkedal, T., and Alveberg, P.Ø. (1996). Ten year mortality among Norwegian drug addicts. A comparison of types of intervention. *Norwegian Medical Journal*, 116, 2912–16.

Andreasson, S., Allebeck, P., and Romelsjo, A. (1988). Alcohol and mortality among young men: Longitudinal study of Swedish conscripts. *British Medical Journal*, 296, 1021–5.

Andreasson, S., Romelsjo, A., and Allebeck, P. (1991). Alcohol, social factors and mortality among young men. *British Journal of Addiction*, 86, 877–87.

Babor, T., Caetano, R., Casswell, S. *et al.* (2003). *Alcohol: No ordinary commodity. Research and public policy*. Oxford University Press, Oxford.

Beautrais, A.L., Joyce, P.R., Mulder, R.T., Fergusson, D.M., Deavoll, B.J., and Nightingale, S.K. (1996). Prevalence and comorbidity of mental disorders in persons making serious suicide attempts: A case-control study. *American Journal of Psychiatry*, 153, 1009–14.

Beck, A.T. and Steer, R.A. (1989). Clinical predictors of eventual suicide: A 5–10 year prospective one-year outcome study. *Journal of Affective Disorders*, 17, 203–9.

Benjaminsen, S. (1998). *Suicidal behaviour among alcohol abusers. A guide to risk assessment, treatment and referrals* [Danish text]. Odense University Hospital, Odense.

Berglund, M. and Öjehagen, A. (1998). The influence of alcohol drinking and alcohol use disorders on psychiatric disorders and suicidal behavior. *Alcoholism – Clinical and Experimental Research*, 22, 333S–345S.

Borges, G. and Rosovsky, H. (1996). Suicide attempts and alcohol consumption in an emergency room sample. *Journal of Studies on Alcohol*, 57, 543–8.

Borges, G., Walters, E.E., and Kessler, R.C. (2000). Associations of substance use, abuse, and dependence with subsequent suicidal behaviour. *American Journal of Epidemiology*, 151, 781–9.

Burge, V., Felts, M., Chenier, T., and Parrillo, A.V. (1995). Drug use, sexual activity and suicidal behaviour in US high school students. *Journal of School Health*, 65, 222–7.

Calafat, A., Fernandez, C., Jerez, M.J., *et al.* (2001). *Risk and control in the recreational drug culture.* SONAR project. IREFREA, Valencia.

Cantor, C.H. (2000). Suicide in the Western World. In *The international handbook of suicide and attempted suicide*, (ed. K. Hawton and K. van Heeringen), pp. 9–28. John Wiley & Sons, Chichester.

Cavanagh, J.T.O., Carson, A.J., Sharp, M., and Lawrie, S.M. (2003). Psychological autopsy studies of suicide: a systematic review. *Psychological Medicine*, 33, 395–405.

Conner, K.R., Beautrais, A.L., and Conwell, Y. (2003). Risk factors for suicide and medically serious suicide attempts among alcoholics: Analyses of Canterbury suicide project data. *Journal of Studies on Alcohol*, 64, 551–4.

Cornelius, J., Kirisci, L., and Tarter, R.E. (2001). Suicidality in offspring of men with substance use disorder: Is there a common liability? *Journal of Child and Adolescent Substance Abuse*, 10, 101–9.

Cullberg, J., Wasserman, D., and Stefansson, C.G. (1988). Who commits suicide after a suicide attempt – an 8 to 10 year follow-up in a suburban catchment area. *Acta Psychiatrica Scandinavica*, 77, 598–603.

Darke, S. and Ross, J. (2002). Suicide among heroin users: rates, risk factors and methods. *Addiction*, 97, 1383–94.

Davidson, K.M. and Ritson, E.B. (1993). The relationship between alcohol dependence and depression. *Alcohol and Alcoholism*, 28, 147–55.

Dawson, D.A. (1997). Alcohol, drugs, fighting and suicide attempt/ideation. *Addiction Research*, 5, 451–72.

Dawson, D.A., Harford, T.C., and Grant, B.F. (1992). Family history as a predictor of alcohol dependence. *Alcohol – Clinical and Experimental Research*, 16, 572–5.

Dube, S.R., Anda, R.F., Felitti, V.J., Chapman, D.P., Williamson, D.F., and Giles, W.H. (2001). Childhood abuse, household dysfunction, and the risk of attempted suicide throughout the life span—Findings from the adverse childhood experiences study. *Journal of the American Medical Association*, 286, 3089–96.

Duffy, J. and Kreitman, N. (1993). Risk factors for suicide and undetermined death among in-patient alcoholics in Scotland. *Addiction*, 88, 757–66.

Engstrom, A., Adamsson, C., Allebeck, P., and Rydberg, U. (1991). Mortality in patients with substance abuse. A follow-up in Stockholm county, 1973–1984. *International Journal of the Addictions*, 26, 91–106.

Eskild, A., Magnus, P., Samuelsen, S.O., Sohlberg, C., and Kittilsen, P. (1993). Differences in mortality rates and causes of death between HIV-positive and HIV-negative intravenous drug users. *International Journal of Epidemiology,* 22, 315–20.

Ettlinger, R. (1975). Evaluation of suicide prevention after attempted suicide. *Acta Psychiatrica Scandinavica,* 260, 1–135.

Fergusson, D.M., Horwood, L.J., and Lynskey, M.T. (1996). Childhood sexual abuse and psychiatric disorder in young adulthood. 2. Psychiatric outcomes of childhood sexual abuse. *Journal of the American Academy of Child and Adolescent Psychiatry,* 35, 1365–74.

Fergusson, D.M., Woodward, L.J., and Horwood, L.J. (2000). Risk factors and life processes associated with the onset of suicidal behaviour during adolescence and early adulthood. *Psychological Medicine,* 30, 23–39.

Fombonne, E. (1998). Suicidal behaviours in vulnerable adolescents. Time trends and their correlates. *British Journal of Psychiatry,* 173, 154–9.

Fugelstad, A., Annell, A., Rajs, J., and Ågren, G. (1997). Mortality and causes and manner of death among drug addicts in Stockholm during the period 1981–1992. *Acta Psychiatrica Scandinavica,* 96, 169–75.

Hanna, E.Z. and Grant, B.F. (1997). Gender differences in DSM-IV alcohol use disorders and major depression as distributed in the general population: Clinical implications. *Comprehensive Psychiatry,* 38, 202–12.

Harris, E.C. and Barraclough, B. (1997). Suicide as an outcome for mental disorders. *British Journal of Psychiatry,* 170, 205–28.

Hasin, D., Grant, B., and Endicott, J. (1988). Treated and untreated suicide attempts in substance abuse patients. *Journal of Nervous and Mental Disease,* 176, 289–94.

Hawton, K., Fagg, J., Platt, S., and Hawkins, M. (1993). Factors associated with suicide after parasuicide in young people. *British Medical Journal,* 306, 1641–4.

Hawton, K., Simkin, S., and Fagg, J. (1997). Deliberate self-harm in alcohol and drug misusers: patient characteristics and patterns of clinical care. *Drug and Alcohol Review,* 16, 123–9.

Helzer, J.E. and Pryzbeck, T.R. (1988). The co-occurrence of alcoholism with other psychiatric disorders in the general population and its impact on treatment. *Journal of Studies on Alcohol,* 49, 219–24.

Hjelmeland, H. (1996a). Parasuicide in the county of Sor-Trondelag Norway—General epidemiology and psychological factors. *Social Psychiatry and Psychiatric Epidemiology,* 31, 272–83.

Hjelmeland, H. (1996b). Repetition of parasuicide: A predictive study. *Suicide and Life-Threatening Behavior,* 26, 395–404.

Hufford, M.R. (2001). Alcohol and suicidal behaviour. *Clinical Psychology Review,* 21, 797–811.

Inskip, H.M., Harris, E.C., and Barraclough, B. (1998). Lifetime risk of suicide for affective disorder, alcoholism and schizophrenia. *British Journal of Psychiatry,* 172, 35–7.

Kerkhof, A.J.F.M. (2000). Attempted suicide: patterns and trends. In *The international handbook of suicide and attempted suicide,* (ed. K. Hawton and K. van Heeringen), pp. 49–64. John Wiley & Sons, Chichester.

Lecomte, D. and Fornes, P. (1998). Suicide among youth and young adults, 15 through 24 years of age. A report of 392 cases from Paris, 1989–1996. *Journal of Forensic Sciences,* 43, 964–8.

Lester, D. (1992). Alcoholism and drug abuse. In *Assessment and prediction of suicide,* (ed. R.W. Maris, A.L. Berman, J. Maltsberger, and I. Yufit), pp. 321–36. Guilford Press, New York.

Lewis, G., Hawton, K., and Jones, P. (1997). Strategies for preventing suicide. *British Journal of Psychiatry*, 171, 351–4.

Lindberg, S. and Ågren, G. (1988). Mortality among male and female hospitalized alcoholics in Stockholm 1962–1983. *British Journal of Addiction*, 83, 1193–200.

Lynch, W.J., Roth, M.E., and Carroll, M.E. (2002). Biological basis of sex differences in drug abuse: preclinical and clinical studies. *Psychopharmacology*, 164, 121–37.

Magruder-Habib, K., Hubbard, R.L., and Ginzburg, H.M. (1992). Effects of drug misuse on symptoms of depression and suicide. *The International Journal of Addictions*, 27, 1035–65.

Marx, A., Schick, M.T., and Minder, C.E. (1994). Drug-related mortality in Switzerland from 1987 to 1989 in comparison to other countries. *International Journal of the Addictions*, 29, 837–60.

Merrill, J., Milner, G., Owens, J., and Vale, A. (1992). Alcohol and attempted suicide. *British Journal of Addiction*, 87, 83–9.

Morgan, M., Hibell, B., Andersson, B., Bjarnason, T., Kokkevi, A., and Narusk, A. (1999). ESPAD Study: Implications for prevention. *Drugs: Education, Prevention and Policy*, 6, 243–56.

Murphy, G.E .(1992). *Suicide in alcoholism*. Oxford University Press, New York.

Murphy, G.E. (2000). Psychiatric aspects of suicidal behaviour: Substance abuse. In *The international handbook of suicide and attempted suicide,* (ed. K. Hawton and K. van Heeringen), pp. 135–46. John Wiley & Sons, Chichester.

Murphy, G.E. and Wetzel, R.D. (1990). The lifetime risk of suicide in alcoholism. *Archives of General Psychiatry*, 47, 383–92.

Nelson, C.B., Heath, A.C., and Kessler, R.C. (1998). Temporal progression of alcohol dependence symptoms in the US household population: Results from the national comorbidity survey. *Journal of Consulting Clinical Psychology*, 66, 474–83.

Norström, T. (1988). Alcohol and suicide in Scandinavia. *British Journal of Addiction*, 83, 553–9.

Norström, T. (1995a). Alcohol and suicide: a comparative analysis of France and Sweden. *Addiction*, 90, 1463–9.

Norström, T. (1995b). Prevention strategies and alcohol policy. *Addiction*, 90, 515–24.

Oyefeso, A., Ghodse, H., Clancy, C., and Corkery, J.M. (1999). Suicide among drug addicts in the UK. *British Journal of Psychiatry*, 175, 277–82.

Perucci, C.A., Davoli, M., Rapiti, E., Abeni, D.D., and Forastieri, F. (1991). Mortality in intravenous drug users in Rome: a cohort study. *American Journal of Public Health*, 81, 1307–10.

Pirkola, S.P., Isometsa, E.T., Heikkinen, M.E., and Lönnqvist, J.K. (2000). Suicides of alcohol misusers and non-misusers in a nationwide population. *Alcohol and Alcoholism*, 35, 70–5.

Preuss, U.W., Schuckit, M.A., Smith, T.L. *et al.* (2002). Comparison of 3190 alcohol-dependent individuals with and without suicide attempts. *Alcoholism: Clinical and Experimental Research*, 26, 471–7.

Pridemore, W.A. and Spivak, A.L. (2003). Patterns of suicide mortality in Russia. *Suicide and Life-Threatening Behavior*, 33, 132–50.

Putnins, A.L. (1995). Recent drug use and suicidal behaviour among young offenders. *Drug and Alcohol Review*, 14, 151–8.

Quaglio, G., Talamini, G., Lechi, A., *et al.* (2001). Study of heroin-related deaths in north-eastern Italy 1985–98 to establish main causes of death. *Addiction*, 96, 1127–37.

Reitan, T.C. (2000). Does alcohol matter? Public health in Russia and the Baltic countries before, during, and after the transition. *Contemporary Drug Problems*, 27, 511–60.

Rossow, I. (1994). Suicide among drug addicts. *Addiction*, 89, 1667–73.

Rossow, I. (2000). Suicide, violence and child abuse: Review of the impact of alcohol consumption on social problems. *Contemporary Drug Problems*, 27, 397–434.

Rossow, I. and Amundsen, A. (1995). Alcohol abuse and suicide: a 40-year prospective study of Norwegian conscripts. *Addiction*, 90, 685–91.

Rossow, I. and Lauritzen, G. (2001). Shattered childhood – a key issue in suicidal behaviour among drug addicts? *Addiction*, 96, 227–40.

Rossow, I. and Wichstrom, L. (1994). Parasuicide and use of intoxicants among Norwegian adolescents. *Suicide and Life-Threatening Behavior*, 24, 174–83.

Rossow, I., Romelsjö, A., and Leifman, H. (1999). Alcohol abuse and suicidal behavior in young and middle aged men—differentiating between attempted and completed suicide. *Addiction*, 94, 1199–207.

Roy, A. (2002). Characteristics of opiate dependent patients who attempt suicide. *Journal of Clinical Psychiatry*, 63, 403–7.

Roy, A. and Linnoila, M. (1986). Alcoholism and suicide. *Suicide and Life-Threatening Behavior*, 16, 244–73.

Salander-Renberg, E. and Jacobsson, L. (1994). Parasuicide in Väterbotten county, Umeå, Sweden 1989–1991. In *Attempted suicide in Europe. Findings from the multicentre study on parasuicide by the WHO regional office for Europe*, (ed. A.J.F.M. Kerkhof, A. Schmidtke, U. Bille-Brahe, D. DeLeo, and J. Lönnquist), pp. 87–105. DSWO Press, Leiden.

Schildhaus, S., Gerstean, D., Brittingham, A., Cerbone, F., and Dugoni, B. (2000). Services Research Outcomes Study: Overview of drug treatment population and outcomes. *Substance Use and Misuse*, 35, 1849–77.

Skog, O.-J. (1991). Alcohol and suicide—Durkheim revisited. *Acta Sociologica*, 34, 193–206.

Skog, O.-J. (1993). Alcohol and suicide in Denmark 1911–24—experiences from a 'natural experiment'. *Addiction*, 88, 1189–93.

Skog, O.J. (1999*a*). Alcohol policy: Why and roughly how? *Nordic Studies on Alcohol and Drugs*, 16 (English Supplement), 21–34.

Skog, O.J. (1999*b*). The prevention paradox revisited. *Addiction*, 94, 751–7.

Sørensen, H.J., Jepsen, P.W., and Haastrup, S. (1996). Dødeligheden i en gruppe af 300 intravenøse københavnske stofmisbrugere [Mortality in a group of 300 intravenous drug addicts in Copenhagen] . In *Sundhedsstyrelsen. Dødsfall blant stofmisbrugere 1970–1995,—stigning, stagnation, forandring!* National Directorate of Health, Copenhagen.

Stack, S. (2000). Suicide: A 15-year review of the sociological literature part I: Cultural and economic factors. *Suicide and Life-Threatening Behavior*, 30, 145–62.

Suokas, J. and Lönnqvist, J. (1995). Suicide attempts in which alcohol is involved: A special group in general hospital emergency rooms. *Acta Psychiatrica Scandinavica*, 91, 36–40.

Suominen, K., Isometsa, E., Henriksson, M., Ostamo, A., and Lönnqvist, J. (1997). Hopelessness, impulsiveness and intent among suicide attempters with major depression, alcohol dependence, or both. *Acta Psychiatrica Scandinavica*, 96, 142–9.

Suominen, K.H., Isometsa, E.T., Henriksson, M.M., Ostamo, A.I., and Lonnqvist, J.K. (1999). Treatment received by alcohol-dependent suicide attempters. *Acta Psychiatrica Scandinavica*, 99, 214–19.

Swift, W., Copeland, J., and Hall, W. (1996). Characteristics of women with alcohol and other drug problems: findings of an Australian national survey. *Addiction*, 91, 1141–50.

Thatcher, W.G., Reininger, B.M., and Drane, J.W. (2002). Using path analysis to examine adolescent suicide attempts, life satisfaction, and health risk behavior. *Journal of School Health*, 72, 71–7.

Tunving, K. (1988). Fatal outcome in drug addiction. *Acta Psychiatrica Scandinavica*, 77, 551–6.

Varnik, A., Wasserman, D., Dankowicz, M., and Eklund, G. (1998). Marked decrease in suicide among men and women in the former USSR during perestroika. *Acta Psychiatrica Scandinavica*, 98 (suppl. 394), 13–19.

Vega, A.W., Gil, A., Warheit, G., Apospori, E., and Zimmerman, R. (1993). The relationship of drug use to suicide ideation and attempts among African, American, Hispanic, and white non-Hispanic male adolescents. *Suicide and Life-Threatening Behavior*, 23, 110–19.

Wasserman, D., Varnik, A., and Dankowicz, M. (1998). Regional differences in the distribution of suicide in the former Soviet Union during perestroika, 1984–1990. *Acta Psychiatrica Scandinavica* 98 (suppl. 394), 5–12.

Wichstrom, L. (2000). Predictors of adolescent suicide attempts: A nationally representative longitudinal study of Norwegian adolescents. *Journal of the American Academy of Child and Adolescent Psychiatry*, 39, 603–10.

Windle, R.C. and Windle, M. (1997). An investigation of adolescents' substance use behaviors, depressed affect, and suicidal behaviours. *Journal of Child Psychology and Psychiatry and Allied Disciplines*, 38, 921–9.

Zador, D. and Sunjic, S. (2000). Deaths in methadone maintenance treatment in New South Wales, Australia 1990–1995. *Addiction*, 95, 77–84.

Zilberman, M.L., Tavares, H., Blume, S.B., and el-Guebaly, N. (2003). Substance use disorders: Sex differences and psychiatric comorbidities. *Canadian Journal of Psychiatry*, 48, 5–13.

16

Restriction of access to methods of suicide as a means of suicide prevention

Keith Hawton

Introduction

Suicidal behaviour can result from a wide variety of causes. These include psychiatric disorder (especially depression and substance abuse), psychological characteristics, life events and problems, exposure to role models in a person's family and social environment and in the media, and genetic and biological factors (Hawton and van Heeringen 2000). However, at the point at which a person feels hopeless and potentially suicidal, access to specific methods for suicidal behaviour can be crucial. Availability of a method may be the key factor that leads to translation of suicidal thoughts into an actual suicidal act. Most importantly, the nature of the method that is available may have a vital influence on the outcome, particularly where an act is impulsive— then the person engaging in suicidal behaviour is likely to use the means most easily available to them. If the method has a high risk of being fatal (e.g. firearms, dangerous chemical substances), then there is a strong possibility that the act will result in death, whereas if the method is less likely to be lethal (e.g. certain psychotropic agents), then the act is more likely to result in survival.

Method choice will also reflect other factors. These include, for example, a person's intention, such as whether the primary goal of the act is death or whether it is associated with other intentions, such as to communicate distress, modify the behaviour of other people, etc. However, the availability of specific methods is probably at least as important as intention in determining outcome. Another factor will be the type of method a person favours. For example, males generally favour more violent methods (e.g. guns or hanging), whereas females tend to favour less violent methods (e.g. overdoses of medication). However, this pattern will also be influenced by availability. For example, males will often have greater access to certain violent means, whereas females tend to have more access to medication. Furthermore, where a method is readily available to members of a society then that method is likely to be seen as more acceptable as a means of suicide. This would apply to firearms in the USA, although availability may not be the sole explanation.

Restricting availability to dangerous methods of suicide is a factor common to all national suicide prevention strategies. There are, however, several important questions to address in considering why restricting access to dangerous means of suicidal behaviour is important. The first is whether availability of specific methods of suicidal behaviour affects suicide rates. A second question is whether prevention of suicide during periods of risk is effective in the long term, or whether people simply find some other way of taking their lives. Finally, there is the question of whether there is evidence that deliberately restricting availability of a dangerous means of suicide is effective, first, in reducing the use of that method for suicide, and, second, in terms of affecting overall suicide rates.

Does availability of method affect suicide rates?

Probably the most dramatic example of the change in availability of a dangerous method of suicide having a significant effect on overall suicide rates comes from the UK (Fig. 16.1). This was the change in suicide rates that accompanied the changeover from toxic coal gas in domestic gas supplies to non-toxic natural (North Sea) gas during the late 1950s through to the early 1970s. This followed a period of increasing suicide rates after the Second World War. Natural gas was introduced region by region. Kreitman (1976)

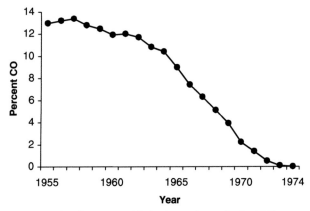

Fig. 16.1 Percentage of carbon monoxide in domestic gas in the UK between 1955 and 1974 (adapted with permission from Kreitman 1976).

estimated the mean percentage of carbon monoxide, the toxic agent in coal gas, in the UK throughout this period. The decrease in the carbon monoxide content began in 1958. At the beginning of the period of changeover, suicide by carbon monoxide poisoning (usually by a person putting his or her head in the gas oven) was the most common method of suicide in the UK, with just under half of all suicides being by this method. As the carbon monoxide content of gas supplies decreased, there was a steady reduction in carbon monoxide suicides in England and Wales in both genders, beginning in 1958 in males and a year or two later in females. The decrease paralleled the reduction in carbon monoxide content of gas supplies. While there was a small increase in use of other methods, the overall net effect was a very large reduction in suicide rates in both genders, the overall suicide rate decreasing by a third (Fig. 16.2). A similar pattern was observed in Scotland. Thus the loss of many thousands of lives through suicide appears to have been prevented by this single measure.

The coal-gas story strongly suggests that availability of a dangerous method of suicide influences risk of completed suicide. What other evidence is there for this? Several studies provide evidence that this is likely to be the case for firearms. Two examples in which a case-control design was used will be

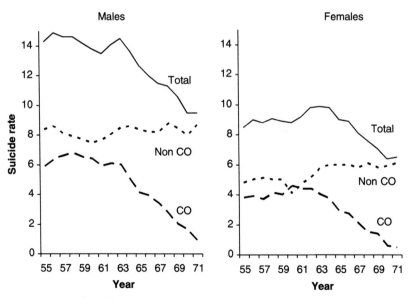

Fig. 16.2 Rates of suicide per 100,000 in males and females in England and Wales between 1955 and 1971, overall, involving carbon monoxide and not involving carbon monoxide (adapted with permission from Kreitman 1976).

summarized here. In the first study, Brent and colleagues (1991) addressed this question in a case-control study involving three groups. The first group was a consecutive series of 47 addescents who died by suicide in western Pennsylvania, 69% of whom had used firearms in their fatal acts. The second group included 47 suicide attempters admitted to psychiatric units, matched for sex and age, and also race and country of origin, with the members of the first group. None of these had used guns in their attempts. The third group also consisted of psychiatric in-patients, but these were individuals who had reported never having had suicidal ideas. Similar matching criteria were used in the selection of this group. Within the group of 47 suicides the use of a firearm for suicide was highly correlated with the presence of a firearm in the home. Thus, where firearms were available in the home, 29 out of 34 (85.3%) individuals used guns for suicide, whereas in those where a firearm was not available in the home only 1 out of 13 (7.7%) used a firearm for suicide.

Brent and colleagues compared the suicides with each of the two control groups separately, regarding firearm availability in the home. Among the suicides, a firearm was available in the household in 72.3% of cases, compared with just 37.0% of the suicide attempters (odds ratio = 4.5, 95% confidence interval 1.9–10.8). Among the control psychiatric in-patients, 38.3% had a firearm available in the home (suicide versus controls: odds ratio = 4.2, 1.8–10.0). These differences were even more marked for *handgun* availability in households, with 55.3% of suicides having a handgun available in the home compared with 19.6% of the suicide attempters (odds ratio = 5.1, 2.0–12.9) and 17.0% of controls (odds ratio = 6.0, 2.3–15.6). There were some differences between the suicides and the attempters in terms of the proportions with a diagnosis of depression and also the degree of suicidal intent involved in the suicidal act, based on scores on the circumstances section of the Beck Suicidal Intent Scale (Beck *et al.* 1974). Brent and colleagues therefore repeated their comparisons regarding presence of firearms in the home after controlling for these two factors. The difference in availability of firearms between the suicides and the attempters was still significant (odds ratio = 2.1, 1.2–3.6). A diagnosis of conduct disorder was somewhat more frequent in the psychiatric controls than in the group of suicides, and therefore the analysis regarding firearm availability in the home was repeated controlling for this factor. Again, a significant difference remained (odds ratio = 2.2, 1.4–3.5). The authors of this study therefore concluded that availability of guns in the home appeared to increase the risk of suicide among adolescents.

In the second study, Kellermann and colleagues (1992) again used a case-control design. They compared 438 people who committed suicide in their homes with control individuals from the general population in Shelby County,

Tennessee, and King County, Washington. The controls were matched with the suicides for gender, race, and age. After controlling for various other factors which differed between the two groups (living alone, psychotropic medication, having been arrested, substance abuse, and not graduating from high school), the suicides more often had firearms in the home (adjusted odds ratio = 4.8, 2.7–8.5). In their report the authors concluded: 'ready availability of firearms appears to be associated with an increased risk of suicide in the home . . . People who own firearms should carefully weigh the reasons for keeping a gun in the home against the possibility that it might someday be used in a suicide.'

The principles underlying reducing availability of methods of suicide as a means of suicide prevention

In order to appreciate the impact of reducing availability of the means of suicide, it is important to be aware of the concept of periods of suicide risk (Fig. 16.3). For most people who become suicidal, the period of real risk is relatively brief, lasting in some individuals for even just a few minutes or a few hours. In others it may last days, but rarely longer. In Fig. 16.3, the pattern A shows someone moving from absence of risk to a period of risk (x–y), and then the risk reducing. This might occur, for example, in a person with depression who is also exposed to a serious life event. In some people (B), a lesser degree of risk is present for a much longer period of time, possibly years, and during that time they may go through periods of added and very high risk. This might occur in someone with a combination of chronic but fluctuating depression and borderline personality disorder or severe substance abuse.

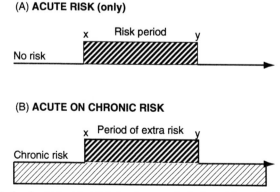

Fig. 16.3 Periods of suicide risk: (A) following a period of no risk; and (B) superimposed on chronic risk.

The concept of periods of risk is very important in understanding the role of altering the availability of methods in prevention, in that if access to a dangerous means of suicide is restricted at such times, then survival until the end of these periods is more likely.

Also relevant to this argument is the nature of psychological processes that may underlie suicidal acts. Although not extensively studied, survivors of near-lethal suicide attempts can be a valuable source of such information. De Moore and colleagues (1994) conducted such a study in Australia when they investigated survivors of self-inflicted firearm injuries. Their sample included 33 consecutive patients admitted to a general hospital after surviving suicide attempts with firearms. Thirty-one were males and 26 were in the 15–35-year age group. Few of them had major psychiatric disorders, the most common diagnosis being adjustment disorder (i.e. stress in response to life events or circumstances). Nearly a third abused alcohol. The most frequent reason given by the individuals for the suicide attempts was interpersonal conflict with a partner or family member. There was often a background of longer-term problems. Most of the patients had shared their suicidal ideas with others before their attempts, but only in the period just before the shooting. Thus there was not usually evidence of long-term suicidal ideas. The actual shooting was relatively impulsive in the vast majority of cases. Most importantly, in all cases firearms were readily available in the home, and availability was usually the reason given for this choice of method for the act. Thus an impulsive response to an acute interpersonal crisis and availability of a firearm in the household were key features leading to suicidal acts by shooting. There was a similar finding in an American study of 30 patients treated in a trauma centre for life-threatening self-inflicted gunshot wounds (Peterson *et al.* 1985). Presumably, if a gun had not been available, at least some of the individuals in these studies would have made suicide attempts by another method, but these may have been potentially less lethal. Indeed, the psychological characteristics of the self-harming behaviour in the sample in this study were very similar to those of people who take overdoses in the UK (Hawton and Catalan 1987), in whom the case fatality rate is relatively low (e.g. Gunnell *et al.* 1997).

Is prevention of suicide during periods of risk effective in the long term?

A crucial question about restricting availability of methods of suicide is whether prevention of suicide during a period of acute risk helps to prevent suicide in the long term, or whether it make no difference, in that a person will seek out and find an effective method in due course (as people sceptical of suicide prevention efforts might suggest). As noted above in relation to the coal-gas story in the UK, there was little evidence of an immediate compensatory increase in the use of other methods of suicide following the reduction in suicides by carbon monoxide poisoning. Two specific examples of strong evidence that survival of acute periods of risk is effective will be provided here. These come from follow-up studies of survivors of serious suicide attempts involving methods that result in death for most people who use them.

O'Donnell and colleagues (1994) studied people who jumped in front of underground (subway) trains in London and survived. Surprisingly, a substantial proportion of individuals do survive what is clearly a method with an apparent high risk of fatality. This is because there is a fairly deep well between the rails and also because the electric rail has been placed furthest from the platform. However, all surviving jumpers report believing with certainty that jumping would kill them. O'Donnell and colleagues studied a consecutive series of 94 individuals who survived jumping in front of underground trains during the three-year period 1977–1979. They followed each of them up for at least 10 years and found that in the group there had been just seven suicides and two probable suicides. Therefore, 9 out of the 94 persons died by likely suicide, a suicide rate of 9.6%. Three of these died by again jumping under subway trains. All the suicides and probable suicides occurred in the first 3 years and 7 months of the follow-up period. There was no evidence of increased risk beyond this time.

The second example comes from a follow-up study of 515 people who were restrained from jumping from the Golden Gate Bridge in San Francisco between 1937 and 1971 (Seiden 1978). Jumping from the bridge is nearly always fatal. During a follow-up period with a median of 26.7 years, only 25, or 4.9%, of the would-be jumpers died by suicide. Eight of these died by jumping from a bridge, all but one from the Golden Gate Bridge. These suicides usually occurred soon after the episodes in which jumping was prevented. In a comparison group of suicide attempters admitted to San Francisco General Hospital in 1956–1957 who were followed up for 15 years, the suicide rate was 7.1%. Thus persons who came close to suicide by jumping from the Golden Gate Bridge had a relatively low long-term suicide rate. Also, such individuals do not necessarily turn to another method.

Examples of suicide prevention by reducing availability of means for suicide

The final consideration in making the case for changing availability of methods of suicide as a means of prevention is to look for examples of where this has been tried. Three examples will be presented. The first concerns firearms used for suicide in the USA, the second self-poisoning with analgesics in the UK, and the final example is use of pesticides and other chemicals for suicide in developing countries.

Firearms

Several studies from North America and other countries have addressed the question of whether reducing firearm availability influences suicide rates. Most have produced evidence that altered availability of firearms does result in reduced rates of suicide. Thus, following adoption of a law banning the purchase, sale, transfer, or possession of handguns by civilians in the District of Columbia in the USA in 1976, accompanied by introduction of registration of firearms, 'fitness' to purchase, and gun safety standards, there was a decline in the rate of suicide by firearms of 23%, with no evidence of substitution of method. No change in suicide rates occurred in the surrounding counties of Maryland and Virginia, where firearm legislation had not changed (Loftin *et al.* 1991). However, the Brady Handgun Violence Prevention Act, implemented across the USA in 1994, had less clear effects. Following this act 32 states with less restrictive laws had to introduce new measures, including background checks on applicants for handgun licences and a 5-day 'cooling off' period before purchase of a gun. Eighteen other states and the District of Columbia already met the requirements of the new act. No difference in changes in rates of suicide were found between the two groups of states, except in persons aged 55 years and over. In this group the reduction in suicide rates was greater in states that had had to implement both the waiting period and background checks than in states only implementing the background checks. There was no change in overall suicide rates (Ludwig and Cook 2000). In Canada, Bill C-SI, which was introduced in 1977, included a complex series of measures aimed at restricting gun availability. This was followed by a decrease in the rate of firearm suicides but with some evidence of method substitution (Lester and Leenaars 1993).

Introduction of firearm legislation has also been evaluated in Australia. Restrictive firearm legislation was introduced in South Australia in 1980. This was followed by a decline in firearm suicide rates in this state but not in the four states where there was no change in legislation (Snowdon and Harris 1992). The state with the least restrictive firearm legislation—Queensland—had a higher firearm suicide rate than the other four states. Subsequently, firearm control legislation was introduced in Queensland, with licences being required for long guns (shotguns and rifles), a 28-day cooling off period, and a safety test for applicants. This was followed by a decline in the rate of firearm suicide in males in metropolitan and provincial cities, but an increase in rural suicides involving firearms. However, there was some evidence of method substitution, with an increase in suicide by hanging and self-poisoning in all areas, except provincial cites, where overall suicide rates declined (Cantor and Slater 1995).

In the UK some further evidence regarding the question of whether altering firearm availability influences suicide rates came from a study of suicide in farmers. Firearms are used in only a small proportion of all suicides in the UK, but in farmers they are used much more frequently, reflecting the availability of shotguns and other firearms on most farms. We studied farmers who died by suicide in England and Wales between 1981 and 1993. Specifically, we examined the most common methods of suicide, namely firearms, hanging, and carbon monoxide poisoning (Hawton et al. 1998). In 1989 the Firearms Amendment Act was introduced in the UK regarding the purchase, registration, and storage of guns. From 1989, firearm suicides in farmers decreased significantly and the overall rates of suicide in farmers also decreased. While there was some increase in the proportion of farming suicides which involved hanging, the absolute rate of hanging suicides in farmers did not change. We also examined firearm suicides in the general population, after excluding farmers. We found a significant decrease of 19% in firearm suicides after the legislation compared with the period beforehand. This study therefore provides further suggestive evidence that availability of firearms can influence overall suicide rates, even in a country where firearms are relatively rarely used for suicide.

Thus, overall, there is reasonably encouraging evidence that reducing availability of firearms, or at least introducing restrictive legislation, not only leads to a reduction in firearm suicides but may also result in a lowering of overall suicide rates.

Analgesics

Between the 1970s and 1990s, rates of both fatal and non-fatal self-poisoning with analgesics sold over the counter, especially paracetamol (acetaminophen), increased dramatically in the UK. By the mid-1990s, between 35% and 50% of all overdose presentations to general hospitals involved paracetamol (Bialas et al. 1996; Hawton et al. 1997), the majority being in very young people. Approximately 220–250 deaths were due to paracetamol poisoning, mainly the result of liver necrosis (O'Grady 1999). Interviews with patients who had taken non-fatal paracetamol overdoses showed that many had used this method of overdose because of the ready availability of the medication in the household, most acting on impulse (Hawton et al. 1995). Interestingly, many patients thought (incorrectly) they would become unconscious as an immediate result of the overdose. Several potential approaches to prevention were considered (Hawton 2002). Reduction in pack sizes, with strict enforcement of the maximum amount of tablets that could be bought per purchase, was chosen as the primary approach, with additional changes to warnings on packs about the danger of overdose. These changes were introduced as legislation in September 1998. The legislation included aspirin as well as paracetamol, because of concerns about possible substitution by aspirin overdose, which is also dangerous.

During the first year following the legislation there were significant changes in sales data, showing that pack size had been reduced and for paracetamol this had been compensated for by increased numbers of packs being bought. The net effect of this would have been that reduced amounts would have been available in households most of the time (Hawton 2002). There were significant reductions in large overdoses of both paracetamol and aspirin, markedly fewer liver transplants due to paracetamol overdose, and, most importantly, a sizeable reduction in deaths due to both paracetamol and aspirin overdoses (Hawton *et al.* 2001). Further evaluation of the impact of the legislation has shown that these changes have largely persisted, and with only limited evidence of substitution of methods involving another over-the-counter analgesic, ibuprofen, but without this itself causing deaths (Hawton *et al.* 2004).

The impact of this measure has clearly been substantial. It has been estimated that it may have resulted in the prevention of approximately 200 deaths during the 3 years since the legislation was introduced (Hawton *et al.* 2004).

Pesticides

Self-poisoning with pesticides is a major cause of suicide deaths in developing countries (Eddleston 2000; Eddleston and Phillips 2004). This is because of ready availability and high levels of toxicity. It has been argued that this is a major reason for the relatively high rates of suicide in countries such as China and Sri Lanka and why, especially in rural areas, patterns of suicide differ markedly from those in Western countries, with reversal of the usual gender patterns for suicide, and peaks in rates in young people (Gunnell and Eddleston 2003). It has been estimated that approximately 300 000 pesticide suicides may occur in China and South-East Asia (Gunnell and Eddleston 2003), with substantial numbers of further deaths from this cause in Africa and South America.

The majority of pesticide suicides in a recent study in China used chemicals stored in the home (Phillips *et al.* 2002). It is reasonable to suppose that, in view of the similarity in gender and age profile to non-fatal self-poisonings in Western countries, many of the deaths would not occur if pesticides were not so readily available, and perhaps if other less toxic substances were more available in households.

Gunnell and Eddleston (2003) have suggested that the problem of pesticide suicides has been little addressed in a practical sense, probably largely for political and commercial reasons. In Western Samoa, reduced use of paraquat (a development driven largely by national financial problems) was followed by fewer fatal pesticide poisonings (Bowles 1995). In Jordan, a decrease in imports of some toxic pesticides and a ban on imports of others was also followed by a reduction in pesticide suicides (Abu al-Ragheb and Salhab 1989). Both initiatives were also accompanied by increasing public awareness of the problem.

Simply restricting imports of certain pesticides to developing countries may not be an acceptable option on a large scale at the present time. Commercial pressure will also mitigate against such a policy until cheap, effective, and less-toxic alternative pesticides are found. There is, however, considerable potential for other initiatives aimed at modifying ease of availability of pesticides, which might help reduce suicides by this means without unduly affecting their availability for use in agriculture. These include ensuring that all pesticides are kept in locked containers, with the key only available to the licensed user, or having a senior person in a village hold the local supplies of pesticides centrally. While both approaches will be associated with some degree of inconvenience and may be difficult to enforce, they require large-scale evaluation.

The potential for suicide prevention in developing countries through tackling the availability of pesticides would appear to be very great. Such an initiative could have a major impact on the global burden of suicide.

Conclusions

Acute suicide risk is generally brief. Suicidal behaviour, including actual suicides as well as attempts, is often impulsive. Most survivors of potentially lethal suicide attempts do not appear to have a very high long-term risk of suicide. There is clear evidence that availability of method influences method choice for suicide. Also changes in availability of popular methods of suicide, as shown in the change from coal gas to natural gas in the UK, can have substantial effects on suicides rates.

Firearms in the home appear to be associated with an increased risk of firearm suicide and an increased absolute risk of suicide. There is limited evidence that modification of firearm availability results in reduced risk of suicide. One awaits major changes in availability of firearms in a country such as the USA, in which suicides by this method are common, to provide clearer evidence of just how effective such a step might be.

Another implication of the evidence presented in this chapter is that it is essential that access to dangerous methods of suicidal behaviour is an integral part of clinical assessment of depressed or suicidal individuals. Dangerous methods should, as far as possible, be removed from the homes of those at risk. There should also be a public education policy regarding the risks associated with having dangerous methods of suicide available in the home. Such a policy should, however, be designed with care, particularly with regard to the potentially negative impact that the provision of such information can have on those who are already suicidal. Finally, serious efforts should be made to substantially reduce the availability of specific methods of suicide, especially from households.

It is quite clear that tackling availability of specific methods of suicide in individual countries must be an important element in national suicide prevention strategies. While not addressing the underlying causes of suicide, it is a policy which may have significant impact on overall suicide rates.

References

Abu al-Ragheb, S.Y. and Salhab, A.S. (1989). Pesticide mortality. A Jordanian experience. *American Journal of Forensic Medicine and Pathology*, 10, 221–5.

Beck, A.T., Schuyler, D., and Herman, I. (1974). Development of Suicidal Intent Scales. In *The prediction of suicide*, (ed. A.T. Beck, H.L.P. Resnik, and D.J. Lettieri). Charles Press, Philadelphia, PA.

Bialas, M.C., Reid, P.G., Beck, P., Lazarus, J.H., Smith, P.M., Scorer, R.C., *et al.* (1996). Changing patterns of self-poisoning in a UK health district. *Quarterly Journal of Medicine*, 89, 893–901.

Bowles, J.R. (1995). Suicide in Western Samoa: an example of a suicide prevention program in a developing country. In *Preventive strategies on suicide*, (ed. R. Diekstra). Brill, Leiden.

Brent, D.A., Perper, J.A., Allman, C.J., Moritz, G.M., Wartella, M.E., and Zelenak, J.P. (1991). The presence and accessibility of firearms in the homes of adolescent suicides. A case-control study. *Journal of the American Medical Association*, 266, 2989–95.

Cantor, C.H. and Slater, P.J. (1995). The impact of firearm control legislation on suicide in Queensland: preliminary findings. *Medical Journal of Australia*, 162, 583–5.

de Moore, G.M., Plew, J.D., Bray, K.M., and Snars, J.N. (1994). Survivors of self-inflicted firearm injury. A liaison psychiatry perspective. *Medical Journal of Australia*, 160, 421–5.

Eddleston, M. (2000). Patterns and problems of deliberate self-poisoning in the developing world. *Quarterly Journal of Medicine*, 93, 715–31.

Eddleston, M. and Phillips, M.R. (2004). Self poisoning with pesticides. *British Medical Journal*, 328, 42–4.

Gunnell, D. and Eddleston, M. (2003). Suicide by intentional ingestion of pesticides: a continuing tragedy in developing countries. *International Journal of Epidemiology*, 32, 902–9.

Gunnell, D., Hawton, K., Murray, V., Garnier, R., Bismuth, C., Fagg, J., *et al.* (1997). Use of paracetamol for suicide and non-fatal poisoning in the UK and France: are restrictions on availability justified? *Journal of Epidemiology and Community Health*, 51, 175–9.

Hawton, K. (2002). United Kingdom legislation on pack sizes of analgesics: background, rationale, and effects on suicide and deliberate self-harm. *Suicide and Life-Threatening Behavior*, 32, 223–9.

Hawton, K. and Catalan, J. (1987). *Attempted suicide: a practical guide to its nature and management.* Oxford University Press, Oxford.

Hawton, K. and Van Heeringen, K. (2000). *The international handbook of suicide and attempted suicide.* Wiley, Chichester.

Hawton, K., Ware, C., Mistry, H., Hewitt, J., Kingsbury, S., Roberts, D., and Weitzel, H. (1995). Why patients choose paracetamol for self poisoning and their knowledge of its dangers. *British Medical Journal*, 310, 164.

Hawton, K., Fagg, J., Simkin, S., Bale, E., and Bond, A. (1997). Trends in deliberate self-harm in Oxford, 1985–1995. Implications for clinical services and the prevention of suicide. *British Journal of Psychiatry*, 171, 556–60.

Hawton, K., Fagg, J., Simkin, S., Harriss, L., and Malmberg, A. (1998). Methods used for suicide by farmers in England and Wales: the contribution of availability and its relevance to prevention. *British Journal of Psychiatry*, 173, 320–4.

Hawton, K., Townsend, E., Deeks, J.J., Appleby, L., Gunnell, D., Bennewith, O., *et al.* (2001). Effects of legislation restricting pack sizes of paracetamol and salicylates on self poisoning in the United Kingdom: before and after study. *British Medical Journal*, 322, 1203–7.

Hawton, K., Simkin, S., Deeks, J.J., Cooper, J., Johnston, A., Waters, K., *et al.* (2004). United Kingdom legislation on analgesic packs: before and after study of long-term impact on poisonings. *British Medical Journal*, 329, 1076–9.

Kellermann, A.L., Rivara, F.P., Somes, G., Reay, D.T., Francisco, J., Banton, J.G., *et al.* (1992). Suicide in the home in relation to gun ownership. *New England Journal of Medicine*, 327, 467–72.

Kreitman, N. (1976). The coal gas story: United Kingdom suicide rates 1960–1971. *British Journal of Preventive and Social Medicine*, 30, 86–93.

Lester, D. and Leenaars, A. (1993). Suicide rates in Canada before and after tightening firearm control laws. *Psychological Reports*, 72, 787–90.

Loftin, C., McDowall, D., Wiersema, B., and Cottey, T. J. (1991). Effects of restrictive licensing of handguns on homicide and suicide in the District of Columbia. *New England Journal of Medicine*, 325, 1615–20.

Ludwig, J. and Cook, P.J. (2000). Homicide and suicide rates associated with implementation of the Brady Handgun Violence Prevention Act. *Journal of the American Medical Association*, 284, 585–91.

O'Donnell, I., Arthur, A. J., and Farmer, R.D.J. (1994). A follow-up study of attempted railway suicides. *Social Science and Medicine*, 38, 437–42.

O'Grady, J. (1999). Acute liver failure. *Medicine*, 27, 80–2.

Peterson, L.G., Peterson, M., O'Shanick, G.J., and Swann, A. (1985). Self-inflicted gunshot wounds: lethality of method versus intent. *American Journal of Psychiatry*, 142, 228–31.

Phillips, M.R., Yang, G., Zhang, Y., Wang, L., Ji, H., and Zhou, M. (2002). Risk factors for suicide in China: a national case-control psychological autopsy study. *Lancet*, 360, 1728–36.

Seiden, R.H. (1978). Where are they now? A follow-up study of suicide attempters from the Golden Gate Bridge. *Suicide and Life-Threatening Behavior*, 8, 203–16.

Snowdon, J. and Harris, L. (1992). Firearm suicides in Australia. *Medical Journal of Australia*, 156, 79–83.

17

Media influences on suicidal behaviour: evidence and prevention

Keith Hawton and Kathryn Williams

Introduction

Suicidal behaviour can result from a range of interacting factors, including psychiatric disorder, personality and psychological characteristics, socio-economic and interpersonal problems, and genetic and biological influences (Hawton and van Heeringen 2000). A further factor is exposure to suicidal behaviour, either via direct contact with suicidal individuals or indirectly via media portrayals and reporting. According to the stress:diathesis model of suicidal behaviour (Mann *et al.* 1999), some factors (e.g. genetic factors, early upbringing) may increase long-term vulnerability to suicidal behaviour (diathesis) and others (e.g. life events) may increase risk at a particular time (stressors). Media influences are usually viewed as acting as facilitators, in an acute sense. There is preliminary evidence that they may also increase vulnerability to suicidal behaviour in a longer-term sense.

There has been longstanding interest in the extent to which suicidal behaviour in the media can influence certain people who are exposed to it. This has relevance to national suicide prevention initiatives (Taylor *et al.* 1997; US Department of Health and Human Services, Public Health Service 2001; Department of Health 2002).

In order to be confident that media stimuli have influenced suicidal behaviour there should ideally be:

(1) evidence of changes in rates of suicide or attempted suicide, or in the nature of suicidal behaviour, following the media stimulus;

(2) control for seasonal and other factors which might influence suicidal behaviour when changes in the behaviour following a media stimulus are being investigated;

(3) evidence that individuals who engaged in suicidal behaviour following a media event were actually exposed to it; and

(4) further evidence of an effect if the media stimulus is repeated.

In order to show a possible prevention effect on suicidal behaviour the same criteria should apply. However, the main focus in prevention is on modification of media stimuli to see if this produces a change (reduction) in levels of suicidal behaviour.

A systematic review of the evidence regarding media influences on suicidal behaviour

Recently we conducted a systematic review, with the aim of assembling all the available evidence on media and suicidal behaviour, in order to address the following questions:

- Is there a media effect on suicidal behaviour?
- If so, how strong is the effect? What is the timing of the effect?
- Under what conditions are effects most likely?
- Which specific features of the message, medium, and audience promote suicidal behaviour?
- Can suicidal behaviour be prevented by changing media presentations, or through specific initiatives in the media?

We used a comprehensive approach in searching for information for the review. We searched several electronic databases (British Nursing Index; RCN Journals Database; EMBASE; Medline Express, PsychLIT/PsychInfo; Sociological Abstracts). Researchers in 26 countries were contacted to seek articles in local languages, published and unpublished. We assembled an advisory group of international experts who provided peer review of the draft of our report, commented on the conclusions, and endorsed the final version.

The literature search identified almost 200 articles, including natural experiments, case studies, anecdotal reports, studies based on content analysis and investigations of reactions to different types of media reports among volunteers. Here we summarize the findings, beginning with news reports of suicide and attempted suicide, and then going on to fictional suicidal behaviour. We also consider music and literature, the Internet, and suicide instructions. We then go on to consider evidence about whether changes in media reporting of suicide can be beneficial, and the potential contrasting influences of public education via the media and facilitation of suicidal behaviour.

Suicide in the news

We divided the studies of suicide in the news into three groups: first, newspaper reports; secondly, reports on TV; and, thirdly, studies which examined multiple media channels.

Newspaper reports

We identified 34 studies examining the impact of newspaper reports on completed suicide. In 22 of these there was an increase in suicides following the reports. One early influential example was the demonstration by Phillips (1974) that national suicide rates in the USA rose after 26 suicide stories appeared on the front page of the *New York Times* between 1948 and 1968. Stories that received more publicity were associated with greater increases in suicide rates than less prominent stories.

While the majority of studies of the possible influence of newspaper reports on suicide were conducted in the USA, there have also been studies in Australia, Germany, Japan, Switzerland, and the UK. In 10 studies there was some evidence that a causal link had been established between news reports and subsequent suicides. Since we completed our review we have become aware of a most dramatic example of how newspaper reporting of a specific method of suicide can lead to an increase of people choosing to die by that method. This comes from Hong Kong. In November 1998 there was a newspaper report of the first known example of someone killing themselves by carbon monoxide poisoning, using the fumes from a barbecue inside a sealed room or apartment. The pictures in the newspaper reports of the first case showed a 35-year-old dead woman looking very peaceful, and also showed the barbecue by her toilet in the adjoining room. This event started a remarkable 'epidemic' of this method of suicide (Lee *et al.* 2002). Nine further charcoal burning suicides occurred in Hong Kong during the following month. By the end of 1998 charcoal burning had become the third most common method of suicide in Hong Kong. The incidence of suicide by this method continued to rise in subsequent years, such that by 2001 it had become the second most common method of suicide, and represented a quarter of all suicides (Chan *et al.* 2003). It appears to have spread to Macau and Taiwan via the Internet (Chan *et al.* 2003). An analysis of coroners' records from the first 100 deaths by charcoal burning revealed that victims were mainly middle-aged, unmarried people with no history of substance abuse or mental disorders (Lee *et al.* 2002). About 80% had experienced one or more recent stressors, particularly debt. Media reports presented charcoal burning as 'a legitimate way out of the person's financial predicament' (Chan *et al.* 2003).

Fewer studies of the potential impact of news reports of suicidal behaviour have focused on newspapers reports of attempted suicide. A statistically significant increase in deliberate self-poisoning with ethylene glycol (anti-freeze) occurred in the UK following a newspaper report of such an episode (Veysey *et al.* 1999).

Television news

Most of the evidence concerning the possible impact of television news reports of suicides comes from a series of studies in the USA. In 10 of 13 such investigations, an increase in completed suicide was identified following news reports that appeared on at least two of the three national television networks. Statistically significant rises in general population suicide rates were observed nationally in three studies. Five studies showed an impact among teenagers. One example was an increase in teenage suicides following 38 TV news reports of suicides in the USA (Phillips and Carstensen 1986). Changes in teenage suicide rates were positively correlated with the number of news programmes that carried each story, suggesting a dose–response effect. One study also showed an effect in elderly people (Stack 1990b). In addition, an increase in suicide following stories of murder-suicides was also found in one study (Stack 1989).

Just one study was identified from outside America: nine people attempted suicide—seven fatally—on the Austrian railways in the week following a TV news story about the stress of train drivers worrying about railway suicides (Deisenhammer et al. 1997). This represented a statistically significant increase in suicide attempts on the railways. Interestingly, the news report did not mention a specific incident but drew attention to a suicide method likely to be perceived as quick and lethal.

News coverage by more than one medium

Although the studies mentioned above focused exclusively on either newspaper or television news, it is of course very likely that some of the news reports would have occurred in multiple media. Stories appearing in more than one news medium were examined specifically in 12 studies, and in 7 of these an increase in suicide rates was identified. In this group of studies there was particularly strong evidence of causal links between reports and suicidal behaviour. For example, the heart drug used in the highly publicized suicide of Miss Hungary in 1986 was chosen as the method of poisoning suicide by 25 other individuals in Hungary during the following 6 months (Fekete and Macsai 1990), compared with just three in the previous 6 months. Although the medical use of that drug declined by almost 40% in the next 3 years, the use of the drug for suicide continued to increase, particularly among young women. Peaks in suicides using the drug were observed following renewed publicity. Interviews with relatives in one county in Hungary revealed that in 11 of 13 cases, the suicidal individual had read the biography of Miss Hungary immediately before their death.

Another example was the suicide in Japan of the popular 18-year-old singer, Yukiko Okada. Two hours after cutting her wrists she jumped to her death from a seven-storey building. This event was widely reported on TV and in newspapers. This was followed by a big increase in suicide by jumping in teenagers, especially girls. There was clear evidence of a link to Yukiko Okada's death in several cases, including one female victim who said before her death by jumping that she wanted to become like Yukiko Okada, and a boy who jumped from the same building as the popstar (Takahashi 1998).

Fictional suicides

Film and TV portrayals

Fictional suicides in films and television dramas were the subject of 13 studies. Of these, five demonstrated an increase in completed suicide following the broadcasts. For example, Schmidtke and Häfner (1988) found that the railway suicide of a 19-year-old man, which was shown at the start of all six episodes of a German television series, *Death of a student,* was associated with a marked increase in suicides by this method during and following the series. Railway suicides by teenage males increased 175% compared with expected figures, based on the previous 5 years and the subsequent 2 years. Increases were also observed among young men and women (aged 15–29 years) but not among older people. Small increases in railway suicides occurred following a second showing of the series, which was in keeping with the lower viewing figures. No evidence was found of a change in methods of suicide by other means, suggesting an absolute increase in suicides overall.

A further four studies demonstrated a significant increase in attempted suicide following television and film portrayals of suicidal behaviour. Particularly convincing evidence of a media effect was found for an episode of a British hospital drama, *Casualty,* in which a man took a presumed fatal overdose of paracetamol (Hawton *et al.* 1999). This episode, which was viewed by more than 12 million people, was followed by a significant increase in self-poisoning during the subsequent 2 weeks, particularly with paracetamol. Interviews with self-poisoning patients before and after the episode showed that the proportion taking paracetamol (versus other substances) was considerably greater among patients who saw that episode compared with patients who had seen previous *Casualty* episodes and presented to hospital because of overdoses before the broadcast.

Music and literature

The potential impact of exposure to certain types of music remains an open question. One study demonstrated that suicide rates were higher in American cities where country music was played more often on the radio (Stack and

Gundlach 1992). However, this finding was challenged due to methodological problems (Maguire and Snipes 1994; Snipes and Maguire 1995). Preference for heavy metal music has been linked with self-harm (Martin *et al.* 1993), reckless behaviour (Arnett 1991), and weaker 'reasons for living' (Scheel and Westefeld 1999). The association with suicide risk factors appears especially strong among female fans of heavy metal (Arnett 1991; Martin *et al.* 1993; Lacourse *et al.*, unpublished). Nevertheless, no conclusions regarding cause and effect can be drawn from such studies. Rather, it appears that some individuals who like heavy metal music also tend to have other risk factors for suicidal behaviour, such as substance abuse, poor relationships with parents, depression, and alienation.

There is also preliminary evidence that listeners' perceptions of music may be altered by labelling it as either 'suicide-inducing' or 'life-affirming' (North and Hargreaves 2005). When exposed to songs with ambiguous lyrics, young people who were told this music had been implicated in the deaths of several teenagers tended to describe it as 'suicide-inducing', while those who were told it contained positive messages about working through one's problems tended to see it in this more hopeful light. The authors suggested that the most effective way to prevent negative effects of so-called 'suicide-inducing' music may be to 'censor the censors' (North and Hargreaves 2005).

Operas often include suicides, but their potential effects have not been studied systematically. Similarly, there is an absence of research investigating the impact of suicides in literature and mythology, although there are anecdotal reports. In fact, one name given to media influence on suicidal behaviour (the 'Werther effect') is based on the apparent epidemic of suicides by shooting after the publication in 1774 of Goethe's book, *The sorrows of young Werther*, in which the hero died by shooting himself when his love for a woman was not reciprocated (Phillips 1974). The novel was said to be the most widely read book in Europe at the time, was influential in the movement towards Romanticism in art and literature, and even inspired male fashions, based on the outfit Werther adopted. A recent study, which examined suicide reports following the book's publication, confirmed that at least a few imitative suicides did indeed occur, but questioned whether this constituted a real 'epidemic' (Thorson and Öberg 2003).

Characteristics of influential presentations

There appear to be links between suicidal behaviour and specific aspects of media presentations. Thus, media impacts appear most likely or most extreme when:

(1) the method of suicide is specified, especially when details are provided (Ashton and Donnan 1981; Schmidtke and Häfner 1988; Fekete and Macsai 1990; Hawton *et al.* 1999; Veysey *et al.* 1999);

(2) the story is repeated (Phillips 1974; Phillilps and Carstensen 1986; Stack 1987);

(3) the story is reported dramatically and prominently, for example with photographs of the deceased or large headlines in newspaper reports (Stack 1987; Kopping *et al.* 1989);

(4) celebrity suicides are reported (Wasserman 1984; Stack 1987, 1990a; Fekete and Macsai 1990).

Vulnerability to media influences

Younger people appear to be more vulnerable to media effects than older adults, as they are to 'contagious' suicidal behaviour in general, as reflected in suicide clusters (Gould *et al.* 1990). There is limited evidence that the elderly may also be more vulnerable, especially to stories about people their own age (Stack 1990b, 1991). Media influences appear greater when there is close similarity between the media stimulus or model and the observer, in terms of age, gender, and nationality. Nevertheless, in many other cases the suicidal individual appears to have had little in common with the media model, yet apparently identified with him or her sufficiently to trigger suicidal behaviour.

Biases in media reporting or portrayal of suicide

Reports or portrayals of suicidal behaviour usually oversimplify the causes. Thus suicide may be represented as the result of a single factor, such as financial difficulty, exam failure, or loss of a relationship. Importantly, the links with mental health problems, which occur in approximately 90% of suicides (Foster *et al.* 1997), are often missing (Fishman and Weimann 1997). Such biases may not only mislead the public about the nature of suicide, but may also possibly encourage suicidal acts in response to the types of stresses represented in the media.

The Internet

Searching the Internet using search terms such as 'suicide' identifies many thousands of sites (Baume *et al.* 1997; Mehlum 2001). One group of these is concerned with provision of constructive and useful information aimed at providing greater understanding of the reasons for suicidal behaviour. Others provide advice and information for people seeking help with dealing with suicidal thoughts. A third category of site includes 'chatrooms' or newsgroups;

the former allow discussions between individuals, and the latter enables people to post messages on electronic news boards to which anyone may respond (Baume *et al.* 1997, 1998). Finally, there are sites that provide instructions on suicide methods (Alao *et al.* 1999) or even encourage suicide, including by pairing up suicidal individuals.

There has been very little research on the impact of such sites. For example, we do not know if some sites may transmit suicide in a contagious manner. The fact that the Internet crosses national boundaries makes investigation of this very difficult. Mehlum (2001) suggests that this may come about because sites may present suicide as a solution to difficulties rather than as itself being a problem. Chatrooms and newsgroups attract young people who are encouraged to discuss their suicidal feelings and the desirability (or otherwise) of suicide. For many people some Internet sites may be helpful, especially those concerned with self-help (Prasad and Owens 2001). But for others, especially those entering sites that encourage suicide, the risk may be increased. Such sites may directly increase risk, such as by putting suicidal individuals in touch with each other as a means of supporting and encouraging suicidal impulses (Baume *et al.* 1997), or indirectly add to risk simply by exposure to their content. They may also be used by suicidal individuals to post suicide notes, including serial notes that document the progression of a person's suicidal ideas and activities. Others may respond to such notes by further encouraging suicide (Baume *et al.* 1997). It is likely that isolated individuals are more vulnerable to such influences from the Internet.

What impact can others have on the potential role of the Internet in suicide prevention? One important task is for organizations concerned with suicide prevention to ensure that there are high-quality Internet sites aimed at provision of support, help, and preventive advice. A second possibility is for feedback to be provided to poor or dangerous sites. However, individual sites are not subject to external regulations outside the country from which they originate. Thirdly, there is the possibility of developing Internet counselling, especially by email. Such an initiative has been established by Samaritans in the UK.

Since we have little or no information about the role of the Internet in contributing to suicide or to suicide prevention, there are clearly major research challenges in this area.

Suicide instructions

Information on methods of suicide is widely available on the Internet, through newsgroups and the World Wide Web. However, the impact of these is difficult to study and we did not identify any scientific investigations in this area, although there was anecdotal evidence of individuals using methods of suicide found on the Internet (Alao *et al.* 1999).

Following publication in America of *Final exit*, a suicide manual with instructions on a fast and pain-free method of suicide, there was a 30% increase in suicides in the USA by the main method described, namely the use of plastic bags (Marzuk *et al.* 1994*a*). There was a further 5.4% increase in suicides using the medication recommended in the book. A study by the same authors in New York found that of 144 people who died using plastic bags and/or the recommended medication, 15 left evidence of exposure to the book, such as it being found by their bodies (Marzuk *et al.* 1994*b*). However, there was no apparent overall effect on suicide rates.

Long-term influences of media

There has been little research on the potential long-term effects of exposure to suicide via the media. Research in Canada suggests that this exposure takes place very early in a child's life—by the age of seven for more than half of the children in one study (Mishara 1999, 2003). All of the older children in the study could report at least one death by suicide that they had witnessed in a television programme. Along with conversations with other children, television was the main source of information about suicide for children of all ages (Mishara 1999). It has been suggested that the understandings of suicide that children develop through media messages remain with them throughout their lives, and may be expressed in actions later in adolescence or adulthood (Mishara 2003).

Preliminary evidence for this theory comes from a recent pilot study in which 12 young people who had recently self-harmed were interviewed about their exposure to suicide in the media and elsewhere (Zahl and Hawton 2004). More than half were able to identify specific media portrayals that had influenced their attitudes or behaviour regarding suicide or self-harm. Some recognized that they had first heard about suicide via the media, even though this had happened many years previously. Suicide stories presented on film or television were most likely to be recalled, and some patients were able to link such stories to strong visual images they experienced before or during an episode of self-harm.

Modification of newspaper reporting of suicides

In our review of the literature we found only three studies in which attempts were made to modify news reporting of suicides. In the first study, newspaper editors in Switzerland changed their policies on suicide reporting following consultation and collaboration with researchers. After the new policies were implemented, the researchers observed a reduction in the 'imitation risk score' of reports, including, for example, the length of reports, dramatic reporting, and use of pictures of the individuals who died by suicide or sites of their deaths (Michel *et al.* 2000). However, the possible impact of this initiative on suicidal behaviour was not assessed.

Studies conducted in Toronto and Vienna demonstrated that voluntary restrictions on newspaper reporting of subway suicides resulted in a decreased number of suicides by this method (Littmann 1983; Etzersdorfer and Sonneck 1998). While the number of suicides on Toronto's subway system doubled from 15 in 1970 to 30 in 1971, the number of newspaper reports about subway suicide increased even more. A voluntary 6-month moratorium on reporting was introduced in response to concerns that an epidemic was developing; after this, the number of subway suicides (and stories) returned to baseline levels (Littmann 1983). Dramatic and sensational reporting of subway suicide in Vienna ceased abruptly with the introduction of media guidelines in July 1987. The number of subway suicides fell by 75% in the second half of 1987 (Sonneck *et al.* 1994) and a similar drop was observed for suicide attempts (Etzersdorfer *et al.* 1992). The reduction in both reporting and incidence of subway suicide was maintained over the next 9 years; researchers responded immediately to any new report by sending the journalist a copy of the guidelines (Etzersdorfer and Sonneck 1998).

Potential educational influences of media

So far we have largely focused on how media reporting and portrayal of suicidal behaviour may facilitate suicide and attempted suicide. In the study of the British hospital drama, *Casualty*, that was described earlier, a questionnaire survey of members of the BBC viewing panel was also conducted to assess their knowledge of the dangers of various types of overdoses (O' Connor *et al.* 1999). Members of the panel were surveyed twice: first, immediately following the episode, and, secondly, 8 months later. After adjusting for differences in age, gender, social group, region, interest in medical matters, medical knowledge (tested by three multiple choice questions), and reported viewing of medical dramas, those who had seen the episode of *Casualty* were markedly better informed about the dangers of taking too much paracetamol than were those who had not seen it. There were no major differences with regard to knowledge of the dangers or otherwise of overdoses of other common substances. Eight months later this difference persisted, with only a small reduction in its size.

A finding such as this highlights a major dilemma. While a TV programme can influence suicidal behaviour in a minority of the population, it also has the potential to provide valuable public health information to the majority.

Conclusions

There is clear evidence that media reporting and portrayal of suicidal behaviour can lead to increases in suicidal behaviour under certain circumstances. The potential impact of the media is more marked where methods of suicide are specified, there is prominent and/or repetitive news coverage, and where celebrity suicides are reported. Young people, in particular, appear to be more vulnerable to media effects. The causes of suicide are often misleadingly represented. These conclusions are supported by the findings of others who have reviewed the literature (Pirkis and Blood 2001).

There is preliminary evidence that modified reporting of suicides can be achieved, leading in turn to fewer suicides by specific methods. This suggests there is considerable potential for dialogue with the media to address the issues identified in this review. Longer-term impacts of media presentations on attitudes to, and knowledge of, suicide have hardly been explored, and this is an area in which further research is needed.

The issue of media influence on suicidal behaviour is an important one, which should be addressed as part of broader suicide prevention policy. Benefits in this area are most likely to be achieved through close collaboration with media personnel in order to explore ways of tackling the issue of suicide responsibly while respecting and protecting media freedoms.

Informing media personnel of the now reasonably strong research findings in this area is clearly a necessary step. Guidelines prepared in collaboration with the media to assist journalists, TV producers, and film makers when dealing with suicide are also important (Centre for Disease Control *et al.* 2002). Ensuring that this topic is included in the curricula of media studies and journalism courses is an essential investment for the future. A further possibility is the establishment of a watchdog body, as has been the case in Australia (Mediawatch), to provide feedback to the media on good and bad examples of media reporting and portrayal of suicidal behaviour.

Acknowledgements

We thank the members of our review advisory group: Robert Goldney (Australia), Madelyn Gould (USA), Brian Mishara (Canada), Stephen Platt (Scotland) and Lakshmi Vijayakumar (India). We also thank the many other individuals who helped identify relevant papers, and Chris Bale and Lesley

Bygrave for their advice and support. Financial support for the systematic review was provided by Syngenta.

References

Alao, A.O., Yolles, J.C., and Armenta, W. (1999). Cybersuicide: the Internet and suicide. *American Journal of Psychiatry*, 156, 1836–7.

Arnett, J. (1991). Heavy metal music and reckless behaviour among adolescents. *Journal of Youth and Adolescence*, 20, 573–92.

Ashton, J.R. and Donnan, S. (1981). Suicide by burning as an epidemic phenomenon: An analysis of 82 deaths and inquests in England and Wales in 1978–9. *Psychological Medicine*, 11, 735–9.

Baume, P., Cantor, C.H., and Rolfe, A. (1997). Cybersuicide: the role of interactive suicide notes on the Internet. *Crisis*, 18, 73–9.

Baume, P., Rolfe, A., and Clinton, M. (1998). Suicide on the Internet: a focus for nursing intervention? *Australian and New Zealand Journal of Mental Health Nursing*, 7, 134–41.

Centers for Disease Control and Prevention, National Institute of Mental Health, Office of the Surgeon General, Substance Abuse and Mental Health Services Administration, American Foundation for Suicide Prevention, American Association of Suicidology, and Annenberg Public Policy Center (2002). Reporting on suicide: Recommendations for the media. *Suicide and Life-Threatening Behavior*, 32, viii-xiii.

Chan, K.P., Lee, D.T., and Yip, P.S. (2003). Media influence on suicide. Media's role is double edged. *British Medical Journal*, 326, 498.

Deisenhammer, E.A., Kemmler, G., De Col, C., Fleischhacker, W.W., and Hinterhuber, H. (1997). Eisenbahnsuizide und—suizidversuche in Österreich von 1990–1994. Erweiterung der Hypothese medialer Vermittlung suizidalen Verhaltens. *Nervenarzt*, 68, 67–73.

Department of Health (2002). *National suicide prevention strategy for England*. Department of Health, London.

Etzerdorfer, E., Sonneck, G., and Nagel-Kuess, S. (1992). Newspaper reports and suicide. *New England Journal of Medicine*, 327, 502–3.

Etzersdorfer, E. and Sonneck, G. (1998). Preventing suicide by influencing mass media reporting. The Viennese experience, 1980–1996. *Archives of Suicide Research*, 4, 67–74.

Fekete, S. and Macsai, E. (1990). Hungarian suicide models, past and present. In *Suicidal behaviour and risk factors*, (ed. G. Ferrari, M. Bellini, and P. Crepet), pp. 149–56. Monduzzi Editore, Bologna.

Fishman, G. and Weimann, G. (1997). Motives to commit suicide: statistical versus mass-mediated reality. *Archives of Suicide Research*, 3, 199–212.

Foster, T., Gillespie, K., and McClelland, R. (1997). Mental disorders and suicide in Northern Ireland. *British Journal of Psychiatry*, 170, 447–52.

Gould, M.S., Wallenstein, S., Kleinman, M.H., O'Carroll, P., and Mercy, J. (1990). Suicide clusters: an examination of age-specific effects. *American Journal of Public Health*, 80, 211–12.

Hawton, K. and Van Heeringen, K. (2000). *The international handbook of suicide and attempted suicide*. Wiley, Chichester.

Hawton, K., Simkin, S., Deeks, J.J., O'Connor, S., Keen, A., Altman, D.G. *et al.* (1999). Effects of a drug overdose in a television drama on presentations to hospital for self poisoning: time series and questionnaire study. *British Medical Journal*, 318, 972–7.

Kopping, A.P., Ganzeboom, H.B.G., and Swanborn, P.G. (1989). Verhoging van suicide in navolging van kranteberichten. *Nederlands Tijdschrift voor de Psychologie en haar Grensgebieden*, 44, 62–72.

Lacourse, E., Claes, M., and Villeneuve, M. Heavy metal music and adolescent suicidal risk, unpublished manuscript.

Lee, D.T.S., Chan, K.P.M., Lee, S., Tin, S., and Yip, P.S.F. (2002). Burning charcoal: a novel and contagious method of suicide in Asia. *Archives of General Psychiatry*, 59, 293–4.

Littmann, S.K. (1983). The role of the press in the control of suicide epidemics. *Proceedings of the International Association for Suicide Prevention and Crisis Intervention*, pp. 166–70. Pergamon Press, Paris.

Maguire, E.R. and Snipes, J.B. (1994). Reassessing the link between country music and suicide. *Social Forces*, 72, 1239–43.

Mann, J.J., Waterman, C., Haas, G.L., and Malone, K.M. (1999). Toward a clinical model of suicidal behaviour in psychiatric patients. *American Journal of Psychiatry*, 156, 181–9.

Martin, G., Clarke, M., and Pearce, C. (1993). Adolescent suicide: music preference as an indicator of vulnerability. *Journal of the American Academy of Child and Adolescent Psychiatry*, 32, 530–5.

Marzuk, P.M., Tardiff, K., and Leon, A.C. (1994a). Increase in fatal self-poisonings and suffocations in the year Final Exit was published: a national study. *American Journal of Psychiatry*, 151, 1813–14.

Marzuk, P.M., Tardiff, K., Hirsh, C.S., Leon, A.C., Stajic, M., Hartwell, N. *et al.* (1994b). Increase in suicide by asphyxiation in New York City after the publication of Final Exit. *Publishing Research Quarterly*, 10, 62–8.

Mehlum, L. (2001). The Internet and suicide prevention. In *Suicide risk and protective factors in the new millennium*, (ed. O.T. Grad) pp. 223–7. Ljubljana, Cankarjev dom.

Michel, K., Frey, C., Wyss, K., and Valach, L. (2000). An exercise in improving suicide reporting in print media. *Crisis*, 21, 1–10.

Mishara, B. (1999). Conceptions of death and suicide in children aged 6 to 12 and their implications for suicide prevention. *Suicide and Life-Threatening Behavior*, 29, 105–18.

Mishara, B. (2003). How the media influences children's conceptions of suicide. *Crisis*, 24, 128–30.

North, A.C. and Hargreaves, D.J. (2005). Labelling effects on the perceived deleterious consequences of pop music listening. *Journal Adolescence*, 28, 433–40.

O'Connor, S., Deeks, J.J., Hawton, K., Simkin, S., Keen, A., Altman, D.G., *et al.* (1999). Effects of a drug overdose in a television drama on knowledge of specific dangers of self poisoning: population based surveys. *British Medical Journal*, 318, 978–9.

Phillips, D.P. (1974). The influence of suggestion on suicide: substantive and theoretical implications of the Werther effect. *American Sociological Review*, 39, 340–54.

Phillips, D.P. and Carstensen, L.L. (1986). Clustering of teenage suicides after television news stories about suicide. *New England Journal of Medicine*, 315, 685–9.

Pirkis, J. and Blood, R.W. (2001). *Suicide and the media: a critical review.* Commonwealth Department of Health and Aged Care, Canberra.

Prasad, V. and Owens, D. (2001). Using the internet as a source of self-help for people who self-harm. *Psychiatric Bulletin*, 25, 222–5.

Scheel, K.R. and Westefeld, J.S. (1999). Heavy metal music and adolescent suicidality: an empirical investigation. *Adolescence*, 34, 253–73.

Schmidtke, A. and Häfner, H. (1988). The Werther effect after television films: new evidence for an old hypothesis. *Psychological Medicine*, 18, 665–76.

Snipes, J.B. and Maguire, E.R. (1995). Country music, suicide and spuriousness. *Social Forces*, 74, 327–9.

Sonneck, G., Etzerdorfer, E., and Nagel-Kuess, S. (1994). Imitative suicides on the Viennese subway. *Social Science and Medicine*, 38, 453–7.

Stack, S. (1987). Celebrities and suicide: a taxonomy and analysis. *American Sociological Review*, 52, 401–12.

Stack, S. (1989). The effect of publicised mass murders and murder-suicides on lethal violence, 1968–1980. *Social Psychiatry and Psychiatric Epidemiology*, 24, 202–8.

Stack, S. (1990a). Media impacts on suicide. In *Current concepts of suicide*, (ed. D. Lester) pp. 107–20. Charles Press, Philadelphia.

Stack, S. (1990b). Audience receptiveness, the media and aged suicides. *Journal of Ageing Studies*, 4, 195–209.

Stack S. (1991). Social correlates of suicide by age: media impacts. In *Life span perspectives of suicide: time-lines in the suicide process*, (ed. A.A. Leenaars), pp. 187–213. Plenum Press, New York.

Stack, S. and Gundlach, J. (1992). The effect of country music on suicide. *Social Forces*, 71, 211–18.

Takahashi, Y. (1998). Suicide in Japan. What are the problems? In *Suicide prevention*, (ed. R.J. Kosky *et al.*) pp. 121–30. Plenum Press, New York.

Taylor, S.J., Kingdom, D., and Jenkins, R. (1997). How are nations trying to prevent suicide? An analysis of national suicide prevention strategies. *Acta Psychiatrica Scandinavica*, 95, 457–63.

Thorson, J. and Öberg, P.A. (2003). Was there a suicide epidemic after Goethe's *Werther?* *Archives of Suicide Research*, 7, 69–72.

US Department of Health and Human Services, Public Health Service (2001). *National Strategy for Suicide Prevention: Goals and objectives for action.* Public Health Service, Rockville, MD.

Veysey, M., Kamanyire, R., and Volans, G.N. (1999). Antifreeze poisonings give more insight into copycat behaviour (letter). *British Medical Journal*, 319, 1131–2.

Wasserman, I.M. (1984). Imitation and suicide: a re-examination of the Werther effect. *American Sociological Review*, 49, 427–36.

Zahl, D.L. and Hawton, K. (2004). Media influences on suicidal behaviour: an interview study of young people. *Behavioural and Cognitive Psychotherapy*, 32, 189–98.

18

Suicide and suicide attempts in prisons

Jo Paton and Rachel Jenkins

Introduction

Suicide is the leading cause of death in prisons systems in most Western countries (Bureau of Justice Statistics 1993; Aardema *et al.* 1998; Dalton 1999). Resulting long-standing concerns have led to a considerable body of research, mainly from Western Europe, the USA, Canada, and Australia. However, the field is bedevilled by a variety of methodological problems that reduce the validity of the studies and limit the value of international comparisons. This chapter outlines the methodological issues, summarizes key findings about suicide and suicide attempts in prison settings, reports one major study in detail and then reviews what is known about prison suicide prevention programmes, evidence of their effectiveness, and prisoner views about them.

In this chapter, unless otherwise specified, we use the term 'prisoner' and 'prison' to refer to all of pre-trial/remand prisoners, convicted but un-sentenced prisoners, and sentenced prisoners, and to the institutions which hold them. Remand and sentenced prisoners are reported to have very different suicide rates, but only in the USA are they held in separate establishments, with studies reporting on them separately. We use the term 'suicide attempt' and 'self-injury' to mean, respectively, incidents of self-harm where the individual has indicated that their motivation was to die and incidents where their motivation was other than to die. The section on suicide prevention programmes focuses on interventions and strategies that aim to prevent suicide.

Methodological issues

A wide range of problems is involved in studying suicides and attempted suicides in prisons. The following list is indicative not exhaustive:

The opinions expressed in this chapter are those of the authors and do not represent the views of HM Prison Service.

1. *Suicide, even in prisons, is a rare event and many prison systems contain small numbers of prisoners.* The number of suicides reported is often too small to make the calculation of rates meaningful unless averaged over several years. Studies that report trends based on wildly fluctuating annual rates may mislead, and the use of such rates to demonstrate the effectiveness of a particular suicide prevention programme may be flawed.

2. *Data collection problems.* For example, national US studies rely on self-report questionnaires being returned by different federal and state prison and jail systems. Response rates vary (Hayes 1995).

3. *Who decides what is included as a 'suicide' and the definition used.* In England, Wales, Scotland and Australia the decision is made by an independent lawyer (coroner). Most early UK studies contain only deaths that received a verdict of 'suicide' although some include verdicts of both 'suicide' and 'undetermined cause' (open verdicts) (Lloyd 1990; Towl and Crighton 1998). More recently, official statistics in England and Wales and Australia, and studies based on those statistics, have broadened their definition to also include deaths that receive verdicts of 'accident' and 'misadventure' where deaths are by hanging (Australia) or where there is an absence of strong evidence that the prisoner did not intend to die (England and Wales). These are termed 'apparent suicides' or 'self-inflicted deaths'. By contrast, US statistics do not include deaths by 'unspecified causes' (17% of total deaths reported to Bureau of Justice Statistics in 1992) or accidents (Bureau of Justice Statistics 1993). Reported suicide rates in the general population in England and Wales include deaths with verdicts of 'suicide' and 'undetermined' in cases of poisoning or injury only. Some have argued that this underestimates the community suicide rate (O'Donnell and Farmer 1995). The differences are significant. Dooley points out that up to 35% of deaths in prison in England and Wales in the 1970s and 1980s with verdicts of 'undetermined' or 'misadventures' were probably suicides (Dooley 1990*a*). Between 1992 and 2000, an average of 15% of deaths recorded by the English and Welsh Prison Service as suicides received verdicts other than 'suicide' or 'undetermined' (Teers 2004).

4. *The way that suicide rates are calculated.* The most common, but not universal, method used to calculate suicide rates is on the basis of the numbers of deaths per 'average daily population' or ADP. Remand prisoners typically spend much shorter periods in prison than do sentenced prisoners. Each annual prisoner-place is therefore occupied by several prisoners, each of whom is usually only in the prison for weeks or months, at the time (the first day, week, and month in custody) when most suicides occur. So this method may overestimate the rate of suicides, especially in

remand prisoners. Using the number of individual prisoners who enter the prison as the denominator can reduce suicide rates by a factor of five (Camilleri *et al.* 1999). (For a discussion of calculation of prison suicide rates, see O'Mahony 1994.)

5. *Lack of control for prisoner characteristics.* Almost uniformly, studies are not controlled for the differing characteristics of the prisoner population—mainly young males from lower socio-economic groups, and with black and indigenous ethnic minority groups over-represented (Liebling 1999). Neither are they controlled for rates of mental disorder or drug dependence (Gore 1999).

6. *Identification of psychiatric and substance misuse disorders.* Reports of the proportions of prisoners who kill themselves who had mental disorder or substance dependence are usually reports of service use rather than the prevalence of disorder, and reflect access to mental health services outside prison and the adequacy, or otherwise, of prison mental health screening (Shaw *et al.* 2003; Kovasznay *et al.* 2004).

7. *Prison systems differ.* For example, US 'prisons' hold those sentenced to more than 1 year and 'jails' hold people awaiting trial or sentenced to less than a year. The two types of facility have very different suicide rates. In other countries, quoted prison suicide rates include all types of prisoners.

Prevalence of suicide

Suicide rates among prisoners

Taking remand and sentenced prisoners together and using un-standardized rates, reported suicide rates in Europe are higher than rates in the general population by a factor of 2 (Poland), 7 (France), 9 (The Netherlands), 10 (Ireland), and 13 (Greece) (Aardema *et al.* 1998). In Australia, quoted rates are higher by a factor of 2.5 (using prisoners received into the system) or 15 (using ADP) (Temby 1990). In US jails (remand prisoners) and prisons (sentenced prisoners) rates are reported to average 9 times and 1.5 times the general population rate, respectively (Hayes and Kajdan 1981; Hayes 1995). Studies that use standardized mortality ratios report that suicide rates are higher in prison than in the general male population by a factor of 3.5 (Canada), 6 (England and Wales), 2 (Austrian sentenced prisoners), and 8 (Austrian remand prisoners and those with a diagnosed mental illness) (Ramsay *et al.* 1987; Fruehwald *et al.* 2002*a*; Snow *et al.* 2002).

Suicide rates among offenders under community supervision

Those few studies that consider suicide rates among offenders under community supervision indicate that the rates for male prisoners are not higher than rates among male offenders outside prison. In England and Wales, the suicide rates in the two groups were found to be similar, despite use of a method to calculate the rates of community offender deaths (total persons starting supervision—a count of individual people) that might be expected to result in a lower rate than the method used to calculate rates of prisoner deaths (ADP—a count of average annual places) (Sattar 2001). In Australia and New Zealand, a total mortality rate for non-custodial offenders of 5.6 times that of prisoners was found, with 21% of the deaths self-inflicted (Flemming *et al.* 1992).

Suicide rates among ex-prisoners

A recent finding from England and Wales showed that the number of suicides by convicted prisoners in the year following release from prison was more than double the number in prison. Between April 1996 and March 2000, 354 convicted prisoners died by suicide in the year following release from prison, 23% of whom died in the first month after release and 12% in the first week (Shaw *et al.* 2003). This compares with a total of 167 convicted prisoners who killed themselves in prison during this period (Safer Custody Group statistics). The definition of suicide used for deaths of prisoners was more inclusive than the definition used for released prisoners. No figures are available for the number of unconvicted prisoners, in those years, who killed themselves following release from prison.

Trends in prison suicide rates over time

Prisoner suicide rates are reported to have risen in Austria (from 1967 to 1996), France (1977–1997), England and Wales (1983–1997), and Scotland (1977–1999); to have remained broadly steady in Australia (1980–1998), the Irish Republic (1990–1999), The Netherlands, and the US jail system, which holds mainly remand prisoners (1982–1988); and to have decreased in the US prison system nationally, which holds mainly sentenced prisoners (1984–1992), and in the New York State Correctional System, which holds mainly newly arrested and remand prisoners (1984–1997) (Clavel *et al.* 1987; Hayes 1989, 1995, 1998; Liebling and Krarup 1993; Aardema *et al.* 1998; Blaauw *et al.* 1999; Williams 2001; Fruehwald *et al.* 2002*b*; Royal College of Psychiatrists 2002; Snow *et al.* 2002; Power *et al.* 2003).

The reasons for the changes are unknown or at least unproven. In England and Wales, Scotland, and Australia the trends in prison suicide rates have paralleled reported trends in community rates (Gunn 1996; Dalton 1999; Royal College of Psychiatrists 2002; Brock and Griffiths 2004). An increase in the consumption of drugs associated with suicide risk, especially cocaine and crack, has also been reported in England and Wales over this period (Ramsay et al. 2001). Other explanations offered include the rapid rise in prisoner numbers that occurred. Harvey and Liebling (2002) hypothesized that the speed of this rise had a disproportionate and negative impact on prisoner care, resulting in, for example, prisoners being moved frequently around the country to find a prison with bed-spaces and being located further from home. However, in Austria, the rise in prison suicide rate occurred during a period when the prison population decreased (Fruehwald et al. 2002b).

In England and Wales and Australia, the introduction of significant suicide prevention programmes was not followed by a drop in suicide rate. In the US prison system, the drop in rate occurred during a period when suicide prevention programmes were being introduced, following the setting of national standards. However, it is reported that only 15% of prison systems actually implemented the programmes as advised (Hayes 1995). In the New York State Correctional System, the drop in suicide rate does appear attributable to a consistently implemented suicide prevention programme (Cox and Morschauser 1997).

Patterns in prison suicides
Method of suicide

Most deaths by suicide of both male and female prisoners occur by hanging: 90%+ in England and Wales, Scotland, Australia, and the USA (Hayes and Kajdan 1981; Dooley 1990a; Dalton 1999; Snow et al. 2002; Power et al. 2003). This reflects the lack of availability of other methods of suicide in the prison setting.

In England and Wales, the most commonly used ligature point is a window and the most commonly used ligature is bedding, followed by shoelaces and then clothing. The great majority of deaths by hanging occur through asphyxiation as the ligature point is usually below head height, and this gives some small opportunity for intervention. In 2003 in England and Wales, 83 prisoners killed themselves by hanging and 50 prisoners attempted to hang themselves and were found and resuscitated (three individuals on two occasions) (Safer Custody Group 2004). In the general population in England and

Wales, suicide by hanging has increased over the past 30 years, although this method still accounts for just under half of male and a quarter of female suicides (Brock and Griffiths 2004).

Associated risk factors

Many studies have examined factors associated with suicides in order to guide prevention, but findings often conflict (for detailed reviews see Lloyd 1990; Camilleri *et al.* 1999; Liebling 1999). Several authors, most notably Liebling (Liebling and Krarup 1993), have argued that there is no one profile of the 'high-risk prisoner', but that it is possible to differentiate several different subtypes.

Age

Newly arrested and remand prisoners in the USA are reported to be more likely to be young, and sentenced prisoners more likely to be older (Hayes and Kajdan 1981; Hayes 1995). The prison population in all countries is made up primarily of socio-economically deprived young men, who make up the largest at-risk group in the community.

Gender

Female deaths have been relatively little studied because of their small numbers (females comprise an average of 4–5% of the prison population in all countries, although this is rising) (Liebling 1999).

Studies that include only deaths receiving a coroner's verdict of 'suicide' have found women to be under-represented in prison suicides (e.g. Dooley 1990*a*; Bogue and Power 1995). In the USA, where narrow definitions of suicide are used, no female suicides were reported in the federal prison system between 1970 and 1995, despite women forming 7% of the prison population (White and Schimmel, 1995).

Some studies that use a broader definition of suicide have found broadly similar rates of male and female deaths, and occasionally higher rates of female deaths (Hatty and Walker 1986; Liebling 1994; Towl and Fleming 1997; Mackenzie *et al.* 2003). Several studies indicate that proportionately fewer apparent suicides by women prisoners receive suicide verdicts at inquests (Dooley 1990*b*; Liebling 1994; Towl and Crighton 1998). As women outside prison are 3–4 times *less* likely to kill themselves than men, a similar or higher rate among women prisoners is very unexpected (Office for National Statistics 2003). A possible explanation is that in prison over 90% of women who kill themselves used the same lethal methods as men (hanging), whereas in the community only around a quarter do so (Department of Health 2002*a*). Other explanations that have been offered include the greater levels of mental health and drug problems in female prisoners and the specific impact of imprisonment on women (Liebling 1999).

Ethnicity

Suicide rates are higher in whites and lower in Afro-Caribbeans and black Americans (Snow *et al.* 2002; Kovasznay *et al.* 2004; New York State Department of Correctional Services 1994). A disproportionately low suicide rate by Afro-Caribbean people has also been reported in mental hospitals (Department of Health 2001, quoted in Gordon 2002) and elsewhere (Neeleman *et al.* 1997). In the USA, African-American prisoners are under-represented in self-harm figures (Livingston 1997). In contrast, suicides by indigenous minorities in Australia and New Zealand are reported to be in line with their (high) proportion of the prison population (Camilleri *et al.* 1999). Suicides by prisoners in Tanzania and Kenya are extremely rare (personal communications, Commissioners of Prisons).

Mental disorder and substance misuse

Many studies have noted high levels of diagnosis of mental disorder and drug misuse in cohorts of prison suicides (Topp 1979; Bogue and Power 1995; Shaw *et al.* 2003; Kovasznay *et al.* 2004). However, in the absence of a control group, they have not been able to show that these high levels of diagnosed disorder are different from those found in the general prisoner population. Furthermore, the studies reported the level of identification and treatment of disorders rather than the prevalence of disorders as such. As a result, several influential UK researchers have suggested that 'broadly defined mental disorder is not an indicator of increased risk of suicide in the prison population' (Towl and Crighton 1998; Liebling 2001). A case-control study of prison suicides in England and Wales is currently under way.

Stage of custody

Reports in England and Wales from 1911 onwards have shown consistently that suicides occur disproportionately in the early stages of custody (Smalley 1911; Topp 1979; Shaw *et al.* 2003). Between 1996 and 2003, 27% of suicides occurred in the first week and almost half of deaths (47%) occurred in the first month of custody (Safer Custody Group 2004). This pattern is remarkably similar to the pattern in in-patients in mental hospitals, where 24% of suicides occurred in the first week of admission (Department of Health 2001, quoted in Gordon 2002). In the USA, as many as 51–52% of new arrestees and unsentenced people in police lock-ups and jails who die by suicide kill themselves in the first 24 hours (Hayes and Kajdan 1981; Hayes 1989). An Austrian study found that risk is greater for these groups of prisoner in the early days, but that risk increased slightly for sentenced prisoners the longer they were in prison (Frottier *et al.* 2002).

Status of prisoner and type of prison

Suicide rates are higher in remand populations and in prisons (local prisons in the UK, jails in the USA) that hold mainly or solely remand prisoners, although this may be partially the result of the way rates are calculated (Backett 1988; Hayes, 1989; Dooley 1990a; Bogue and Power 1995; Morrison 1996).

Type of offence and length of sentence

Most studies find an association between suicide and being charged or convicted of a violent offence, especially homicide (Dooley 1990a; Kerkhof and Bernasco 1990; New York State Department of Correctional Services, 1994; Bogue and Power 1995; Morrison, 1996; Nock and Marzuk 2000). The main exceptions are studies of police lock-ups and jails in the USA, where most suicides occur among intoxicated, first time, non-violent offenders (Hayes 1989). The link between violence and self-destructive behaviour is well established (Plutchik and van Praag 1990).

Closely linked to this finding (and a mutually confounding variable) is the finding that, among sentenced prisoners, those on long sentences, and especially life sentences, are more likely to kill themselves (Topp 1979; Hatty and Walker 1986; Dooley 1990a; Lloyd 1990). Most people serving life sentences have been convicted of murder. Among lifers in England and Wales, two groups can broadly be identified: those who killed themselves relatively early in custody, most of whom had killed a close family member and were openly suicidal from their arrival in the prison; and those who killed themselves more than a year into custody, whose suicides appeared to have been triggered by setbacks in their custodial careers, such as failed appeals and licence failures (Borrill 2002).

Quality of prison life

There is some evidence of a relationship between the quality of prison life and suicides and suicidal thoughts. Rates of suicides in prisons that provide lower levels of purposeful activity are higher, irrespective of prison type (Leese 2003). In a study of 12 prisons in England and Wales, psychological distress and self-reported suicidal thoughts were higher in prisons where (using a Quality of Life survey of 100 randomly selected prisoners in each prison) prisoners reported more experiences of unfairness, feeling physically unsafe, and lower levels of assistance for particularly vulnerable individuals (Liebling *et al.* 2003).

Isolation/segregation

In the USA, suicides and attempted suicides are reported to be strongly associated with location, in the form of special locked units, such as segregation or psychiatric seclusion units (Bonner 1992; White and Schimmel 1995; Goss *et al.* 2002). In other countries, the relationship with special accommodation is either not found or has not been studied (Lloyd 1990; Camilleri *et al.* 1999). Research has shown consistently that most suicides occur where the prisoner is alone (Hayes 1989; Biles 1992; Camilleri *et al.* 1999).

Suicide clusters

In the closed environment of a prison, one prisoner suicide may encourage others. In Australia, at the height of the media debate about Aboriginal deaths in custody that was prompted by a Royal Commission investigation, there was an eightfold increase in the number of Aboriginal deaths by hanging in custody (Biles *et al.* 1992).

There is some evidence from both outside prison (Eisenberg 1986; Phillips and Carstensen 1986) and inside prison (Liebling 1992; Lester and Danto 1993) that this is particularly likely to be the case where young people who are themselves undergoing a crisis are exposed to the suicide of someone they see as similar to themselves. An evaluation of 'safer cells', which are designed to be as near ligature-free as possible, found that once one prisoner had discovered an innovative way to hang himself in a safer cell (using the door upper hinge as a ligature point), two more deaths swiftly occurred using the same method (Burrows *et al.* 2003).

Suicidal thoughts and suicide attempts in prisons

The national psychiatric morbidity survey in prisons in England and Wales provides the first comprehensive national survey of prison suicidal behaviour (Singleton *et al.* 1998). It is large enough to analyse for effects of gender and prisoner status, it gives comparative figures for prisoners who have never attempted suicide, it uses standardized measures of mental disorder and substance misuse, and it differentiates between suicide attempts and self-harm for other reasons. It therefore avoids many of the methodological limitations of studies of completed suicides and is important for the light it sheds on the psychiatric and social contribution to the high rate of suicide and on opportunities for prevention in prisons.

Prevalence of suicidal thoughts and attempts in prisoners

The study found that the lifetime prevalence of suicidal thoughts in prisoners, compared to people living at home, is increased by a factor of 3, the last year prevalence by a factor of 5–12, and the last week prevalence by a factor of more than 20. Over a quarter of male remand prisoners had attempted suicide in their lifetime, and one-sixth in the previous year. For female remand prisoners the figures were even higher, with nearly one-half having attempted suicide in their lifetime and over a quarter in the past year. The proportions of male and female sentenced prisoners who had tried to kill themselves were less than in the remand population (one-twelfth of male and one-sixth of female sentenced prisoners had tried to kill themselves in the past year), but none the less much higher than in the general population living in their own homes, where only 1% of both men and women had tried to kill themselves in the past year.

Prisoners who had had suicidal thoughts and attempted suicide in the past week, the past year, and over the course of their lifetime tended to be young, white, single, born in the UK, and to have left school early and be more poorly educated than non-suicidal prisoners.

Prisoners who had had suicidal thoughts and attempted suicide in the past week, past year, and over their lifetime were more likely to have very small primary support groups, to report a severe lack of social support, and to have experienced a variety of adverse life events, particularly violence or sexual abuse.

Between a third and a quarter of all prisoners have been in local authority care as a child. Prisoners who had attempted suicide in the past year were twice as likely to have been placed in care as a child than the non-suicidal prisoners.

Mental disorders in the general prisoner population

The National Psychiatric Morbidity studies used the same measures to estimate prevalence rates for mental disorders in the general population, in prisons, in mental institutions, and in homeless populations (Meltzer *et al.* 1994, 1995; Gill *et al.* 1996; Singleton *et al.* 1998). The figures from these studies, summarized in Table 18.1, show that prisoners in England and Wales have higher rates of morbidity than do residents in homeless hostels, and higher neurosis but lower psychosis levels than residents in psychiatric institutions.

Mental disorders in prisoners who think about and attempt suicide

Although mental disorders are very common in the general prisoner population, the study found that they are even more common in prisoners who think about or attempt suicide. The percentage of prisoners with neurotic disorder (depression, anxiety, obsessive–compulsive disorder, and/or

Table 18.1 Rates of mental disorders in different settings

Population	Psychosis	Neurosis	Alcohol dependence[b]	Drug dependence[c]
Residents of general households	0.4%	12.3% male; 19.5% female	7.5% male; 2.1% female	2.9% male; 1.5% female
Residents in homeless hostels	8%	38%	16%	6%
Male prisoners[a]	6–11%	40–59%	30%	34–43%
Female prisoners[a]	13–15%	63–76%	19–20%	36–52%
Residents in psychiatric institutions	78%	8%	Not available	Not available

[a]Lower figures in range represent percentage of sentenced prisoners, higher figures the percentage of remand prisoners with these disorders.
[b]Defined as Audit (Alcohol Use Disorder Identification Test) score of 30 or above.
[c]Defined as dependence on opiates, stimulants, or both.

phobias), psychosis, multiple personality disorders, and alcohol and drug dependence rose stepwise amongst those who had either thought about or attempted suicide in their lifetime, the past year, and the past week, compared to those prisoners who had never thought about or attempted suicide (Tables 18.2 and 18.3).

The disorders that most distinguished the suicidal from the non-suicidal groups of prisoners were psychosis and neurosis, with 41% of prisoners who had attempted suicide in the past week having a psychotic disorder, nearly 23 times the percentage of those who had never attempted suicide. It is of particular interest that the suicidal group were four or five times more likely to

Table 18.2 Psychiatric diagnoses of prisoners who have suicidal thoughts

Diagnosis	Percentage of prisoners who have thought about suicide			
	Past week	Past year	Lifetime	Never
Psychosis	26.1	16.3	12.0	1.6
Neurotic disorder	95.5	80.8	66.5	30.4
Heavy drinking (Audit score 16 or above)	40.5	37.3	37.1	25
Dependence on opiates, stimulants, or both	21.7	17.2	14.4	9.3
Diagnosis of antisocial personality disorder + another PD	54.9	55.7	51.6	26.1

PD, personality disorder.

Table 18.3 Psychiatric diagnoses of prisoners who attempt suicide

Diagnosis	Percentage of prisoners who have attempted suicide			
	Past week	Past year	Lifetime	Never
Psychosis	41.2	27	19.2	1.8
Neurotic disorder	85.1	83.9	68.7	37.6
Heavy drinking (Audit score 16 or above)	54.6	39.5	39.2	27
Dependence on opiates, stimulants, or both	33.5	19	15	10
Diagnosis of antisocial personality disorder + another PD	67.3	57	51.4	31.6

PD, personality disorder.

have extensive co-morbidity (i.e. four or five categories of psychiatric disorder simultaneously) than the non-suicidal prisoners. Indeed, 94% of those attempting suicide in the past week had three or more psychiatric disorders.

On the key question of whether suicidal thoughts occur in the absence of psychiatric disorder, only 0.5% of those with suicidal thoughts in the past week, 2.1% of those with suicidal thoughts in the past year, and 3% of those with suicidal thoughts in their lifetime had no identifiable disorder at the time of the interview. There were no actual suicide attempts in the past week in the absence of psychiatric disorder. Of those making an attempt in the past year, 2% had no current disorder, and of those who had ever made an attempt, only 3% had no current disorder. Thus, to all intents and purposes, suicidal attempts do not occur in the absence of broadly defined mental disorder in prisoners, and the risk of suicide attempts in the presence of mental disorder is increased still further by co-morbidity.

Motivations and precipitating factors

Problems with relationships with relatives, staff, or other inmates, trial-related concerns, bullying, bereavements, traumatic events occurring in custody, a lack of activities to distract them from painful thoughts and memories, and lack of access to prescribed medication have all been reported to precipitate suicide attempts (Reiger 1971; Kerkhof and Bernasco 1990; Blaauw et al. 2002; Borrill et al. 2005). Poor relationships with other inmates and staff (being a loner), a lack of social support, and an absence of anything to do are also reported as important issues in studies of broadly defined self-harming behaviour (Liebling and Krarup 1993; Dear et al. 1998b quoted in Camilleri et al. 1999).

Researchers have attempted to distinguish between prisoners' motivations for attempting suicide and those for self-injury. One hundred and forty-three prisoners who self-harmed in a range of male and female adult and young offender institutions in England and Wales were interviewed (Snow 2002). Those who said they had intended to kill themselves explained their actions in terms of grief or bereavement, hopelessness, homesickness, relationship problems, and actual or expected lengthy sentence. Those who had not intended to die gave explanations related to alternatives to outwardly expressed emotion, such as anger towards others, relieving stress or tension, a wish to see blood or to experience physical pain, and an alternative to the use of drugs or alcohol. Most prisoners reported more than one reason for their self-injury or attempted suicide. Men were more commonly motivated by what they perceived to be concrete events, such as the end of a relationship, while women were more likely to report being motivated by negative emotions such as anger, frustration, or tension.

Dear and colleagues describe three categories of motivation in prisoners who self-harm: escape, psychological relief, and 'manipulative motives' (Dear et al. 2000). While suicidal intent and medical lethality of method are reported to be higher in those reporting escape as a motivation, a significant minority of those reporting that they self-harmed in order to control their environment did so in ways that would have resulted in death if intervention had not been provided immediately (Dear et al. 2000; Power et al. 2003).

'Manipulative motives' are better conceived, as they are by both Power and Snow, as 'attempts to gain support and care or to avoid unpleasant circumstances by use of maladaptive means': for example 'I was too scared to come out from behind my door and I couldn't stand another day being alone so I cut up to get moved out of the hall'... 'The only time they do give a toss about you is when you're going to hurt yourself' (Power et al. 2003).

Suicide prevention strategies in prisons, their rationale, evidence of effectiveness, and prisoner views
Reduction of access to means of suicide

The earliest and still most common approach to suicide prevention in prison is to reduce access to the means of suicide. Wire netting to prevent prisoners jumping from galleries, adapted gas lighting to prevent suicide by inhalation of gas, and specially adapted furniture and utensils were all in place in English prisons near the beginning of the twentieth century (Hobhouse and Brockway 1922).

This approach predates both the evidence base (from post-1960 studies outside prisons of the effect of restricting access to lethal means of suicide such as domestic gas, guns, car exhausts, and medications) and the theoretical rationale—the 'decision' theory of suicide developed by Clarke and Lester, who view suicide as the combined result of deep but possibly temporary despair, the weakening of moral restraints, and the availability and acceptability of a method of suicide (Clarke and Lester 1989; Lester and Danto 1993).

However, access to means of suicide is already restricted in prison (and almost certainly contributes to the very high use of hanging as a method) and reducing it further may come at a high price in terms of human dignity and isolation. Most 'suicide-proof' conditions are bare, undignified, and depressing (Lloyd 1990; Liebling and Krarup 1993). Hancock and Snow (2001) describe practice in some US prisons thus: 'Prisoners wore leg irons or were chained to beds or wore heavy gloves that precluded the use of hands to aid self-harm'.

Interviews with prisoners in Scotland and England and Wales confirm that they dislike the lack of human interaction that may accompany being placed in 'suicide proof' accommodation (Power 1997; Borrill et al. 2005). Prison systems are liable to legal challenge on the grounds of having taken insufficient precautions to prevent a suicide. However, in Europe, the European Human Rights Act raises the potential for legal challenge on the grounds that the steps taken have constituted inhuman or degrading treatment. This has added further pressure to find a workable alternative to isolating prisoners and stripping them of their clothes and possessions (Council of Europe 2001).

To respond to these concerns, the English and Welsh prison service has developed a range of designs of 'safer cells' and 'crisis suites' which aim to make suicide as difficult as possible, while providing an environment that is as light, open, supportive, and calming as possible (Safer Custody Group 2002). Similar approaches have been described in Scotland and Australia (Gunn 1996; McArthur et al.,1999).

An evaluation of the English and Welsh safer cells programme found that three prisoners (out of 54 interviewed) said that they would have killed themselves had they not been in a safer cell at the time (Burrows et al. 2003). In addition, the self-harm data available suggested that a higher proportion of prisoners in safer cells compared to those in normal cells used less lethal methods of self-harm (notably cutting) instead of more lethal methods such as hanging. The researchers concluded that spontaneous suicides may be prevented by the use of safer cells.

In the female prison that was studied, the women disliked the single safer cells as they wanted the companionship of another prisoner when they were distressed. In the Young Offenders Institution included in the survey, where the safer cells were spread around the prison, stigmatization was an issue, as occupying a safer cell clearly marked out the young person as different and potentially vulnerable to bullies.

Another study of prisoners' views about having their shoelaces removed in police or prison custody also found that the potential for stigmatization is an important issue for young offenders (Borrill 2001). In particular, it was key that alternative footwear be acceptable (for example, trainers with velcro fasteners as opposed to slippers) and that it was given to all prisoners on the unit to avoid stigmatization and fears of bullying. Around 23% of prisoners who kill themselves in English and Welsh prisons use shoelaces as a ligature.

Identification of risk

Most prison suicide prevention strategies include both a screen to try to identify those at risk of suicide at the point of reception into prison and procedures for identifying prisoners thought to be at risk later in the custodial experience. However, many researchers have pointed out the limitations of this approach, given the state of the art of risk assessment and the fact that prisoners, in general, are a high-risk population (Lloyd 1990).

Identification of risk takes place on reception and later. Two studies investigated whether prison staff succeed in identifying and selecting for care those prisoners who are at highest risk. In Scotland, prisoners identified 'at risk' were more likely than controls to have mental health problems, a history of self-injury or suicide attempts, and a history of physical abuse, emotional abuse, and relationship difficulties (Power et al. 2003). In England and Wales, prisoners identified as 'at risk' were nine times more likely to be suicidal than those not so identified, but only about half of those prisoners who were suicidal at the time of the study had been identified (Senior et al. 2002). The researchers therefore recommended that assessment and care be provided for a broader group of prisoners—that is all who have mental health, substance misuse problems, and/or a history of self-harm, instead of seeking to identify solely those currently intending to kill themselves.

Supervision/monitoring

Suicide prevention programmes in the USA, England and Wales, and Scotland include specific requirements about different levels of observation and the frequency with which prisoners identified as suicidal must be monitored. While the rationale seems obvious, an ongoing study of suicides in mental hospitals in England and Wales has reported that frequent but intermittent observations (e.g. five times an hour) were ineffective in preventing suicides (Department of Health 2001, quoted in Gordon 2002).

In addition, researchers who have asked prisoners how they feel about these systems uniformly report that they strongly dislike being observed, where that observation occurs without emotional support and respect, perceiving this approach to constitute 'back-watching' for the staff rather than care for them (Liebling and Krarup 1993; Power 1997; Power et al. 2003).

A leading US programme, that of the Federal Bureau of Prisons, operates only two levels of supervision—one where the prisoner is not considered to be at immediate risk and is offered counselling and/or medication, and the other where the prisoner is considered to be at imminent risk and is placed on constant supervision (White and Schimmel 1995). Seventy-two percent of all 'watch hours' in federal prisons during 1992 were reported to be performed by paid inmate companions, instead of (or supplementing) staff. These 'inmate observation aides' interact with the suicidal person and are given training in understanding suicidal behaviour, empathic listening, and other techniques for building communication.

Ethical concerns have been expressed about the use of prisoners in this role (National Center on Institutions and Alternatives 2003). The views of the suicidal prisoners themselves and whether they find the inmate companions more or less acceptable than staff have not been reported.

Risk management/care planning systems

England and Wales, Scotland, and Australia have developed multidisciplinary care planning systems in order to plan and deliver care to prisoners identified as 'at risk'. Care plans recommended by the teams may include increased supervision and also increased social support via more contact with families, increased staff or peer support, special placements in crisis care units (Australia), counselling, help in resolving practical and social and other problems, and special accommodation, including shared cells and dormitories.

Evaluations in four studies showed that, where working well (especially in the second-generation Scottish system), prisoners reported benefits of feeling cared for and respected, having less chance to harm themselves, and getting out of stressful situations, such as being bullied (Power 1997; Senior et al. 2002; Western Australian Department of Justice Suicide Prevention Taskforce 2002; Power et al. 2003). Prisoner-reported disadvantages included being placed in an anti-ligature cell (most preferred dormitory, shared, and normal accommodation, although a few disliked the lack of privacy of sharing a cell), staff keeping them awake at night carrying out routine observations, and the stigma reported to accompany being placed on the system.

All four studies reported that individual responsibility for making sure the care plan was implemented was unclear and that staff tended to place greater emphasis on close supervision of the prisoner than on other types of interventions. Achieving good multidisciplinary working and staff training emerged as of key importance in overcoming these problems and providing better-quality care.

Peer support schemes

Prisoners who attempt suicide are more likely than others to have impoverished social networks, as already noted above and elsewhere (Biggam and Power 1997). In order to increase the level of social support available to prisoners, the majority of prisons in England and Wales, Scotland, and some in Canada and Australia, operate peer-support schemes (usually known as 'listeners'), trained and supported by Samaritans (a national charity) and based on their model of the provision of confidential, non-judgemental support. The largest evaluation carried out (of 2224 listener contacts) found that the service was well used by prisoners, with a high proportion of self-referrals, accepted by staff, and used by both suicidal prisoners (most but not all of whom had also been identified by staff) and by those who were not suicidal (Power *et al.* 2003). Prisoners expressing suicidal thoughts consulted their peers most commonly to seek help with emotional difficulties, relationship difficulties, uncertainty about the future, and problems coping with imprisonment. Smaller evaluations report that the majority of users of the service were satisfied with the help received, that being a listener was of benefit to the peer-supporters themselves, and that many prisoners consulted their peers for relatively 'minor problems' such as help to read or write letters or make applications (Snow 2000; Syed and Blanchette 2000; Southgate and Southgate 2001).

A variant is a scheme in Rhode Island, USA, where the role of the 'inmate aides' includes giving information to newly arrived inmates about what to expect in prison, as well as befriending potentially suicidal inmates, assessing suicide risk, and informing officers of which inmates are at risk (Lester and Danto 1993). A similar model has recently been introduced in England and Wales ('insiders'). Seventy-eight per cent of the 60 prisoners who used the service during the pilot period reported that they found their conversation with the insider useful, and over half said they felt much, or a bit, better after talking to them. Prisoners who were in prison for the first time were more likely to find the service useful (Teers 2002).

However, there are some indications that those who most need social support may find it hardest to ask for help. Some female prisoners who had survived a suicide attempt reported that they found it difficult to confide in others, including listeners, or to ask for help, derived in some cases from their own personal histories of abuse and lack of trust (Borrill *et al.* 2005). They wanted to be able to choose a person they trusted to talk to, and some wanted to have contact with friends instead of a peer-supporter. The researchers conclude that support should be offered pro-actively and in accordance with the individual's preferences where possible.

Shared accommodation

A method of simultaneously providing companionship and of reducing the opportunity for suicide is to place prisoners at risk in shared cells or dormitory accommodation. This approach is used in England and Wales, Scotland, and many Australian states. It has not been formally evaluated, although there are some indications that the use of dormitory accommodation in the Northern Territory of Australia has reduced distress among young Aboriginal inmates (McArthur *et al.* 1999).

The use of shared accommodation may also provide an explanation for the reported very low suicide rates in prisons in sub-Saharan Africa, e.g. Tanzania and Kenya (three suicides in whole of Tanzanian prisons in 2003, and none in 2000–2002) and in Hungary (prison suicide rate marginally lower than that in the community and an average of 3.67 prisoners to a room) (Aardema *et al.* 1998). This relationship deserves further investigation. Countries with high use of dormitory accommodation, for example, may well also have high rates of assaults. Prisoner views may also vary between cultures and genders.

Promoting closer staff–prisoner relationships

There are some indications that good relationships with staff have an important role to play in preventing suicide, especially in young offenders. In a study of Scottish young offenders, levels of hopelessness and suicidal thoughts were reported to correlate with the perceived social and emotional support available to the individual from family, friends, and staff, with the quality of the relationship with the Personal Officer being the best predictor of hopelessness (Biggam and Power 1997). The authors suggest that this shows that hopelessness is increased by the young men's belief that they had no adequate personal contact for emotional help should they require it. However, in one maximum security prison, prisoners were reported to be reluctant to approach prison officers for emotional support (Hobbs and Dear 2001).

The introduction of 'Unit Management' (creating small, manageable units with greater personal interaction between prisoners and staff) forms part of the suicide prevention strategy in Victorian prisons in Australia (McArthur *et al.* 1999). In the USA, both Unit Management and jail design are credited with facilitating better staff knowledge of prisoners, closer relationships, and therefore improving suicide prevention (Atlas 1989; Hayes 1995). No evaluations have been reported.

Staff training

Staff training is frequently reported as a critical element in suicide prevention in European countries, the USA, Canada, and Australia (Hayes 1995; Cox and Morschauser 1997; Aardema *et al.* 1998; Camilleri *et al.* 1999).

ASIST (Applied Suicide Intervention Skills Training) has been evaluated in part of the Canadian prison system. Provided in a 2-day workshop, the training covers attitudes, knowledge, and skills using video and role play. In a follow-up study 6 months after training, staff who had been trained were found to be more aware of suicide, felt more confident in approaching a person at risk, reported using the competencies learned in the training, and continued to rate ASIST as a helpful or very helpful learning experience (Crookal and McLean 1986). Psychologists in the prisons reported a much higher number of referrals. A key factor in the success of the training was considered to be ensuring that all relevant staff received it.

A similar model of skills training (STORM or Skills Training in Risk Management) is currently being piloted and evaluated in some English prisons. The interim evaluation found statistically significant differences before and after the training in attitude to suicide prevention and confidence in dealing with a suicidal person (Hayes 2004). A longer-term follow-up is under way to see if the improvements remain at 6 months and if the officers have used the skills they have learned.

The New York State Correctional System programme also provides training for mental health staff in crisis intervention and suicide prevention, and gives them information about working in prison. The aim is to promote mutual respect and understanding between uniformed staff and health-care staff, and to promote good communication and multidisciplinary working. It is reported that this emphasis on training and multidisciplinary working is critical to the success of this programme (Cox and Morschauser 1997).

Organizational leadership

Underpinning all types of strategy are prison policies, standards, and organizational leadership. For example, all prisons in England and Wales have Suicide Prevention Teams, and Suicide Prevention Co-ordinators (usually prison officers) have been appointed in all high-risk prisons. In federal prisons in the USA, prevention programmes are led by dedicated, qualified staff (usually psychologists) with full accountability for the management of suicidal prisoners (White and Schimmel 1995). No evaluations of these different arrangements have been reported.

Treatment for mental health and drug/alcohol disorders

The rationale for mental health provision forming a core part of prison suicide prevention is set out above. Significantly higher levels of major mental disorder than in the general population have been reported in prison and jail inmates in the USA, Finland, Ireland, The Netherlands, Scotland, and Denmark, as well as in England and Wales (Teplin 1994; Jordan *et al.* 1996; Aardema *et al.* 1998).

The New York State Correctional System, which is the only large jail system (holding pre-trial prisoners) claiming to have produced a significant fall in the rate of prisoner suicides, operates an extensive mental health service delivery system (and has put particular emphasis on promoting close relationships between jails and police lock-ups and community mental health services) (Cox and Morschauser 1997; Kovasznay *et al.* 2004).

A study of suicides in English and Welsh prisons found that 57% of the suicides studied had shown signs of mental disorder at reception, and of these 72% were referred to a health-care professional. Thirty per cent had a history of psychiatric treatment and, of these, 70% were referred to a health-care professional. Where the prisoner had received mental health treatment outside prison, in less than half of cases was information sought from the provider of care (Shaw *et al.* 2003).

In England and Wales more mental health staff and more clinical treatment of drug withdrawal have recently been introduced at the prisons considered to have highest levels of need, including suicide risk (Department of Health 2002*b*). Except in the case of violent or dangerous offenders, it is not necessary for the required services to be provided in a prison setting. In Scotland, in response to the finding that drug withdrawal played an important role in the majority of female prisoner suicides, a non-custodial treatment centre has been established in Glasgow to house and treat female offenders whose offending is associated with drug dependence (Fairweather and Skinner 1998; Jamieson 2004).

Psychosocial interventions

Individual psychological factors may interact with stressful aspects of prison life to lead to self-harm and suicide (Zamble and Porporino 1990). Broadly defined, self-harm has been shown to be associated with the use of particular types of coping strategies by the prisoners concerned (Dear *et al.* 1998*a*). Problem-solving therapy has been shown to reduce depression and hopelessness in studies outside prison settings (Townsend *et al.* 2001). However, as yet, psychosocial interventions to reduce suicidal thoughts and depression or improve coping strategies are not widely reported to form part of prison suicide prevention programmes.

An adaptation of dialectical behaviour therapy, specifically designed for use in a prison setting, produced promising results with inmates with a diagnosis of borderline personality disorder who are at raised risk of suicide (Eccelston and Sorbello 2002). Teaching coping skills followed by the provision of ongoing support resulted in significant changes in a group of eight inmates at high risk of suicide, as measured by the Reasons for Living Inventory (Jackson 2003). A controlled trial (23 in each group) of a short-term intervention, teaching social problem-solving to vulnerable young offenders, including those identified at risk of suicide, was associated with reductions in anxiety, depression, and hopelessness, and an improvement in problem-solving abilities (Power *et al.* 2003).

Minimizing the impact of prison-specific stressors on all prisoners

Several countries, including England and Wales, The Netherlands, Scotland, and Western Australia, include broad strategies that aim to reduce stress for all prisoners, or for prisoners on remand, as part of their approach to suicide prevention.

For example, the Western Australian suicide prevention strategy includes increased access to recreational activities, and radio and television, for prisoners on remand, and improved standards for punishments for prisoners in order to avoid unnecessary use of punishment cells (McArthur *et al.* 1999). The strategy in England and Wales stresses that 'a supportive culture based on good staff/prisoner relationships, a constructive regime in all prisons and a physically safe environment' are at the core of its approach (HM Prison Service 2001). In a number of prisons in England and Wales, the Prison Service is also piloting initiatives to reduce stress on entry into custody, including more welcoming physical environments, 'first night packs' containing tobacco and phone cards to allow a call home, 'first night centres' made up of 100% 'safer cells' with reduced ligature points, TVs in cells, specially selected staff with good interpersonal skills and attitudes, and a peer-support scheme whereby an established prisoner meets all newly arrived ones and gives them support and information. An evaluation of this initiative is in progress.

These approaches are based on the deprivation theory of prison suicide, where suicide is viewed as being caused by prison-specific factors such as loss of autonomy, inactivity, fears for physical safety, and loss of family support

(Sykes 1958; Bonner 1992; Shneidman 1993). Bonner posits a 'stress–vulnerability model', where stressors such as loss of outside relationships and victimization within the prison interact with psychosocial vulnerabilities such as psychiatric illness to produce hopelessness.

No formal evaluations have been reported. There is also some evidence that the intended strategies may not be fully implemented (HM Chief Inspector of Prisons for England and Wales 1999).

Conclusions and recommendations

Suicidal thoughts and attempts are highly related to a combination of early life experiences, together with current social, psychiatric, and drug/alcohol-related factors. These experiences and characteristics are found in offenders, whether inside or outside of prison, and thus offenders as a group are particularly vulnerable to suicide wherever they are located. All these factors are highest in remand facilities and in female prisoners, and some in young prisoners. The early days of custody and the period following release are the times of highest risk.

Strategies to prevent prisoner suicides therefore need to address the longitudinal pathways in and out of prison, as well as the period in prison. In the time before prison, Local Authority care is clearly a major risk factor, and improvement of the quality of that care is of key long-term importance to suicide prevention in young people, both within and outside the prison environment .

Services for offenders, both inside and especially outside prison, are required for all types of mental disorder, for drug/alcohol dependence, self-injurious behaviour, bereavement, and abuse. Particular attention needs to be given to providing support for those who have recently been released from prison.

Within prisons, we need an approach that recognizes the great importance of both psychiatric and social risk factors, and hence of both health and social care. There is no place for the unhelpful debate that has characterized research and policy, at least in England and Wales, between the respective merits of a 'medical' versus 'social' model. Services need to be available within an overall context of positive and respectful staff–prisoner relationships and access to constructive activities. Particular attention should be paid to promoting good multidisciplinary working between health and discipline staff. In addition, careful attention needs to be paid to how strategies are implemented, with staff and prisoners themselves consulted about any potential for unexpected negative impacts, and how these can be avoided. This is especially true in relation to ways of reducing access to means of suicide, and levels of suicide supervision.

In terms of research, larger and higher-quality studies are needed, with careful use of terminology, of proxy measures for suicide that have a higher base rate (e.g. suicide attempts) and with 'time at risk' used as the denominator for suicide rates. Careful evaluations of particular elements of preventive strategies are needed, and these should include prisoners' views. There are particular gaps in knowledge about:

- what kind of staff–prisoner relationships and 'constructive activity' are effective in reducing hopelessness and suicidal behaviour, and how these can best be promoted;
- psychosocial interventions to reduce suicidal behaviour;
- how to provide supervision for suicidal prisoners in ways that are both effective in preventing suicide and provide emotional support in a way acceptable to the individual concerned; and, finally,
- to what extent, and for which types of prisoner, is the use of shared accommodation an acceptable preventive measure.

References

Aardema, A., Blaauw, E., Gatherer, A., Kerkhof, A., and Themeli, O. (1998). *Mental health in European prisons.* Department of Clinical Psychology, Vrije Universiteit, Amersterdam.

Atlas, R. (1989). Reducing the opportunity for inmate suicide: a design guide. *Psychiatric Quarterly,* **60**, 161–71.

Backett, S. (1988). Suicide and stress in prison. In *Imprisonment today,* (ed. S. Backett, J. McNeil and A. Yellowless). MacMillan, London.

Biggam, F. and Power, F. (1997). Social support and psychological distress in a group of incarcerated young offenders. *International Journal of Offender Therapy and Comparative Criminology,* **41**, 213–30.

Biles, D. (1992). International review of deaths in custody, research paper no 15. In *Deaths in custody, 1980–1989: the research papers of the Criminology Unit of the Royal Commission into Aboriginal Deaths in Custody,* (ed. D. Biles and D. McDonald), pp. 351–80. Australian Institute of Criminology, Canberra.

Biles, D., McDonald, D., and Flemming, J. (1992). Australian deaths in custody 1980–1988: An analysis of Aboriginal and non-Aboriginal deaths in prison and police custody. In *Deaths in custody, 1980–1989: The research papers of the Criminology Unit of the Royal Commission into Aboriginal Deaths in Custody,* (ed. D. Biles and D. McDonald), pp. 213–37. Australian Institute of Criminology, Canberra.

Blaauw, E. and Kerkhof, A.J.F.M. (1999). Suicides in detentie. Quoted in *Suicide policy for prisons, working group report 1999.* Available at website http://www.hipp-europe.org/resources (last accessed in July 2005).

Blaauw, E., Kraij, V., Arensman, E., Winkel, F.W., and Bout, R. (2002). Traumatic life events and suicidal risk among jail inmates: the influence of types of events, time period and significant others. *Journal of Traumatic Stress,* **15** (1), 9–16.

Bogue, J. and Power, K. (1995). Suicide in Scottish prisons 1976–1979. *British Journal of Forensic Psychiatry,* **6**, 527–40.

Bonner, R.L. (1992). Isolation, seclusion and psychological vulnerability as risk factors for suicide behind bars. In *Assessment and prediction of suicide*, (ed. R. Maris *et al.*). Guilford Press, New York.

Borrill, J. (2001). *Prisoners' attitudes to removal of shoelaces and to alternative forms of footwear*. Report to Safer Custody Group, HM Prison Service.

Borrill, J. (2002). Self-inflicted deaths of prisoners serving life sentences: 1988–2001. *British Journal of Forensic Practice*, 4 (4), 30–8.

Borrill, J., Snow, L., Medlicott, D., Teers, R., and Paton, J. (2005). Learning from near misses: interviews with women who survived an incident of severe self harm. *Howard League Journal*, 44, 57–69.

Brock, A. and Griffiths, C. (2004). *Trends in suicide by method in England and Wales, 1979–2001*. Office for National Statistics, London.

Bureau of Justice Statistics (1993). *Jail inmates 1992*. US Department of Justice, Washington DC.

Burrows, T., Brock, A., Hulley, S., Smith, C., and Summers, L. (2003). *Safer cells evaluation*. Report to the Prison Service, The Jill Dando Institute of Crime Science.

Camilleri, P., McArthur, M., and Webb, H. (1999). *Suicidal behaviour in prisons: a literature review*. School of Social Work, Australian Catholic University, Canberra.

Clarke, R.V. and Lester, D. (1989). *Suicide: closing the exits*. Springer-Verlag, New York.

Clavel, J., Benhamou, S., and Famant, R. (1987). Decreased mortality among male prisoners. *Lancet*, 2, 1012–14.

Council of Europe (2001). 11th General report on the CPT's activities covering 1 January to 31 December 2000. Available at website http://cpt.coe.int/en/annual/rep-11.html (last accessed July 2005)

Cox, J. and Morschauser, P. (1997). A solution to the problem of jail suicide. *Journal of Crisis Intervention and Suicide Prevention*, 18, 178–84.

Crookal, P. and McLean, T. (1986). *Evaluation of the suicide prevention training program in the Atlantic Region*. Correctional Service Canada, Ottawa.

Dalton, V. (1999). Prison deaths 1980–1997: national overview and state trends. *Trends and Issues in Crime and Criminal Justice, 81*. Australian Institute of Criminology, Canberra.

Dear, G., Thomson, D., Hall, G., and Howells, K. (1998a). Self inflicted injury and coping behaviours in prison. In *Suicide prevention: the global context*, (ed. R. Kosky, H. Esh Kevari, R. Goldney, R. Hassan), pp. 189–99. Plenum Press, New York.

Dear, G., Thompson, D., Hall, G., and Howells, K. (1998b). Self-harm in Western Australian prisons: an examination of situational and psychological factors. School of Psychology, Edith Cowan University, Western Australia.

Dear, G.E., Thomson, D.M., and Hills, A.M. (2000) Self harm in prison. *Criminal Justice and Behaviour*, 27, 160–75.

Department of Health (2001). *Safety first: five year report of the National Confidential Inquiry into Suicide and Homicide by People with Mental Illness*. HMSO, London.

Department of Health (2002a). *National suicide prevention strategy for England*. HMSO, London.

Department of Health (2002b). *Health services for prisoners*. HMSO, London.

Dooley, E. (1990a). Prison suicide in England and Wales, 1972–87. *British Journal of Psychiatry*, 156, 40–5.

Dooley, E. (1990b). Non-natural deaths in prison. *British Journal of Criminology*, 30, 229–34.

Eccelston, L. and Sorbello, L. (2002). The RUSH program – real understanding of self-help: a suicide and self-harm prevention initiative within a prison setting. *Australian Psychologist*, 37, 237–444.

Eisenberg, L. (1986). Does bad news about suicide beget bad news? *New England Journal of Medicine*, 315, 705–7.

Fairweather, C. and Skinner, A. (1998). *Women offenders – a safer way.* Social Work Services and Prisons Inspectorate for Scotland, Edinburgh.

Flemming, J., McDonald, D., and Biles, D. (1992). Self inflicted harm in custody. Research paper no.16. In *Death in custody, 1980–1989: the research papers of the Criminology Unit of the Royal Commission into Aboriginal Deaths in Custody*, (ed. D. Biles and D. McDonald), pp. 381–416. Australian Institute of Criminology, Canberra.

Frottier, P., Fruehwald, S., Ritter, K., Eher, R., Schwaerzler, J., and Bauer, P. (2002). Jailhouse blues revisited. *Social Psychiatry and Psychiatric Epidemiology*, 372, 68–73.

Fruehwald, S., Frottier, P., Ehar, R., Gutierrez K., and Ritter, K. (2002a). Prison suicides in Austria: 1975–1997. *Suicide and Life-Threatening Behavior*, 30, 360–9.

Fruehwald, S., Frother, P., Ritter, K., Eher, R., and Gutierrez, K. (2002b). Impact of overcrowding and legislative change on the incidence of suicide in custody experiences in Austria: 1967–1996. *International Journal of Law and Psychiatry*, 25, 119–28.

Gill, B., Meltze, R.H., and Hinds, K. (1996.). *The prevalence of psychiatric morbidity among homeless adults.* OPCS, London.

Gordon, H. (2002) Suicide in secure psychiatric facilities. *Advances in Psychiatric Treatment*, 8, 408–17.

Gore, S.M. (1999). Suicide in prisons: reflection of the communities served, or exacerbated risk? *British Journal of Psychiatry*, 175, 50–5.

Goss, R., Peterson, K., Smith, L., Kalb, K., and Brodey, B. (2002). Characteristics of suicide attempts in a large urban jail system with an established suicide prevention program. *Jail Suicide/Mental Health Update*, 11 (3), 1–6.

Gunn, J. (1996). Suicide prevention in Scottish prisons: a brief review. Report to Scottish Prison Service, unpublished.

Hancock, N. and Snow, L. (2001). Suicide prevention in North America: fewer deaths but at what cost? *Prison Service Journal*, 138, 24–6.

Harvey, J. and Liebling, A. (2002). *Prison population increase, psychological distress and suicidal behaviour: some possible mechanisms.* Report to HM Prison Service, London.

Hatty, S.E. and Walker, J.R. (1986). *A national study of deaths in Australian prison.* Australian Centre of Criminology, Canberra.

Hayes, A. (2004). An evaluation of STORM suicide prevention training in HM Prison Service. Unpublished report to HM Prison Service.

Hayes, L.M. (1989). National study of jail suicides: seven years later. *Psychiatric Quarterly*, 60, 7–29.

Hayes, L.M. (1995). *Prison suicide: an overview and guide to prevention.* US Department of Justice, National Institute of Corrections.

Hayes, L.M. (1998). Model suicide prevention programs. *Jail suicide/mental health update*, 8 (1–4), 1–20.

Hayes, L.M. and Kajdan, B. (1981). *And darkness closes in: a national study of jail suicides.* National Centre on Institutions and Alternatives, Washington DC.

HM Chief Inspector of Prisons for England and Wales (1999). *Suicide is everyone's concern: a thematic review.* Home Office, London.

HM Prison Service (2001). *Prevention of suicide and self harm in the Prison Service: an internal review.* HM Prison Service, London.

Hobbs, G.S. and Dear, G.E. (2001). Prisoners' perceptions of prison officers as sources of support. *Journal of Offender Rehabilitation,* 31, 127–42.

Hobhouse, S. and Brockway, F. (1922). *English prisons today.* Longmans, Green and Co, London.

Jackson, J. (2003). Outcome research with high-risk inmates. *Behaviour Therapist,* 26, 215–16.

Jamieson, C., Scotland's Justice Minister, cited in the *Guardian* 19 February 2004.

Jordan, B.K., Schlenger, W.E., Fairbank, J.A., and Caddell, J.M. (1996). Prevalence of psychiatric disorders among incarcerated women. *Archives of General Psychiatry,* 53, 513–19.

Kerkhof, J.F.M. and Bernasco, W. (1990). Suicidal behaviour in jails and prisons in the Netherlands: incidence, characteristics and prevention. *Suicide and Life-Threatening Behavior,* 20, 123–37.

Kovasznay, B., Miraglia, R., Beer, R., and Way, B. (2004). Reducing suicides in New York State Correctional Facilities. *Psychiatric Quarterly,* 75, 61–70.

Leese, M. (2003). *Rate of self-inflicted death and associated factors in prisons in England and Wales 2000–2002.* Report for the Safer Custody Group.

Lester, D. and Danto, B. (1993). *Suicide behind bars: prediction and prevention.* Charles Press, Philadelphia.

Liebling, A. (1992). *Suicides in prison.* Routledge, London.

Liebling, A. (1994). Suicides amongst women prisoners. *Howard Journal,* 33, 1–9.

Liebling, A. (1999). Prison suicide and prisoner coping. In *Prisons, crime and justice: An annual review of research,* Vol. 26, (ed. M. Tonry and J. Petersilia), pp. 283–360. University of Chicago Press, Chicago.

Liebling, A. (2001). Suicides in prison: ten years on. *Prison Service Journal,* 138, 35–41.

Liebling, A. and Krarup, H. (1993). *Suicide attempts and self injury in male prisoners.* Home Office, London.

Liebling, A., Durie, L., van Den Beuckel, A., and Tait, S. (2003). Legitimacy, prison suicide and the moral performance of prisons. Paper presented to the American Society of Criminology Conference Roundtable, Denver, 13 November 2003.

Livingston, M. (1997). A review of the literature on self-injurious behaviour among prisoners. *Issues in Criminology and Legal Psychology,* 28, 21–35.

Lloyd, C. (1990). *Suicide and self injury in prison: a literature review.* Home Office Research Study No. 115, Home Office, London.

Mackenzie, N., Oram, C., and Borrill, J. (2003). Self-inflicted deaths of women in custody. *British Journal of Forensic Practice,* 5 (1), 27–35.

McArthur, M., Camilleri, P., and Webb, H. (1999). Strategies for managing suicide and self-harm in prisons. Australian Institute of Criminology. *Trends and Issues in Crime and Justice,* Paper no. 125. Canberra. Available at www.aic.gov.uk, accessed July 2005.

Meltzer, H., Gill, B., and Petticrew, M. (1994). *The prevalence of psychiatric morbidity among adults aged 16–64 living in private households in Great Britain.* OPCS, London.

Meltzer. H., Gill, B., Petticrew, M., and Hinds, K. (1995). *The prevalence of psychiatric morbidity among adults living in institutions.* OPCS, London.

Morrison, S. (1996). Custodial suicide in Australia: a comparison of different populations. *Medicine, Science and Law,* 36, 167–77.

National Center on Institutions and Alternatives (2003). Use of 'no-harm' contracts and other controversial issues in suicide prevention. *Jail Suicide and Mental Health Update,* 12, 1–9.

Neeleman, J., Mak, V., and Wessely, S. (1997). Suicide by age, ethnic group, coroners' verdict and country of birth: a three-year survey in inner London. *British Journal of Psychiatry,* 171, 463–7.

New York State Department of Correctional Services (1994). *Characteristics of suicide victims in NYSDOCS between 1986–1994.* New York State Department of Correctional Services, Albany, NY.

Nock, M.K. and Marzuk, P.M. (2000). Suicide and violence. In *The international handbook of suicide and attempted suicide,* (ed. K. Hawton and K. van Heeringen). Wiley, Chichester.

O'Donnell, I. and Farmer, R. (1995). The limitations of official suicide statistics. *British Journal of Psychiatry,* 166, 458–61.

Office for National Statistics (2003). *Health Statistics Quarterly,* No. 20. The Stationery Office, London.

O'Mahony, P. (1994). Prison suicide rates: what do they mean? In *Death in custody: international perspectives,* (ed. A. Liebling and T. Ward). Whiting and Birch, London.

Phillips, D.P. and Carstensen, L.L. (1986). Clustering of teenage suicides after television news stories about suicide. *New England Journal of Medicine,* 315, 685–9.

Plutchik, R. and van Praag, H.M. (1990). Psychosocial correlates of suicide and violence risk. In *Violence and suicidality: perspective in clinical and psychobiological research,* (ed. H.M. van Praag, R. Plutchik, and A. Apter). Brunner Mazel, New York.

Power, K.G. (1997). *Evaluation of the Scottish Prison Service Suicide Prevention Strategy.* Scottish Prison Service. Edinburgh

Power, K., Swanson, V., Luke, R., Jackson, C., and Biggam, F. (2003). *Evaluation of the Revised Scottish Prison Service Suicide Risk Management Strategy.* Scottish Prison Service Occasional Paper Series 01/2003. Edinburgh.

Ramsay, M., Baker, P., Goulden, C., Sharp, C., and Sondhi, A. (2001). *Drug misuse declared in 2000: results from the British Crime Survey.* Home Office Research Study No. 224. Home Office, London.

Ramsay, R.F., Tanner, B.L., and Searle, C.A. (1987). Suicide prevention in high-risk prison populations. *Canadian Journal of Criminology,* 29, 295–307.

Reiger, W. (1971). Suicide attempts in a federal prison. *Archives of General Psychiatry,* 24, 532–5.

Royal College of Psychiatrists (2002). *Suicide in prisons: Report of Council Working Party.* Royal College of Psychiatrists, London.

Safer Custody Group. HM Prison Service, statistics, 2004.

Safer Custody Group (2002). *Suicide prevention strategies: guidance on preventing prisoner suicides and reducing self-harm, the role of the Samaritans and safer custody cell protocols.* HM Prison Service, London.

Sattar, G. (2001). *Rates and causes of death among prisoners and offenders under community supervision.* Home Office Research Study 231, London.

Senior, J., Shaw, J., Bowen, A., Hayes, A., Pratt, D., Taylor, G., *et al.* (2002). *An assessment of the F2052SH system for the monitoring of self-harm in five prisons.* Report to HM Prison Service.

Shaw, J., Appleby, L., and Baker, D. (2003). *Safer prisons: a national study of prison suicides 1999–2000 by the National Confidential Inquiry into Suicides and Homicides by People with Mental Illness.* Department of Health, London.

Shneidman, E. (1993). *Suicide as Psychache: a clinical approach to self-destructive behaviour.* Jason Aronson, Northvale, New Jersey.

Singleton, N., Meltzer, H., Gatward, R., Coid, J., and Deasy, D. (1998). *Psychiatric morbidity of prisoners in England and Wales*. Office for National Statistics, London.

Smalley, H. (1911). Report by the medical inspector. In the *Report by the Prison Commissioners*. HMSO, London.

Snow, L. (2000). The role of formalised peer-group support in prisons. In *Suicide in prisons*, (ed. G. Towl, L. Snow, and M. McHugh). British Psychological Society. Leicester.

Snow, L. (2002). Prisoners' motives for self-injury and attempted suicide. *British Journal of Forensic Practice*, 4 (4), 18–29.

Snow, L., Paton, J., Oram, C., and Teers, R. (2002). Self-inflicted deaths during 2001: an analysis of trends. *British Journal of Forensic Practice*, 4 (4), 3–17.

Southgate, P. and Southgate, G. (2001). *Peer support schemes for suicide and self harm prevention in prisons*. Report to Safer Custody Group, HM Prison Service.

Syed, F. and Blanchette, K. (2000). *a) Results of an evaluation of the Peer Support Program at Joliette Institution for Women b) Results of an evaluation of the Peer Support Program at Grand Valley Institution for Women c) Results of an evaluation of the Peer Support Program at Noval Institution for Women*. Correctional Service of Canada, Ottawa.

Sykes, G. (1958). *The society of captives*. Princeton University Press, Princeton.

Teers, R. (2002). Insiders: first night peers support evaluation. Unpublished report to Safer Custody Group, HM Prison Service.

Teers, R. (2004). Self inflicted deaths in 2001 with non-suicide verdicts. Unpublished report to the Prison Service Safer Custody Group.

Temby, I. (1990). Neglected to death. *Criminology Australia*, 19–20 July/August.

Teplin, L. (1994). Psychiatric and substance abuse disorders among male urban jail detainees. *American Journal of Public Health*, 84, 290–3.

Topp, D.O. (1979). Suicide in prison. *British Journal of Psychiatry*, 134, 24–7.

Towl, G. and Fleming, C. (1997). Self inflicted deaths of women prisoners. *Forensic Update*, 51, 5–8.

Towl, G.J. and Crighton, D.A. (1998). Suicide in prisons in England and Wales from 1988–1995. *Criminal Behaviour and Mental Health*, 8, 184–92.

Townsend, E., Hawton, K., Altman, D., Arensman, E., Gunnel, D., Hazel, P., House, A., and Van Heeringen, K. (2001). The efficacy of problem-solving treatments after deliberate self harm: a meta-analysis of randomised controlled trials with respect to depression, hopelessness and improvement in problems. *Psychological Medicine*, 31, 979–88.

Western Australian Department of Justice Suicide Prevention Taskforce (2002). *Suicide in prison*. Available at www.justice.wa.gov.au, accessed July 2005.

White, T.W. and Schimmel, D.J. (1995). Suicide prevention in federal prisons: a successful five-step programme. In *Prison suicide: an overview and guide to prevention*, (ed. L.M. Hayes). US Department of Justice, National Institute of Corrections.

Williams, P. (2001). Deaths in custody: 10 years on from the Royal Commission. Australian Institute of Criminology, *Trends and Issues in Crime and Criminal Justice*, Paper no. 203 Canberra. Available at www.aic.gov.uk, accessed July 2005.

Zamble, E. and Porporino, F.J. (1990). Coping imprisonment and rehabilitation: some data and their implications. *Criminal Justice and Behaviour*, 17, 53–70.

19

Volunteer perspectives on suicide prevention

Lakshmi Vijayakumar and Simon Armson

Introduction

Do volunteers prevent suicide? How many suicides do they actually prevent? What is the evidence for their effectiveness? Are volunteers knowledgeable and capable? These are simple but difficult questions which need to be addressed to understand volunteers' perspectives on suicide prevention.

Suicide and suicidal behaviour as a separate and different area of research and clinical significance became apparent in the early 1960s, but the idea that suicides should be prevented, rather than could be prevented, originated in the volunteer sector and infused hope, whereas previously suicide was generally thought to be inevitable.

The importance of volunteers in suicide prevention

In the past three decades international organizations and governments have become aware of the value and importance of the voluntary sector. The United Nations General Assembly proclaimed the year 2001 as the International Year of the Volunteer, the aim of which was to enhance the recognition, facilitation, networking, and promotion of voluntary services. The following are some points regarding the importance of volunteers in suicide prevention.

1. It is estimated that there are about 100 000 volunteers working specifically in suicide prevention worldwide, compared to about 10 000 professionals. Thus volunteers constitute the largest entity worldwide in suicide prevention.

2. Volunteers are available in areas where professional services are unavailable. The World Health Organization (2001) *Atlas of Mental Health Resources in the World* reveals that Africa, South-East Asia, and China, which account for 89% of the world population, have the smallest professional mental health resources (two persons per 100 000 population). But 88% of these countries have NGOs in mental health.

3. Volunteers bridge the treatment gap in services, as the majority of suicidal persons do not access mental health services. Furthermore, in developing countries such as India, Sri Lanka, China, and African countries, the crisis centres run by volunteers often function as an entry point for the needed health services.
4. Volunteers are cost effective, innovative, and flexible, and since they function as the eyes and ears of the society, are often the first to recognize changing trends in suicidal behaviour and the first to react with new initiatives in confronting new needs.

Organizations in the volunteer sector, such as Samaritans, Lifeline, Befrienders International, and the Suicide Prevention Advocacy Network (SPAN), have carried out pioneering work in suicide prevention advocacy and awareness.

Despite the importance of the volunteer sector, there is a paucity of information on its merits and faults, successes and failures, strengths and weaknesses, problems and innovations.

Do volunteers prevent suicide?

There have been two types of evaluative studies of suicide prevention centres (Table 19.1):

(1) ecological studies that compare the suicide rates for a number of regions (states, countries, or cities) with and without centres, either at one specific time, or over two time periods separated by an interval;
(2) time-series studies that examine changes in suicide rates over time in one region or nation before and after introduction of a centre or centres.

Table 19.1 Suicide prevention centres and suicide rates

Type of study	Investigators	Country	Preventive effect
Ecological studies			
Single year	Bridge et al. (1977)	USA	No
	Medoff (1984)	USA	Yes
Correlational	Lester (1993)	USA	Yes
	Leenaars and Lester (1995)	Canada	No
	Miller et al. (1984)	USA	Yes
Time series			
Without control	Weiner (1969)	USA	No
	Riehl et al. (1988)	Germany	No
With control	Lester (1994)	England	Yes
	Huang and Lester (1995)	Taiwan	Yes
	Lester et al. (1996)	Japan	Yes

In England, Bagley (1968) compared suicide rates in 15 towns with suicide prevention centres with the rates in two samples of towns which were matched for socio-demographic variables and did not have such centres. He also compared the rates during the 3 years before and 3 years after the establishment of the centres. He found that there was a decline in suicide rates in the towns with suicide prevention centres compared to control towns, which experienced an increase in suicide rate. Barraclough and colleagues (1977) repeated Bagley's study using four samples of towns which were more accurately matched with regard to suicide rates, proportion of single-person households, and other factors, and found that there was no significant difference in suicide rates between towns with Samaritan centres and towns without them.

In the USA, Lester (1974a,b) found no evidence of an impact of suicide prevention centres on the suicide rate of American cities, whereas Miller *et al.* (1984) found that suicide prevention centres appeared to have a positive effect on suicide rates. Dew *et al.* (1987) examined five studies and concluded that there was no overall preventive effect.

In 1997, Lester conducted a meta-analysis of studies that presented data as to whether suicide prevention centres prevented suicides in the

Table 19.2 Results of a meta-analysis of studies of effectiveness of suicide prevention centres (Lester 1997)

Study	Pearson *r*	Degrees of freedom
Bridge *et al.* (1977)	−0.05	194
Huang and Lester (1995)	−0.35	15
Jennings *et al.* (1978)	+0.08	97
Leenaars and Lester (1995)	−0.22	96
Lester (1974*a,b*)	−0.11	22
Lester (1980)/Bagley (1968)	−0.35	54
Lester (1990)	−0.18	18
Lester (1993)	−0.10	405
Lester (1994)	−0.13	90
Lester *et al.* (1996)	−0.22	183
Medoff (1984)	−0.11	462
Riehl *et al.* (1988)	no data	
Weiner (1969)	−0.31	2
Average	−0.16	2549, *P* = 0.002

communities served (Lester 1997) (Table 19.2). It can be seen that 12 of the 13 studies reported a preventive effect, although the effect failed to reach statistical significance in one and in many the size of the effect was small. Lester averaged the results of the 12 analyses and found a significant preventive effect ($r = -0.16$, $P = 0.002$). Overall it can be surmised that suicide prevention centres, which are mostly staffed by volunteers, do have a preventive effect, although the size of the effect is small. A preventive effect has also been found in Asian countries such as Taiwan and Japan (Huang and Lester 1995; Lester *et al.* 1996). The only study to have found suicide prevention centres being associated with an increase in suicide rate was by Riehl and colleagues (1988) in Germany. An increase in rates occurred in 3 of the 25 cities with centres.

The concept of 'befriending' in the context of suicide prevention was first introduced by the Samaritans in the UK. This form of intervention relies heavily on the interpersonal and empathetic skills of volunteers, and does not require training or qualification. It can be argued that this model follows the Rogerian concept of person-centred, non-directive counselling, although the befriending relationship typically does not have boundaries to be found in more formalized counselling relationships. It is a more open-ended arrangement whereby the user of the service is able, at any time of the day or night, to obtain emotional support through the process of befriending offered by the volunteer. Thus there is no 'contract' and therefore little opportunity of affective measurement of change. However, as noted below, there have been a few examples where such measurement has been undertaken, with some positive results.

A detailed investigation of the impact of befriending (emotional support) by volunteers in Sri Lanka was conducted by Marecek and Ratnayeke (2001). Sri Lanka has an extremely high rate of suicide, especially in rural areas. Marecek and Ratnayeke evaluated the Sumithrayo programme. Sumithrayo is a leading suicide prevention NGO in Sri Lanka which has been functioning for over three decades. In 1996 Sumithrayo designed a controlled study to assess the effectiveness of 'befriending' (emotional support) in preventing suicide. Two villages with comparable socio-demographics were identified and one was assigned as the index village, the other the control village. In the index village two experienced Sumithrayo volunteers were recruited for the project and after training they began the intervention. The initial phase was devoted to establishing a presence in the community, by making contact with village leaders and organizing public meetings. Every household was visited for gathering basic information. Families where suicide and attempted suicide had occurred, and those with economic crisis, illness, violence, or interpersonal strife were visited regularly (once a week) and provided with emotional

Table 19.3 Sumithrayo Project in Sri Lanka (Marecek and Ratnayeke, personal communication, 2001)

	Index village	Control village
Population	404 (125 households)	410 (121 households)
Religion	Buddhism	Buddhism
Employment	Farmers/manual labourers	Farmers/manual labourers
Electricity/telephones	Nil	Nil
Before intervention (between 1990 and 1995)		
Number of suicides	13	16
Number of attempted suicides	18	25
After intervention (between 1990 and 1995)		
Number of suicides	0	3
Number of attempted suicides	0 (4 years)	10 (2 years)

support. In addition, Sumithrayo initiated small community projects, such as sewing classes, which enabled the villagers to earn small amounts of money from selling garments and rag rugs. More importantly, it brought the women together in a shared endeavour. The success of the programme is shown in Table 19.3. The sharp decline in suicide and attempted suicide in the index village contrasts with the rates in the control area (and the rest of the area), which showed a 6% increase in suicidal behaviour.

It can be stated categorically that volunteers do prevent suicide, but it is hoped that they could prevent more.

Volunteer characteristics

Personal characteristics

The essential qualification for volunteers in suicide prevention is their basic humanity. Volunteers traditionally do not possess specific qualifications, experience, or expertise. Instead, they offer themselves as human beings who seek to alleviate emotional distress in other human beings by providing them with support. It has often been found that reticent individuals who are likely to take the view that they would be unable to 'rise to the challenge' of offering emotional support to other people in distress have proved themselves to be the most successful in fulfilling this role. It is the fundamental diffidence and willingness to accept that very often there are no easy answers to be found that best equips volunteers for this type of work. Conversely, those who wish to become involved with this work in order to 'solve problems' very often prove to be the least effective, and fail to demonstrate the patience and the skill needed in gently and slowing enabling the distress of another person to be brought to the surface, expressed, and possibly understood.

Additionally, attitudes toward death and suicide and personal suicide behaviour are particularly relevant to suicide intervention skills. A suicide attitude questionnaire (SUIATT), developed by Diekstra and Kerkhoff (1989), which had been used in many centres, was administered to 105 volunteers in the UK and 74 volunteers in India (Vijayakumar and Keir 1998). The centres in India and the UK were affiliated to Befrienders International and functioned according to the guidelines of Befrienders International. Their primary aim was to offer emotional support to suicidal persons in a completely confidential and caring atmosphere. The training that the volunteers underwent to enrol in the suicide prevention centres was similar, although there were minor cultural differences. Volunteers were questioned about whether suicide would be a deliberate or impulsive act for 'myself', 'person most near and dear', and 'someone close'. There were significant differences for all of these categories, with volunteers in India usually perceiving suicide as an impulsive act. Even one's own possible suicide was seen as more impulsive than deliberate. Research from around the world has revealed a strong association between suicide and mental disorders. Unfortunately, 70% of the volunteers in the UK and India were unaware that psychiatric disorders were a risk factor for suicide. This factor needs to be emphasized during the training of the volunteers. The percentage of volunteers reporting previous suicidal ideation was higher in the UK volunteers. Overall, 9.8% of the UK volunteers and 1.2% of the Indian volunteers had themselves attempted suicide. These differences could be due to different criteria used for selecting the volunteers, or more openness on the part of the volunteers in the centres in the UK. It is surprising that although all the respondents were volunteers in suicide prevention centres, only 30% of the UK volunteers and 59% of the Indian volunteers believed in the effectiveness of such centres (Table 19.4).

McClaire (1973) systematically evaluated 125 volunteers working in telephone help services in the USA. The suicide prevention service attracted significantly more volunteers reporting a history of suicide thoughts and attempts than did a hot-line for teenagers. In their study of volunteers in Montreal, Mishara and Giroux (1993) found that 50% of the volunteers had thought of suicide and 13% had attempted suicide. This raises two questions. Are volunteers who themselves appear to be, or have been, emotionally distressed capable of supporting someone else in suicidal crisis? Are volunteers

Table 19.4 Attitude of volunteers to suicide in the UK and India (Vijayakumar and Keir 1998)

	UK ($n = 105$)	India ($n = 74$)
Suicide is usually:		
Deliberate	50%	12%
Impulsive	15%	57%
Not related to mental illness	72%	70%
Volunteers reported:		
Suicidal thoughts	33%	17%
Suicide attempts	9.8%	1.2%
Centres are effective in suicide prevention	30%	57%

more effective and empathetic in suicidal crises because many of them have had similar feelings?

Professional characteristics

In the USA, Reid and Smith (1980) administered a 16-item questionnaire regarding knowledge about suicide to 192 subjects from various professions. The results revealed that medical students, psychologists, volunteers, and general practitioners were more knowledgeable than social workers, students, clergy, and lay people. Rogers *et al.* (2002) showed that the experience and educational level of volunteers led to more accurate suicide risk assessment. Training in intervention skills has been shown to increase competence in suicide counselling (Neimeyer and MacInnes 1981).

Volunteers usually receive specialized training and monitoring so that they perform according to the standards of the organization for which they work. They usually learn to 'actively listen' and intervene in a more active role with those in suicidal crisis. Considering the large number of calls to suicide prevention centres, it is evident that clients obtain some satisfaction from their contacts.

How the volunteers put their training into practice and how they proceed in helping suicidal clients has not been researched vigorously. Thus there has been very little research on the 'process' of suicide prevention by volunteers.

Daigle and Mishara (1995) observed 617 calls to two suicide prevention centres and generated intervention profiles. They identified two styles—non-directive and directive. The identification of these styles with the volunteers suggest that, notwithstanding the debate about their efficacy, their process of intervention is rather similar to intervention by professionals. Further analysis indicated that the particular style of intervention was related more to the characteristics of the clients themselves than to the characteristics of the volunteers.

Talking with a suicidal person is stressful for professionals and volunteers alike. Mishara and Giroux (1993) examined stress perceived by volunteers in a suicide prevention centre. Their study showed that volunteers with more experience were less stressed. Stress was directly related to:

(1) urgency of the caller,
(2) number of calls received, and
(3) coping styles like magical thinking and feeling personally responsible.

Stress was indirectly related to more experience, number of volunteers present, education, and having realistic expectations. These factors should be considered during selection and training. It is suggested that there should be a ceiling on the number of calls received in a shift, that there needs to be a sufficient gap between calls, and that other volunteers should be available for consultation. Training should emphasize expectations and minimizing feelings of personal responsibility.

Cotton and Range (1992) reported that more experienced volunteers gave more adequate response to suicide scenarios than a less-experienced group. Using the Suicide Intervention Response Inventory (SIRI) in professionals, para-professionals (volunteers), and non-professionals, Neimeyer *et al.* (2001) investigated the relationship of professional and personal factors to the ability of counsellors to respond appropriately to suicide verbalization. SIRI was designed to measure competence in choosing appropriate therapeutic response to suicidal individuals (Neimeyer and MacInnes 1981). It contains 25 items, each of which consists of a 'client' remark and a choice between two 'helper' responses, one of which is facilitative and the other non-facilitative from a crisis intervention point of view. The score consists of the number of appropriate options selected, with a higher SIRI score reflecting a better therapeutic response to suicidal individuals. Neimeyer and colleagues found that death acceptance was related to positive SIRI scores, whereas acceptance of suicide as a right to die had a negative correlation. Volunteers who had a history of suicidal thoughts or behaviours had poorer SIRI scores. Of all the various factors related to suicide counselling skills that were investigated, the significant ones were attitude, behaviours, and experiences with suicide *per se*, rather than personal or professional background variables. Thus it can be surmised that the appropriate response to a suicidal crisis is a unique skill, and one that is linked to a person's history with, and reactions to, life-threatening situations.

Outcome of the intervention

Wenz and Papendick (1988) evaluated the effect of a crisis telephone service upon both the suicidal callers and volunteers. Only 19% of the callers felt they were not helped. Mishara and Daigle (1992) studied two telephone services in Quebec and found that many callers benefited from the calls, as indicated by decreased ratings for depression and suicidal urgency, and the fact that the majority made and respected a 'no suicide' contract.

Volunteers are often exposed to horrific accounts of human pain and suffering, which may affect their personal thoughts, feelings and beliefs, and actions. Kinzel and Nanson (2000) suggest that educating and debriefing volunteers are two strategies that may prevent the onset of compassion fatigue, which they argue is the cost of caring. Debriefing is used as an effective strategy for volunteers, as it has been found to be successful in assisting other helpers in many different contexts to cope and deal with the traumatic events that they experience or hear about.

Innovations

The primary goal of suicide prevention centres is to provide emotional support to suicidal persons in the population, through befriending and counselling, in person or by telephone. In many countries they are the NGOs in suicide prevention and they are instrumental in increasing awareness about suicide and its prevention in the local population. They are often the premier or sole agency for suicide prevention in each country and so they have enlarged their perspectives by being proactive in rural and remote areas and in accessing special populations. Many ingenious innovations for raising awareness and increasing help-seeking behaviour have been initiated. Although great strides have been made by these centres, there are also certain drawbacks. There is wide variability in their expertise and services. Quality control measures are inadequate and the majority of their highly publicized programmes are not evaluated.

In the UK, it was recognised by the Samaritans that the average suicide rate in prisons was up to five times higher than that of the rest of the population. It was also recognized that, by definition, prisoners were unable to gain access to emotional support that was available to the rest of the population through the services offered by the Samaritans. As a result of this, initiatives were developed whereby Samaritan volunteers were specifically selected and trained to work in prison establishments. This was only possible on a very part-time basis, and certainly could not match the constant service (24 hours a day, 7 days a week) provided for the rest of the population. However, it became apparent that this limited service in prisons was greatly appreciated and valued by prisoners and prison staff alike. Additionally, in some establishments it was possible to arrange for dedicated telephone lines to be made available so that prisoners could make confidential telephone calls to the Samaritans at specific times of the day.

Local suicide prevention programmes have been developed in several countries. The enormity of the problem and the paucity of services led, in 1986, to the formation of Sneha, a suicide prevention centre in Chennai, India. Since then this has been the flagship centre in India and has helped to set up 10 other centres in the country. India currently has no national plan, policy, or programme for suicide prevention. Apart from functioning as a crisis centre, a decision was taken to initiate nested suicide prevention programmes. The idea behind these programmes is that, since suicide is a multidimensional problem, suicide prevention could be incorporated in other health and social programmes. So relevant, viable successful programmes were identified and the component of suicide prevention introduced:

1. Alcoholism plays a significant role in suicide in India and so, with the Ranganathan Foundation, a leading NGO working in alcoholism rural camps, prevention programmes were conducted concerning the double danger of alcoholism and suicide. (A rural camp is one where, after prior advertising in a rural area, a team of professionals is available for a specific purpose and all the people in the nearby villages can make use of their services, which are usually free of cost.)
2. With women's activist groups, coping strategies were imparted to female construction workers.
3. Along with another NGO involved in health education in the form of street plays in the urban slums, street plays were conducted in all the slums of the city, watched by 60 000 people. The street plays focused on emotional distress, suicidal thoughts, the need to seek help, and the support systems that are available. Subsequent visits were also made to assess the impact of the plays and to offer support in the community.
4. Along with an environment activist group, biopesticides were promoted to counter the high rates of chemical pesticide poisoning deaths (Vijayakumar 2003).

In response to the high number of suicides by young men in Hong Kong, volunteers initiated the SKO life skills project. The project is a collaborative effort of the Samaritans (voluntary suicide prevention centre), Kely Support Group (an agency focusing on developing peer support in local schools and communities to fight drug abuse), and Outward Bound (an agency focusing on self-confidence, leadership, and team work). The aim of the project was to train young students to support those in distress and to teach others how to recognize and respond to people in distress and despair. The programme was considered a huge success by all the agencies. Unfortunately there was no follow up of the students to evaluate its impact on them (Kumaria 2001).

Reaching Young Europe is a project initiated by Befrienders International, with the collaboration of professionals and schools. It teaches problem-solving skills to young children by means of tales and cartoons. The programme has been evaluated and shown to produce a significant improvement in social skills and empathy, but not in coping skills (Mishara and Ystgaard 2000).

Volunteer organizations were the first to use technology such as e-mail for supporting suicidal persons. Even in countries where only letters were used for communication, volunteers had perfected a system of leading support through letters. Marginalized people, people living in rural and remote areas, and vulnerable populations have the focus of attention for these initiatives.

Relative strengths of volunteers and professionals

The major strengths of volunteers are their easy availability, accessibility, affordability, unconditional acceptance, and their flexibility. Professionals, on the other hand, are more knowledgeable and experienced, have greater frustration-tolerance, and have more knowledge of how to deal with co-morbid conditions and how to treat suicidal persons. Both volunteers and professionals need to be empathetic while dealing with suicidal clients. This suggests that volunteers are ideally suited to handle the short-term risk of suicide, while professionals are more proficient in handling longer-term suicide risk.

An example of collaboration

Mrs X is a young mother with two children. She is overwhelmed with the routine work of keeping a home and caring for her children and the family, along with a husband who needs to travel a lot at work. She has seriously contemplated suicide several times, and the last time she came close to the point of attempting suicide. One morning she happened to see an advertisement of a help centre in the local newspaper, with an accompanying phone number. The advertisement said that people who are having thoughts about ending their lives could call and there would be somebody to talk to and share their feelings with.

On seeing this information Mrs X called the centre and spoke to a volunteer, who listened to her patiently. After speaking to the volunteer Mrs X felt a little better and that she could now handle her life situation. But after a couple of days she called back again. The volunteer who spoke to Mrs X felt that her thoughts about ending her life were deep rooted and needed more professional help. So the volunteer asked Mrs X to go to a psychiatrist. Mrs X's initial reaction was rejection of even the idea of taking such a step. But the volunteer spoke to her at length and convinced her that it would be for her own good, and going to a professional would give her the necessary strength to face the challenges in her life. Finally, after considerable discussion, Mrs X agreed to go to the psychiatrist, but only with the volunteer. She saw an understanding friend in the volunteer who provided the required moral support to go to the professional.

The psychiatrist conducted a detailed assessment of Mrs X and also spoke to her at length about her problems. He then prescribed her medication. Mrs X took the medication, but very reluctantly. She felt that both her family and society would consider her a mentally unbalanced person. Keeping her on medication itself required a lot of support and encouragement, and the professional collaborated with the volunteer to ensure compliance.

When she became a little more confident, Mrs X wanted to reduce the dosage of the medication. A few days after the medication was reduced she once again started feeling suicidal. She called the volunteer who, after talking to her, sought her permission to call the psychiatrist. The psychiatrist and the volunteer decided to work together to help Mrs X. This was an instance where the close interaction between the professional and the volunteer helped the client to overcome her suicidal crisis.

This kind of interaction between the concerned parties would go a long way in preventing suicide. The patient feels assured that there are knowledgeable people who care for her, and she receives a more holistic style of care. The volunteer is reassured that even if there is a relapse, there is an expert to turn to. The doctor knows that his diagnoses and treatment are being followed, along with the necessary emotional support, without which individuals may become suicide statistics.

It would be interesting to find out:

+ how many suicidal clients willingly seek professional help;
+ the reactions of the spouse and other family members once the suicidal patient starts treatment;
+ the level of ease with which suicidal patients are integrated within the family;
+ the implications once the client starts treatment with a volunteer or professional; and
+ how many well-structured programmes there are for caring for suicidal clients where professionals and volunteers work together collaboratively.

Conclusions

When individuals contemplate suicide, it is because they have reached the end of their mental and emotional resources. It is obvious that not everyone attempts suicide only because they are overwhelmed with life's challenges—brain chemistry also plays a role in increasing the risk of suicidal behaviour, along with pathological causes and genetic influences, as well as the mental and emotional make-up of the individual, together with environmental factors. Where there are multiple reasons for suicidal behaviour, effective care may also need to be multifaceted. This requires cooperation, collaboration, and commitment.

Until now, volunteer action toward suicide prevention was based on the needs of the client and what the volunteer could offer within the domain of their functioning. The need of the moment is to structure programmes undertaken by volunteers in the area of suicide prevention on scientific principles, constantly evaluate and study the efficacy of such programmes, and incorporate necessary changes, thereby establishing a 'science to practice' approach.

The psychological skills of the professionals, along with their knowledge of psychopharmacology, may enable them to handle the psychopathology of an individual with suicidal tendencies. Often, however, the professional does not have the extended time and accessibility required for these clients. The volunteer has the time, accessibility, and the skills to provide the necessary emotional support. When all these specialized skills are brought together, prevention of suicide can become more effective and meaningful to suicidal persons, volunteers, and professionals.

References

Bagley, G. (1968). The evaluation of a suicide prevention scheme by an ecological model. *Social Science and Medicine*, 2, 1–14.

Barraclough, B.M., Jennings, C., and Moss, J.R. (1977). Suicide prevention by the Samaritans. *Lancet*, i, 237–9.

Bridge, T., Potkin, S., Zung, W., and Soldo, B. (1977). Suicide prevention centers. *Journal of Nervous and Mental Disease*, 164, 18–24.

Cotton, C.R. and Range, L.M. (1992). Reliability and validity of the Suicide Intervention Response Inventory. *Death Studies*, 16, 79–86.

Daigle, M.S. and Mishara, B. (1995). Intervention styles with suicidal callers at two suicide prevention centres. *Suicide and Life Threatening-Behavior*, 25, 261–75.

Dew, M.A., Bromet, E.J., Brent, D.F., and Greenhouse, J.B. (1987). A quantitative literature review of the effectiveness of suicide prevention centers. *Journal of Counselling and Clinical Psychology*, 55, 239–44.

Diekstra, R.F.W. and Kerkhoff, A.J.F.M. (1989). Attitudes towards suicide: the development of a suicide attitude questionnaire (SUIATT). In *Suicide and its prevention, the role of attitude and imitation*, (ed. R.F.W. Diekstra, R. Maris, S. Platt, A. Schmidtke, and G. Sonneck), pp. 91–107. Britt, Leiden.

Huang, W.C. and Lester, D. (1995). Have suicide prevention centers prevented suicide in Taiwan? *Chinese Journal of Mental Health*, 8 (3), 27–9.

Jennings, C., Barraclough, B.M., and Moss, J.R. (1978). Have the Samaritans lowered the suicide rate? *Psychological Medicine*, 8, 413–22.

Kinzel, A. and Nanson, J. (2000). Education and bebriefing: Strategies for preventing crisis in crisis line volunteers. *Crisis*, 21 (3), 126–34.

Kumaria, S. (2001). Training young befrienders. *Crisis*, 22, 87–8.

Leenaars, A.A. and Lester, D. (1995). Impact of suicide prevention centers on suicide in Canada. *Crisis*, 16, 39.

Lester, D. (1974a). Suicide prevention centers. *Journal of the American Medical Association*, 229, 394.

Lester, D (1974b). Effect of suicide prevention centres on suicide rates in the U.S. *Health Services Psychological Reports*, 89, 37–9.

Lester, D. (1980). Comment. Suicide prevention by the Samaritans. *Social Science and Medicine*, 14A, 85.

Lester, D. (1990). Was gas detoxification or establishment of suicide prevention centers responsible for the decline in the British suicide rate? *Psychological Reports*, 66, 286.

Lester, D. (1993). The effectiveness of suicide prevention centers. *Suicide and Life-Threatening Behavior*, 23, 263–7.

Lester, D. (1994). Evaluating the effectiveness of the Samaritans in England and Wales. *International Journal of Health Sciences*, 5, 73–4.

Lester, D. (1997) Effectiveness of suicide prevention centres—A review. *Suicide and Life-Threatening Behavior*, 27 (3), 304–10.

Lester, D., Saito, Y., and Abe, K. (1996). Have suicide prevention centers prevented suicide in Japan? *Archives of Suicide Research*, 2, 125–8.

McClaire, J.N. (1973). Volunteers in a suicide prevention service. *Journal of Community Psychology*, 4, 397–8.

Medoff, M.H. (1984). An evaluation of the effectiveness of suicide prevention centers. *Journal of Behavioral Economics*, 15, 43–55.

Miller, M., Coomber, D., Leeper, J., and Barton, S. (1984). An analysis of the effects of suicide prevention facilities on suicide rates in the US. *Americal Journal of Public Health*, 74, 340–3.

Mishara, B.L. and Daigle, M. (1992). The effectiveness of telephone intervention by suicide prevention centers. *Canada's Mental Health*, 40 (3), 24–9.

Mishara, B.L. and Giroux, G. (1993). The relationship between coping strategies and perceived stress in telephone intervention counseling at a suicide prevention centre. *Suicide and Life-Threatening Behavior*, 23 (3), 221–9.

Mishara, B. and Ystgaard, M. (2000). Exploring the potential for primary prevention. Evaluation of Befrienders International Reaching Young Europe pilot programme in Denmark. *Crisis*, 21, 4–6.

Neimeyer, R.A. and MacInnes, W.D. (1981). Assessing paraprofessional competence with the Suicide Intervention Response Inventory. *Journal of Counseling Psychology*, 28, 206–9.

Neimeyer, R.A., Fortner, B., and Melby, D. (2001). Personal and professional factors and suicide intervention skills. *Suicide and Life-Threatening Behavior*, 31 (1), 71–82.

Reid, P. and Smith, H. (1980). Knowledge about suicide among members of helping agencies in Ireland. *Journal of the Irish Medical Association*, 73, 117–19.

Riehl, T., Marchner, E., and Moller, H.J. (1988). Influence of crisis intervention telephone services ('Crisis hotlines') on the suicide rate in 25 German cities. In *Current issues of suicidology*, (ed. H.J. Moller, A. Schmidtke, and R. Welz), pp. 431–6. Springer-Verlag, New York.

Rogers, J.R., Lewis, M.M., and Sublich, L.M. (2002). Validity of the Suicide Assessment Checklist in an emergency crisis center. *Journal of Counselling and Development*, **80**, 493–502.

Vijayakumar, L. (2003) Sneha – Working with suicide. In *Meeting the mental health needs of developing countries*, (ed. V. Patel and R. Thara), pp. 261–72. Sage Publications, New Delhi.

Vijayakumar, L. and Keir, N. (1998). Volunteer attitude to suicide. *Befriending Worldwide*, **3**, 4–5.

Weiner, I.W. (1969). The effectiveness of a suicide prevention program. *Mental Hygiene*, **53**, 357–63.

Wenz, F.R. and Papendick, K.M. (1988). How telephone crisis counselors perceive suicidal callers. *Proceedings of the Annual Meeting of the American Association of Suicidology*, pp. 71–2. American Association of Suicidology, Washington DC.

World Heath Organization (2001). *Atlas of Mental Health Resources in the World*. World Health Organization, Geneva.

20

Suicide survivorship: an unknown journey from loss to gain—from individual to global perspective

Onja Grad

> The loss of a loved person is one of the most intensely painful experiences any human being can suffer, and not only is it painful to experience, but also painful to witness, if only because we are so impotent to help.
> (*Bowlby 1991*)

Introduction

The terms 'suicide survivor' or 'survivor of suicide' used to be confusing and ambiguous, and sometimes still are. They were used for two kinds of individuals: those who attempted suicide and survived the act and those who lost somebody they were close to by suicide. Lately, the second meaning has been fully adopted by various organizations helping these people. It has also been used in the professional and lay literature, and bereaved individuals themselves have identified with it. 'Survivors of suicide are the family members and friends who experience the suicide of a loved one' (McIntosh 1993).

When suicide survivors started to attract attention in both the clinical and scientific fields, and the number of publications about this issue started to increase, it became clear how difficult it was to do methodologically well-planned, evidence-based, and controlled studies. Pfeffer's statement that 're-search data is not conclusive or extensive enough to provide reliable and valid perspectives on the issue of suicide survivors' (Pfeffer 2002) reflects the present state of the art. Many theories, conclusions, and therapeutic suggestions derive from anectodal evidence, usually based on studies of individuals seeking help. The results of these studies may not be accurate, for at least three reasons:

(1) individuals in the studies are selected—either by their own judgement that they need help or through being referred by their GP or others in their close environment;

(2) the studies are usually based on small samples, mostly without matched, or often any, controls; and

(3) if a caregiver or a therapist is performing the research, which is often the case, there is a danger of a biased view, contaminated by transference and counter-transference.

Bearing these shortcomings of past research in mind, we can better understand the diversity of findings about the reactions and needs of suicide survivors and models of suicide survivorship. Clark (2001) talks about two kinds of models of grieving in the literature: passive models, such as disease models and those that emphasize the passage of bereavement through various stages; versus active approaches, involving work, tasks, participation, growth, and fulfilment.

Conclusions from studies vary between those claiming that bereavement after suicide is similar or that it is different to the bereavement after other kinds of death. Many authors have argued that grief after suicide takes longer, is more difficult and ambigious, brings some expected and even more unexpected feelings or mood changes (Farberow 1991, 1992; Cleiren 1993; Cleiren et al. 1996; Grad and Zavasnik 1996, 1999). Grief after suicide, although sharing much in common with sadness after other modes of death, does appear to have several features that distinguish it from the grief following from other types of death (Barret and Scott 1990; Bailey et al. 1999; Harwood et al. 2002; Silverman et al. 1995). As Clark (2001) says:

> In light of evidence that the grieving process may last several years and of the increased risk of mortality as well as physical, psychological and social morbidity associated with bereavement, the cumulative effects of completed suicide are far reaching indeed. Concern with the issue of bereavement after suicide is therefore of prime importance, not only because of our humanitarian responsibility toward alleviating the collective distress, but also to prevent complications arising from the aftermath of completed suicide, one of which, importantly, is further suicide.

Individual level of grief

Grief is a reaction to extreme damage to a social bond. If we recall Freud's views—to love someone is to place in that person a part of one's self, therefore when that person dies, so does the part of the self (Freud 1934)—then the death of a loved one is linked to damage to a secure sense of self (Seale 1998). Bereavement that follows is a long-term, multidimensional process (Lund and Caserta 1998), in which bereaved people show certain similarities, yet may be very different at the same time. Even though some phases and feelings of bereavement are largely universal across cultures and individuals, mourning also seems to be one of the most unique and individual behaviours of human beings.

The process of bereavement depends on many factors, one of the most important being the way in which the person died. The process is more complicated when the death was unexpected, violent, and traumatic (Jordan 2001; Merlevede *et al.* 2004). Suicide is definitely that kind of death. It starts and ends with pain. A person commits suicide when his or her inner pain is so unbearable that he or she cannot stand it any more. This inner pain may derive from various combinations of biological and genetic factors, as well as environmental factors. The unbearable pain is also very often provoked and triggered by the loss of something or someone that this person had, wished or hoped for, needed, was promised, or thought that he/she had been entitled to. Some of these things might be: a happy childhood, a good relationship or marriage, intact physical or mental health, position in society, etc. Each of these things may have been essential to the person, but one or more was not achieved for a variety of reasons, so they decided that it was impossible to live without them (Grad 2002). When suicide occurs, the bereaved person may be part of this failure, or is at least aware of the unfulfilled wishes of the deceased. The bereaved is left with the question, 'What was my share in his/her decision-making?'

This crucial question of the bereaved person's own involvement with the deceased's decision to comit suicide makes suicide different to most other deaths, and can make the event extremely difficult to survive. So how do bereaved people feel and react afterwards? According to Freud's (1934) and Bowlby's (1991) views, definitely not as being intact any more. Not only do they report feelings of rejection, self-blame, guilt, shame, anger, lowered self-esteem, and anxiety (Picton *et al.* 2001), but also often fear that they somehow did not stop certain behaviour or try to influence the person not to end their life. Certain differences in reactions are found in the controlled studies comparing bereavement after suicide with other violent modes of death (accidents, murders) and with natural, expected deaths (Cleiren *et al.* 1996; Grad and Zavasnik 1996; Jordan, 2001; Harwood *et al.* 2002) (Table 20.1). Jordan (2001) talks about three distinctions between bereavement after suicide and other modes of death: (1) the thematic content of grief, (2) the social processes surrounding the survivor, and (3) the impact suicide has on the family system. While scientific studies do not necessarily indicate that bereavement after suicide is more painful than bereavement after other modes of death, the writings of survivors themselves suggest that it is (Bolton 1983; Dunne 1987; Wertheimer 1997).

Even though many authors showed some differences in bereavement after suicide compared with other types of death, more overall similarities were found between different modes of death, especially when comparing sudden

Table 20.1 Differences found in bereaved individuals after different modes of death

Alexander (1991)	Suicide survivors more frequently reported experiencing feelings of rejection and abandonment
Bailey *et al.* (1999)	Feelings of rejection and abandonment, feelings of responsibility for the death by suicide, more embarrassment and shame, more rumination about why
Barret and Scott (1990)	Larger number of grief reactions, more rejection, concealment of the cause of death from others, sensitivity to media coverage, more stigmatization and shame
Clark and Goldney (1995)	Even though grief after suicide is quantitatively similar, it is qualitatively different
Cleiren (1993)	Less depressed than bereaved after traffic accidents, different pace of detachment and depression.
Cleiren *et al.* (1996)	Cross-cultural comparison between two countries—Slovenia and The Netherlands—and three modes of death: suicide bereaved felt more abandoned by both societies and more blamed and avoided by others than bereaved by traffic fatalities and terminal illness
Demi (1984)	Widows after suicide of their husbands better off than widows after other modes of death?accustomed to the mental illness and other problems of deceased spouse before suicide
Farberow (1991)	Less qualitative social support (men), slower recuperation from depressed state (more fluctuation in men) in people bereaved by suicide compared with people bereaved by natural death
Farberow *et al.* (1992)	Poorer mental health and higher levels of depression in spouses bereaved by suicide compared with spouses bereaved by other types of death 12 months after the deaths; differences largely disappeared 30 months after the deaths
Grad and Zavasnik (1996)	The bereaved examined 2 months after their spouse's death by suicide and those after traffic accidents—the former had significantly more difficulties in accepting the death, but thought more often that 'death seemed a good solution'
Grad and Zavasnik (1999)	Spouses bereaved after suicide, traffic accident, terminal illness—suicide group expressed more shame (after 2 months, but not after 14), more feelings of being abandoned by the deceased; after 14 months better recovery for those grieving suicide
Harwood *et al.* (2002)	Higher scores (on the GEQ) on stigmatization, shame, rejection, and unique reactions subscales in people bereaved by suicide compared to those bereaved by deaths due to illness
Osterweis *et al.* (1984)	More social stigmatization than following other modes of death
Range and Calhoun (1990)	Social reactions more condemning after suicide than after accidental deaths

Table 20.1 (continued) Differences found in bereaved individuals after different modes of death

Rudestam (1992)	Less social support for suicide survivors than those who have experienced other types of death
Reed and Greenwald (1991)	People bereaved by suicide show more feelings of guilt, shame and rejection, but less emotional distress and shock than people bereaved by accidental deaths
Thompson and Range (1993)	Suicide bereavement involved most variability in social support in comparison with bereavement after four other modes of death

deaths or bereavement process over time, when previous differences between the groups tended to disappear (Barret and Scott 1990; Ellenbogen and Gratton 2001; Grad and Zavasnik 1999; McIntosh 1993).

If we summarize the possible differences between groups grieving after different modes of death, we find suicide survivors to be more ashamed and to feel more stigmatized, rejected, and abandoned. The crucial conclusion is what Jordan (2001) so clearly observed: 'that there is an apparent contradiction between the perceptions of people who are bereaved by suicide and the clinicians who work closely with them, and researchers who study survivors from a greater distance with the tools of social science'. This was supported by the study by Grad and Zavasnik (1999), who expected differences in level of depression (BDI scores) between the groups of suicide survivors and survivors of traffic accidents, but found little or none. Their previous assumptions were based on the clinical experiences with the bereaved who had searched for psychotherapeutic help, while the randomly selected sample proved to be different.

History of bereavement after suicide

Throughout history the phenomenon of suicide has triggered a variety of studies, involving a range of sciences, and also religious and philosophical explanations, as well as often appearing in novels. In addition, much attention has been paid to how best to help suicidal individuals and to a range of preventive measures.

Yet, the enigma persists as to why—in spite of all this interest in suicide and suicidal people—surviving individuals and families struck by suicide of someone close have received so much social punishment, stigma, pain, and scars, and received so little scientific or therapeutic interest and help. That was the case at least until very recently. Before the middle of the twentieth century the bereaved were not only robbed of their loved one, of their pride, self-esteem, and property, they were also punished. Survivors often lost their position in society, their property was confiscated, and, with this act, they were also robbed of the prospect for future life (Parkes *et al.* 1997). They were proclaimed sinners without committing a sin. In addition, and most importantly, they were often rejected and had no voice to speak up for themselves.

Did this happen because of some sort of belief that those left behind had in some way been involved in the decision of the deceased for his or her chosen death? Or was the purpose of this attitude to protect society from inner fears that something like this might happen to anybody? A very plausible explanation is that this ignorant behaviour towards the survivors simply provided a defence, namely that suicide happens to others, to those sinful, insane people, who are probably also genetically vulnerable and deserve to be ignored, stigmatized, or even punished. Of course, another possible explanation is that this absolutely inappropriate treatment of the survivors might serve as a (rather unsucessful) suicide prevention measure—both for potentially suicidal people and their relatives—through encouraging people not to commit suicide because of social control and social fear.

After each death, society offers, demands, and expects some rituals to be followed, with the purpose of these being to help the bereaved. The suffering of the bereaved is acute after any death, but the grief inflicted by suicide may be the hardest of all to cope with. Survivors of other kinds of death can depend on the rituals civilization has developed to support them in their grief. But for thousands of years survivors of suicide have suffered alone and in silence. In fact, the best treatment they could hope for was to be ignored. Although the corpses of persons who have committed suicide are no longer dragged through the streets and their property is not confiscated, survivors still face a legacy of anti-suicidal attitudes that have evolved over centuries (Colt 1987). This 'mark of Cain', though much more disguised and hidden than before, is still an additional source of pain for the survivors of suicide. Today's attitudes toward suicide are the product of centuries of condemnation, religious and ethical imperatives, medical opinions, and personal experience with suicidal behaviour (Stillion and Stillion 1999).

> Suicide is not socially acceptable way to die under any circumstances – without socially acceptable reasons for death, how can the loss be socially acceptable?
>
> (Wallace 1977)

The present state of suicide survivorship

When we look at the countries that officially recognize the problem, and offer help to this group of suffering individuals, we find only a small number of them, mainly limited to the most developed countries of Western Europe, North America, and Australia (Clark 2001). Countries with some of the highest rates of suicide (Eastern Europe, some Asian countries), or where suicides are not officially registered (some developing countries), have very little or no service for suicide survivors whatsoever. In Europe, a recently published directory for suicide survivors services reveals that only 17 countries have some services available for the bereaved, and that this number presents a fourfold increase within the 5 years since 1997 (Farberow and Andriessen 2002). Even in those countries where suicide survivor movements are active— like the USA and Scandinavia—it is estimated that only a quarter, at most, of the bereaved seek help of any kind after their loss (Saarinen *et al.* 1999).

There are several possible explanations why so few suicide survivors get involved in any kind of help or support:

◆ Some survivors simply do not need help other than from their family and friends.
◆ Some suppress or deny difficult feelings and reactions to avoid pain or to keep their emotional balance.
◆ Some fear being recognized as a survivor and try to avoid public reactions, such as pity, blame, condemnation, stigmatization, etc.
◆ Suicide survivors with certain personality traits may feel uncertain about their own need for help because they fear this might lower their self-esteem, make them more insecure, and unbalance their fragile inner homeostasis.
◆ Some do not believe in the notion of obtaining any help from the outside and keep their pain and problems inside (especially men), or try to find another way to relieve their feelings (substance abuse, overworking, etc.).
◆ There is no organized help available in their environment, even though needed.
◆ Unfavourable attitudes and public opinions or rules on how to behave towards the survivors of suicide mitigate against help being offered.

It would be interesting to know how the level of suicide in a society relates to the attitudes towards survivors. Does the frequency of suicide help or hinder positive reactions towards suicide survivors? And what is the impact of the level of suicide on the language we use when talking about suicide? Could what the immunologist Ihan (2001) proposed be possible, namely that there is an inner protocol for committing suicide incorporated in the human brain that has been transmitted from mother to child through coded language based on local culture, and that this is triggered by specific signals from the culture? Similar social code could probably serve survivors as well.

There are some possible explanations why there has been so little scientific pressure to perform methodologically sound research, thus placing so much reliance on more anecdotal or case-based evidence:

1. It is difficult to get survivors to co-operate in research. The findings are mostly based on reports of those survivors that are willing to co-operate. We lack information on those who decline, who, in most studies, comprise between 20 and 50% of potential subjects (Kissane *et al.* 1996; Grad and Zavasnik 1999; Herkert 2000). Therefore generalization from the results of these kind of studies is problematic (Brownstein 1992). In a recent British study on bereavement following suicide, the authors were able to provide limited information on non-participants (Harwood *et al.* 2002).

2. This research poses ethical and moral dilemmas, especially regarding the potential intrusion of investigators in the family after such a traumatic loss. This may contribute to the relatively high rate of refusal to participate, self-protection or protection of some family members, and negative opinions of ethical committees about such studies. It would be relevant to study also the attitudes and prejudices of members of ethical committees concerning the subject of suicide. There is also a question of the effect of the interview on the phenomenon being studied, and the reliability of data based on a selected group of individuals (Asgard and Carlsson-Bergstrom 1991; Beskow *et al.* 1991).

3. Living in a Western culture, many bereaved, especially those bereaved after suicide, are uneasy with a direct discussion on death and grieving (Herkert 2000), and many researchers agree with the notion that grief and mourning are private, intimate, and highly personal matters, and thus difficult to investigate.

However, to obtain more relevant information on why and how suicide survivors grieve, we have to try to get more survivors to co-operate with studies, so that we can obtain findings that are generalizable to all parts of the target population and not just those that are more readily accessible (Lund and Caserta 1998).

Suicide bereavement at the global level

On the basis of the claims that each suicide has, on average, a major impact on six people (Shneidman 1969, 1972), at least 6 million people worldwide (if not more) each year are affected by the horrifying experience of surviving the suicide of a close relative, friend, school-mate, student, colleague at work, patient, or a therapist. As Shneidman commented, they represent the largest mental health casualty area related to suicide (Shneidman 1972; McIntosh

1993). On the basis of the findings from a Finnish study, only one-quarter of them seek any help (Saarinen *et al.* 1999). However, half of all the interviewees (women more often than men) in this study felt the need for psychiatric counselling and treatment, which means that 25% of all the survivors who admitted the need for help had not received it. This seems to be similar for most Western societies. On the other hand, we can only speculate what is happening in the rest of the world.

Different outcomes of suicide bereavement

The experience of such a traumatic event as loss by suicide is extremely powerful. It is likely to release great emotional energy, whether recognized and allowed expression, or suppressed and denied. The power and direction of these emotions are not possible to foresee or forecast. It is unlikely that any human being is left unaffected in some way by the experience, even though some individuals might seemingly react as if they are.

Before a disastrous and traumatic loss occurs in human life, most persons hold three basic assumptions: that their world seems benevolent, that it has meaning, and that they are themselves worthy (Reisman 2001). Any traumatic and unexpected death (such as suicide) can create a powerful distress and many people suddenly feel that their fundamental assumptions were illusory. This notion is likely to produce changes in a person's attitudes towards the self, others, and the world as a whole.

Several factors influence the course of bereavement (Grad 1996; Clark and Goldney 2000). These include the gender and age of the bereaved, the age of the deceased, the nature of the relationship with them, the time elapsed since the death, exposure to the body immediately after the death, the method of suicide, the extent to which the act was anticipated, social support, and receipt of preliminary help. Because the outcome of the bereavement process after suicide depends on many personal, cultural, and historical factors, it is unpredictable and in some ways mysterious (Fig. 20.1). At the individual level it depends on the personality traits of the bereaved, the relationship with the deceased, past experiences with different losses, and the support of the immediate social network (Fig. 20.2).

At the family level, many specific and combined factors play an important part in the process of bereavement, such as: transgenerational patterns, the stage of the life cycle in which the family is, the role and position of the deceased member inside the family structure and hierarchy, specific beliefs, values and taboos (family scripts) that a family or individual members have, whether the family was functional or dysfunctional before the suicide, the

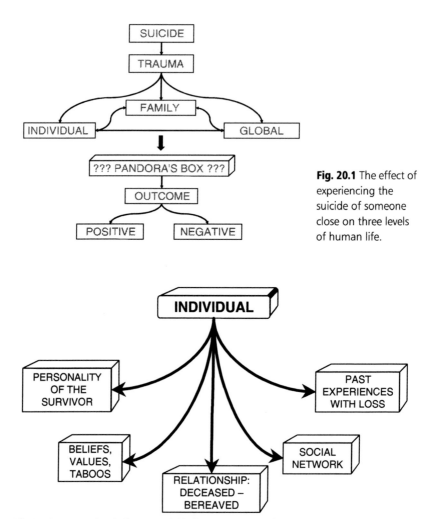

Fig. 20.1 The effect of experiencing the suicide of someone close on three levels of human life.

Fig. 20.2 Factors that influence suicide bereavement at the individual level.

experiences with previous losses and how the family as a system coped with them (Fig. 20.3) (Byng-Hall 1991).

The third, global level of bereavement after suicide is determined by rituals around bereavement, the social network of the bereaved, generally accepted way of raising children (resulting in the so-called national character), social norms, cultural and religious influences, possible stigma or taboo within the society, and political or economic factors (Fig. 20.4). We have relatively little understanding of the importance of each level, how they influence each other and their relevance to possible outcome. This is an area that would benefit from more research, especially cross-cultural comparisons.

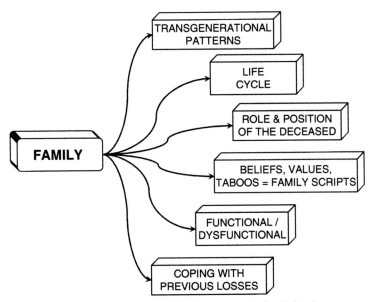

Fig. 20.3 Factors that influence suicide bereavement at the family level.

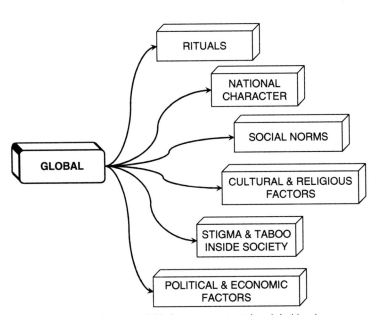

Fig. 20.4 Factors that influence suicide bereavement at the global level.

Therapeutic care for suicide survivors

Help for close relatives, friends, and others witnessing suicide is divided into two parts:

+ immediate help at the spot, or when notifying whoever about the death; and
+ long-lasting help when the bereavement process becomes overwhelming and unbearable for some bereaved.

The immediate help or emotional support on the spot should be offered by a coroner or GP on duty after they are called to examine the body of the deceased. When the suicide has happened somewhere else, and the family has only been notified, the person on duty (in some countries this would be a policeman or coroner, in others this would be a physician, and in others a combination of such individuals) should be trained to help, or at least to refer the most distressed family member to the closest trauma counselling service. If help is given immediately after the body is found, it should predominantly consist of support, understanding, and enabling venting of the feelings of first shock. This depends on who found the body, in what circumstances, and how unexpected the act was. Usually shock protects the next of kin from immediate awareness of the reality, and makes them feel as if they are only witnessing somebody else's experience. However, in cases of severe reaction following the death, the person suffering should be helped on the spot (crisis intervention) or taken to a psychiatrist for help. It is also important for people close to the deceased to have the opportunity to see the body (or at least a part of it, if it is too mutilated) and also to have the oportunity and time to say good-bye.

When bereavement starts and the bereaved encounters some difficulties coping, different kinds of help should be offered. After reassessing relevant literature, Jordan (2001) proposes homogeneous groups, psychoeducational services, and family and social network interventions. As the whole process of bereavement after suicide varies with every individual, and depends on his or her personality, experiences with the deceased, the length and quality of the relationship, the life cycle in which the bereaved is (Grad 2002; Hawton and Simkin 2003), and many other factors mentioned above, it is important that the individual receives help that is as personalized as possible.

There has been some experience with peer and therapist-led groups (Farberow 1992; Clark and Goldney 1995; Grad *et al.*, 2003) and, since Freud, individual therapies have been offered to the bereaved. However, a distinction must be made between pathological grief reactions, where strict professional help is needed, and the time-limited expected problems in mourning that follow most suicides, where lay or professional support may be given. Many suicide survivors need help, because it is difficult to talk about suicide in the family to others, due to their blame and guilt feelings and to real or projected social stigma. Some need more support in understanding and recognizing their own feelings of rejection, abandonment, and guilt, and some need more reassurance for their lowered self-esteem, loss of strength, and motivation for life. Sometimes the physical and emotional problems become unbearable, depression is severe and social isolation dangerous. Most suicide survivors need understanding, support, and to be listened to, sharing brutal details that haunt them after finding the body, and time with a counsellor or other survivors to work through their grief—both in individual and group settings (Table 20.2). Some need more: a skilled therapist who would help them to understand and to work through their own inner images, unexpected emotions and disturbing thoughts, nightmares, and fantasies. The therapist may use different approaches, but psychodynamically oriented psychotherapy with a cognitive–systemic base has proved to be most successful, combined with antidepressant therapy if needed (Worden 1991; Clark and Goldney 2000; Grad 2002).

The aftermath

While the bereavement process often causes much emotional turmoil, the eventual aftermath can vary greatly. Some suicide survivors come out of their

Table 20.2 Key elements in helping suicide survivors

Providing helpful, tolerant, secure, and understanding atmosphere for the bereaved
Going over the details of finding the body and about their feelings when they were notified of the suicide
Going through positive, ambivalent, and negative memories about the deceased
Understanding, venting, accepting, and allowing feelings: sadness, anger, fury, fear, anxiety, guilt, shame, self-blame, regret
Accepting and allowing crying and other behavioural expressions of emotions
Raising self-esteem (Clark and Goldney 2000) and supporting new social skills
Provoking expressions of transitional objects (Worden 1991), symbolizations (Grad and Zavasnik 2003), fantasies, dreams; accepting them and explaining their meaning
Using photos to remember, and writing farewell letters to the deceased, if acceptable and relieving for the bereaved
Talking about different experiences and problems when discussing the deceased's suicide with other people (extended family, colleagues, friends, acquaintances)
Acknowledging and expressing (usually unrealistic) questioning of why and consequent self-blaming for suicide
Follow-up (Dyregrow 2003).

grief with a positive outcome, others with a negative outcome. One of the rare prospective studies of this was a Finnish investigation as part of the National Suicide Prevention Project in Finland. This showed how suicide survivors deal with their grief and life in the long run. Saarinen and colleagues (2000) assessed 104 survivors of suicide with a baseline interview within the first 6 months after suicide and again 10 years later with 64 of the original participants. They found that major life changes associated with suicide were common, and that these could be unfavourable as well as favourable. Personal growth was the term used for the positive outcome in the so-called experimental theory of bereavement (Hogan *et al.* 1996). The interviewed participants mostly claimed that they had become more empathic, caring, and connected to others.

There are some dilemmas about what can be labelled as positive and negative outcomes after a long journey through the emotional ordeal of suicide survivorship. There is an accepted assumption that the bereaved person is 'healed' when they are performing at the same level as before the death, or when 'a person can reinvest his or her emotions back into the life and in the living' (Worden 1991). It is probably as important and significant to know how a person is *feeling* rather than that they are at least apparently functioning as usual.

More often suicide survivorship has been connected to different negative outcomes, which are:

♦ becoming suicidal or even committing suicide;
♦ becoming depressed, and staying depressed for a long period of time, possibly permanently;
♦ functioning poorly in the role of a parent, partner, worker, student (long sick leave, social isolation, invalidity pension as a result of never having finished bereavement);
♦ preserving the taboo connected to suicide through silence and denial and transmitting it to the next generation;
♦ never-ending questioning about the reasons for suicide, and thus not reaching inner peace and acceptance of the reality of the loss;
♦ transmitting the negative outcome to the next generation and thus increasing the risk for suicide via language, silence, prejudice, attitudes, and preserving myths.

A special category of survivors comprises those individuals inside the 'silent' societies, where the suicide itself is never discussed or bereavement after suicide is not recognized. They might not recognize any emotional reaction related to this loss and thus cannot express it and ask for help. But the energy provoked may be bottled up and may lead to disturbed or even violent behaviour.

There are also positive and favourable outcomes, however absurd and paradoxical this might seem to the survivor immediately after the loss. There is no doubt that after surviving suicide nothing seems the same as before. No one other than the survivors themselves can judge at what point they should feel better. After the long passage through the various phases of bereavement—either with or without professional help—we can observe some beneficial outcomes at the individual, family, and global levels.

At the individual level (Lieberman 1996; Lund and Caserta 1998):

♦ After concluding the process of bereavement the survivor says: 'Nothing worse can happen to me, I can handle life if I survived this trauma'. They believe in their own life strength.
♦ The survivor can better cope with life problems.
♦ The survivor becomes more sensitive to suicidal clues in other people.
♦ The survivor gains independence, autonomy, pride, feels more self-sufficient, and grows personally.

At the family level:

♦ The surviving family becomes more connected and more functional.
♦ The family can produce and follow a new family script that will strengthen the whole family system.
♦ The family as a whole can be more sensitive to the signs of potential suicide in others, including family members.

At the global level:

♦ The survivors of suicide are the experts in human suffering related to suicide—usually they know a lot about suicide and they are more aware than the average person of the needs suicidal people have. They can use their knowledge to diminish taboos, to destigmatize, and to educate.
♦ Suicide survivors can help in organizing self-help movements and national programmes, and also prepare publications to help others learn from their experiences.

Conclusions

When suicide occurs we think and talk mainly about the loss. It is difficult to even imagine that a survivor would, or could, see anything else but the negative side of this event. When, as a therapist, one helps survivors to travel through their grief and to conclude this dramatic journey one way or another, and to pick up their lives again, it is a privilege to realize what they gained through their time of suffering. As Frank Campbell recently said (Clark 2001): ' I have had the privilege of working with survivors and watching them climb out of canyons of pain in order to stand on mountaintops, forever changed by this indescribable and complicated bereavement.'

Different help, support, and individual or group therapies offer the bereaved some resolving of grief at the pre-suicide level of functioning, which determines the end of the bereavement process. Sometimes they might even feel better, wiser, and more satisfied. It is quite possible that a bereaved person could remain somewhat depressed but at the same time feel pride in learning how to do something new, and feel motivated to learn other new skills (Yalom and Lieberman 1991; Lieberman 1996; Lund and Caserta 1998). Feeling at peace with oneself, trying to better understand others and their problems, becoming more tolerant and wiser—these are definitely gains after experiencing such an event. Survivors can help to organize actions, associations, and programmes for either preventing suicidal behaviour or helping new survivors. Through these acts the survivor's own suffering might help others. This may change the suicide of someone close from an act that made no sense at all to an act that brought some sense in preventing other similar acts. Survivors' activity and speaking out can help themselves and other survivors, but it can also make a difference in society in terms of changing attitudes about suicide, improve preventive measures, and open up new scientific approaches. As Leo Tolstoy wisely said: 'Silence will not cure a disease. On the contrary, it will make it worse' (Knieper 1999). Silence is usually the enemy of healing. The goal of any society that cares for suffering people should be to offer and allow survivors of suicide to have equal opportunity to stop this unhealthy silence and to gain as many positive outcomes as possible—in any aspect of their lives.

> There is no growth without pain and conflict,
> there is no loss which cannot lead to gain
> (Pincus 1972)

References

Alexander, V. (1991). Grief after suicide: Giving voice to the loss. *Journal of Geriatric Psychiatry*, 24, 277–91.

Asgard, U. and Carlsson-Bergstrom, M. (1991). Interviews with survivors of suicides: Procedures and Follow-Up of Interview Subjects. *Crisis*, 12, (1), 21–33.

Bailey, S.E., Kral, M., and Dunham, K. (1999). Survivors of suicide do grieve differently. Empirical support for a common sense proposition. *Suicide and Life-Threatening Behavior*, 29, 256–71.

Barret, T.W. and Scott, T.B. (1990). Suicide bereavement and recovering patterns compared with non-suicide bereavement patterns. *Suicide and Life-Threatening Behavior*, 20, 1–15.

Beskow, J., Runeson, B., and Asgard, U. (1991). Ethical aspects of psychological autopsy. *Acta Psychiatrica Scandinavica*, 84, 482–7.

Bolton, I. (1983). *My son, my son. A guide of healing after death, loss or suicide*, pp. 5–32. Bolton Press, Atlanta.

Bowlby, J. (1991). *Loss: sadness and depression*, pp. 7–34. Penguin Books, London.

Brownstein, M. (1992). Contacting the family after a suicide. *Canadian Journal of Psychiatry*, 37, 208–12.

Byng-Hall, J. (1991). Family scripts and loss. In *Living beyond loss: Death in the family*, (ed. F. Walsh and M. McGoldrick), pp. 131–43. Norton, New York and London.

Clark, S. (2001). Mapping grief: An active approach to grief resolution. *Death Studies*, 25, 531–48.

Clark, S. and Goldney, R.D. (1995). Grief reactions and recovery in support group for people bereaved by suicide. *Crisis*, 16, 27–33.

Clark, S. and Goldney, R.D. (2000). Impact of suicide on relatives and friends. In *The international handbook of suicide and attempted suicide*, (ed. K. Hawton and K. Van Heeringen), pp. 467–84. Wiley, Chichester.

Cleiren, M.P.H.D. (1993). *Bereavement and adaptation. A comparative study of the aftermath of death*. Hemisphere Publishing Corporation, Washington DC.

Cleiren, M.P.H.D., Grad, O., Zavasnik, A., and Diekstra, R.F.W. (1996). Psycho-social impact of bereavement after suicide and fatal traffic accident: a comparative two-country study. *Acta Psychiatrica Scandinavica*, 94, 37– 44.

Colt, G.H. (1987). The history of the suicide survivor. The mark of Cain. In *Suicide and its aftermath: Understanding and counselling the survivors*, (ed. E.J. Dunne, J.L. McIntosh, and K. Dunne-Maxim), pp. 3–18. Norton, New York and London.

Demi, A.S. (1984). Social adjustment of widows after a sudden death: Suicide and Non-suicide survivors compared. *Death Education*, 8 (suppl.), 91–111.

Dunne, E.J. (1987). Special needs of suicide survivors in therapy. In *Suicide and its aftermath: Understanding and counselling the survivors*, (ed. E.J. Dunne, J.L. McIntosh, and K. Dunne-Maxim), pp. 193–207. Norton, New York and London.

Dyregrow, K. (2003). Micro-sociological analysis of social support following traumatic bereavement: unhelpful and avoidant responses from the commmunity. *Omega*, 48, 23–44.

Ellenbogen, S. and Gratton, F. (2001) Do they suffer more? Reflections on research comparing suicide survivors to other survivors. *Suicide and Life-Threatening Behavior*, 31, 83–90.

Farberow, N.L. (1991). Adult survivors after suicide. Research problems and needs. In *Life-span perspectives of suicide*, (ed. A.A. Leenaars), pp. 259–79. Plenum Press, New York.

Farberow, N.L. (1992). The Los Angeles survivors–after suicide program. *Crisis*, 13, 23–34.

Farberow, N.L. and Andriessen, K. (2002). *European Directory of Suicide Survivors*, pp. 1–68. IASP, Sneha, Chennai.

Farberow, N.L., Gallagher-Thomson, D., Gilewski, M., and Thompson, L. (1992). Changes in grief and mental health of bereaved spouses of older suicides. *Journal of Gerontology*, 47, 357–66.

Freud, S. (1934). Mourning and Melancholia. In *Collected papers*, (S. Freud), pp. 152–70. Leonard and Virgina, London.

Grad, O.T. (1996). Suicide—How to survive as a survivor. *Crisis*, 17, 136–42.

Grad, O. (2002). Psychological pain after suicide in the family. *Duševna bolečina*, 2. Ormoško srečanje (2nd Ormoz meeting), Book of Proceedings 11–14.

Grad, O.T. and Zavasnik, A. (1996). Similarities and differences in the process of bereavement after suicide and after traffic fatalities in Slovenia. *Omega*, 33, 243–51.

Grad, O. and Zavasnik, A. (1999). Phenomenology of bereavement process after suicide, traffic accident and terminal illness (in spouses). *Archives of Suicide Research*, 5, 157–72.

Grad, O. and Zavasnick, A. (2003). Symbolic expressions of loss in suicide survivors. In: *Crossing borders in suicide prevention—from genes to the human soul*. XXII World Congress of the International Association for Suicide Prevention. Stockholm, Sweden. Unpublished abstract.

Grad, O., Clark, S., Dyregrow, K., and Andriessen, K. (2003). Surviving the suicide of someone close. In: *Suicide prevention: Meeting the challenge together*, (ed. L. Vijayakumar), pp. 123–35. Orient Longman, Chennai.

Harwood, D., Hawton, K., Hope, T., and Jacoby, T. (2002). The grief experiences and needs of bereaved relatives and friends of older people dying through suicide: a descriptive and case-control study. *Journal of Affective Disorders*, 72, 185–94.

Hawton, K. and Simkin, S. (2003). Helping people bereaved by suicide. *British Medical Journal*, 327, 177–8.

Herkert, B.M. (2000). Communicating grief. *Omega*, 41, 93–115.

Hogan, N., Morse, J.M., and Tason, M.C. (1996). Toward an experiential theory of bereavement. *Omega*, 33, 43–65.

Ihan, A. (2001). Why do societies need suicide? In *Suicide risk and protective factors in the new millenium*, (ed. O.T. Grad), pp. 33–9. Cankarjev dom, Ljubljana.

Jordan, J.R. (2001). Is suicide bereavement different? A reassessment of the literature. *Suicide and Life-Threatening Behavior*, 31, 91–102.

Kissane, D.W., Block, S., Dowe, D.L., Snyder, R.D., Onghena, P., McKenzie, D.P., *et al.* (1996). The Melbourne family grief study. Perceptions of family functioning in bereavement. *The American Journal of Psychiatry*, 153, 650–62.

Knieper, A.J. (1999). The suicide survivor's grief and recovery. *Suicide and Life-Threatening Behavior*, 29, 353–64.

Lieberman, M.A. (1996). *Doors close, doors open: Widows, grieving and growing*, pp. 5–122. GP Putnam's Sons, New York.

Lund, D.A. and Caserta, M.S. (1998). Future directions in adult bereavement research. *Omega*, 36, 287–303.

McIntosh, J. (1993). Control group studies of suicide survivors: a review and critique. *Suicide and Life-Threatening Behavior*, 23, 146–61.

Merlevede, E., Spooren, D., Henderick, H., Portzky, G., Buylaert, W., Jannes, C., *et al.* (2004). Perceptions, needs and mourning reactions of bereaved relatives confronted with a sudden unexpected death. *Resuscitation*, 61, 341–8.

Osterweis, M., Salomon, F., and Green, M. (1984). *Bereavement: Reactions, consequences and care*. National Academy, Washington DC.

Parkes, C.M., Laungani, P., and Young, B. (1997). *Death and bereavement across cultures*, pp. 3–252. Routledge, London.

Pfeffer, C. (2002). *Suicide survivors*. Available at website www.afsp.org/research/articles/pfeffer2.html, last accessed July 2005.

Picton, C., Cooper, B.K., Close, D., and Tobin, J. (2001). Bereavement support groups: timing of participation and reasons for joining. *Omega*, 43, 247–58.

Pincus, L. (1972). *Death and the family*, pp. 2–6. Pantheon, New York.

Range, L.M. and Calhoun, L.G. (1990). Responses following suicide and other types of death: The perspective of the bereaved. *Omega*, 21, 311–20.

Reed, M.D. and Greenwald, J.Y. (1991). Survivor-vctim status, attachment, and sudden death bereavement. *Suicide and Life-Threatening Behavior*, 21, 385–401.

Reisman, A.S. (2001). Death of a spouse: illusory basic assumptions and continuation of bonds. *Death Studies*, 25, 445–60.

Rudestam, K.E. (1992). Research contributions to understanding the suicide survivor. *Crisis*, 13, 41–6.

Saarinen, P.I., Viinamaki, H., Hintikka, J., Lehtonen, J., and Lonnqvist, J. (1999). Psychological symptoms of close relatives of suicide victims. *European Journal of Psychiatry*, 13, 33–9.

Saarinen, P.I., Viinamaki, H., Lehtonen, J., and Lonnqvist, J. (2000). Is it possible to adapt to the suicide of a close individual? Results of a 10-year prospective follow-up study. *International Journal of Social Psychiatry*, 46, 182–90.

Seale, C. (1998). *Constructing death: The sociology of dying and bereavement*, pp. 123–231. Cambridge University Press, Cambridge.

Shneidman, E.S. (1969) Prologue. In *On the nature of suicide*, (ed. E.S. Schneidman). Jossey-Bass, San Francisco.

Shneidman, E.S. (1972). Foreword. In *Survivors of suicide*, (ed. A.C. Cain), pp. IX–XI. CC Thomas, Springfield.

Silverman, E., Range, L., and Overholser, J. (1995). Bereavement from suicide as compared to other forms of bereavement. *Omega*, 30, 41–51.

Stillion, J.M. and Stillion, B.D. (1999). Attitudes toward suicide: past, present and future. *Omega*, 38, 77–97.

Thompson, K.E. and Range, L.M. (1993). Bereavement following suicide and other types of deaths – why support attempts fail. *Omega*, 26, 61–70.

Wallace, S.E. (1977). On the atypicality of suicide bereavement. In *Suicide and bereavement*, (ed. B.L. Danto and A.H. Kutscher), pp. 44–53. MSS Information Corporation, New York.

Wertheimer, A. (1997). *A special scar*. Routledge, London.

Worden, J.W. (1991). *Grief counseling and grief therapy*. Springer, New York.

Yalom, I.D. and Lieberman, M.A. (1991). Bereavement and heightened existential involvement. *Psychiatry*, 54, 324–45.

Index

Page references to **figures, tables and boxes** are shown in **bold**. Statistical methods and terminology are indexed at their definition and/or first reference.